Comprehensive
Tumour Terminology Handbook

Comprehensive Tumour Terminology Handbook

Edited by

P.H. McKee
C.N. Chinyama
W.F. Whimster
W.V. Bogomoletz
G.S. Delides

Technical Editor
C.J.M. de Wolf

✸WILEY-LISS

A John Wiley & Sons, Inc., Publication
New York • Chichester • Weinheim • Brisbane • Singapore • Toronto

Library of Congress Cataloging-in-Publication Data

Comprehensive tumour terminology handbook / edited by Phillip H. McKee ... [et al.].
    p.   cm.
  Includes index.
  ISBN 0-471-18485-3 (paper)
    1. Tumors—Dictionaries. 2. Tumors—Terminology.   I. McKee, Phillip H.
  RC254.6.C66 2001
  616.99'2'0014—dc21

                                                                00-068054

Printed in the United States of America

10   9   8   7   6   5   4   3   2   1

Contents

Preface   xi

Introduction   xiii

Contributors   xv

Glossary   xix

Section 1

Tumours of the Eye and Adnexa   1
S. Falkmer

Section 2

Tumours of the Central Nervous System   7
P. Iuzzolino and G.M. Mariuzzi

Section 3

Tumours of the Pituitary Gland and Pineal Gland   18
S. Falkmer

Section 4

Tumours of the Thyroid Gland   23
L. David and M. Sobrinho-Simões

Section 5

Tumours of the Parathyroid Gland   33
L. David and M. Sobrinho-Simões

Section 6

Tumours of the Adrenal Cortex, Adrenal Medulla,
and Paraganglia   *36*
   S. Falkmer

Section 7

Tumours of the Exocrine and Endocrine Pancreas   *43*
   G. Zamboni and G.M. Mariuzzi

Section 8

Tumours of the Oral Cavity, Pharynx, and Tongue   *53*
   F. Bonetti, W.M. Tilakaratne, P.R. Morgan, and G.M. Mariuzzi

Section 9

Tumours of the Salivary Glands   *59*
   P. Arapantoni-Dadioti, W.M. Tilakaratne, and P.R. Morgan

Section 10

Tumours of the Oesophagus   *66*
   W.V. Bogomoletz

Section 11

Tumours of the Stomach   *71*
   F. Carneiro

Section 12

Tumours of the Small Intestine Including Duodenum
and Ampulla of Vater   *82*
   W.V. Bogomoletz

Section 13

Tumours of the Large Intestine and Appendix   *88*
   W.V. Bogomoletz

Section 14

Tumours of the Anal Canal and Anus   *95*
   W.V. Bogomoletz

Section 15

Tumours of the Liver and Intrahepatic Bile Ducts   98
    R. Colombari and G.M. Mariuzzi

Section 16

Tumours of the Gall Bladder and Extrahepatic Bile Ducts   109
    R. Colombari and G.M. Mariuzzi

Section 17

Tumours of the Middle and Inner Ear   113
    S. Falkmer

Section 18

Tumours of the Nasal Cavity and Paranasal Sinuses   117
    G. Martignoni and G.M. Mariuzzi

Section 19

Tumours of the Larynx and Hypopharynx   127
    J. Sugar

Section 20

Tumours of the Trachea, Bronchi, and Lungs   132
    M. Sheppard

Section 21

Tumours of the Serous Cavities (Pleura, Pericardium,
Peritoneum)   147
    M. Sheppard

Section 22

Tumours of the Heart   155
    M. Sheppard

Section 23

Tumours of the Bone Marrow and Leukaemia   159
    C. Matsouka, C.N. Chinyama, and M. Kalmanti

Section 24

Tumours of the Lymph Nodes and Spleen 163

P. Kanavaros and C.N. Chinyama

Section 25

Tumours of the Thymus 171

J. Iakovidou and G.S. Delides

Section 26

Tumours of the Mediastinum and Retroperitoneum 176

W.V. Bogomoletz and G.S. Delides

Section 27

Tumours of the Kidney 179

M. Pea and G.M. Mariuzzi

Section 28

Tumours of the Urinary Bladder, Urethra, Ureter, and Renal Pelvis 188

J. Lekka and G.S. Delides

Section 29

Tumours of the Prostate and Seminal Vesicles 195

R. Montironi, C. Parkinson, and G.M. Mariuzzi

Section 30

Tumours of the Testis and Epididymis 203

M. De Nictolis, E. Prete, and G.M. Mariuzzi

Section 31

Tumours of the Penis and Scrotum 208

M. Pea and G.M. Mariuzzi

Section 32

Tumours of the Ovary 212

M. De Nictolis, E. Prete, C.H. Buckley, and G.M. Mariuzzi

Section 33

**Tumours of the Fallopian Tube
and Para-Adnexal Structures**   241
   D.E. Hughes and M. Wells

Section 34

Tumours of the Corpus Uteri   244
   D.E. Hughes and M. Wells

Section 35

Tumours of the Cervix Uteri   249
   D.E. Hughes and M. Wells

Section 36

Tumours of the Vagina   254
   D.E. Hughes and M. Wells

Section 37

Tumours of the Vulva   258
   D.E. Hughes and M. Wells

Section 38

Tumours of the Placenta   262
   D.E. Hughes and M. Wells

Section 39

Tumours of the Breast   263
   P.M. Arapantoni-Dadioti and C.N. Chinyama

Section 40

Tumours of Skin (Melanocytic)   275
   J. Sugar and P.H. McKee

Section 41

Tumours of Skin (Non-Melanocytic)   285
   S.S. Seopela and P.H. McKee

Section 42

Tumours of Soft Tissue   *312*
    C.D.M. Fletcher

Section 43

Tumours of the Bone   *341*
    J.R. Salisbury

Section 44

Tumours of the Jaws and Teeth   *356*
    F. Bonetti, W.M. Tilakaratne, P.R. Morgan, and G.M. Mariuzzi

Preface

Medicine is a rapidly advancing and changing discipline. The input of basic science, applied research, and novel therapeutic modalities has rendered much of our dogma obsolete. The ever-expanding literature has created new entities out of old or given birth to multiple generations of new tumours. However, the continued use of eponyms and multiple synonyms has resulted in an increasingly confused nomenclature, which is becoming more and more difficult to unravel.

The objective of the editors and authors of this book is to provide a readily accessible reference manual designating acceptable terminology and cross-indexing redundant synonyms and eponyms. The resulting book is easy to use and, in addition to recommending appropriate terminology, provides basic information concerning each of the tumours.

This book is particularly aimed at clinicians and other professional staff dealing with the treatment of patients suffering from cancer.

The International Union Against Cancer (UICC) is deeply indebted to the authors for undertaking the difficult task of unravelling the complexities in nomenclature in their particular fields of interest. In addition the valuable contribution of Miss Nicola Kennedy, acting as the editorial assistant in a crucial phase of the editorial process is acknowledged. Also the precious input of Mrs. Anicka Joye and Mrs. Michelle Denogent is recognized. Special thanks are expressed to the Hellenic Cancer Society for its support and, in particular, for providing a quiet, creative atmosphere for the editorial workshops that were necessary to complete this task.

Sadly, one of the original editors, Bill Whimster, passed away during the early stages in the development of this book.

Dr. Miklós Bodó
International Union Against Cancer (UICC)
Detection & Diagnosis Programme Chairman

Introduction

Before the advent of immunocytochemistry and electron microscopy, nomenclature of tumours was based entirely on the morphological description of the reporting pathologist. This resulted in the emergence of descriptive terminology based upon the gross appearances or histological features emphasised by the author(s). Many tumours were described simultaneously, resulting in numerous synonyms, and unawareness of histogenesis sometimes led to the use of eponyms.

The emergence of such a random system of nomenclature has inevitably been extremely confusing. It is against this background that the concept of Comprehensive Tumour Terminology was originally conceived. This book identifies the tumours and tumour-like lesions described to date, highlights the preferred terminology, lists the many synonyms currently in use and, for completeness, many of the now obsolete terms.

Although no attempt has been made to include immunocytochemical, electron microscopic, and molecular observations in this book, these investigative modalities have been taken into account to determine the most appropriate nomenclature for the myriad of tumours that may affect the human body.

The purpose of this book therefore is to provide the reader with a comprehensive index of all the terms applied to any one particular tumour and to recommend the use of the most appropriate nomenclature. Each section is devoted to one organ or organ system. The information is presented in three columns. In the first column are listed, in alphabetical order, all of the names that have been used for the various tumours that may develop within that particular organ. Preferred terms are shown in bold. The second column refers the reader to the synonym term. Brief information concerning the designated entities is included within the third column.

With the history of this book in mind, it is clear that nomenclature and classification of tumours can never be a static phenomenon. It must be adaptable and ready to include the new information derived from state-of-the-art research in this ever-changing field. This book therefore represents the current state of play in the field of neoplasia terminology. Further editions, however, can be anticipated to include the many conceptual revisions that ongoing research observations will inevitably provoke.

The Editorial Committee:

P.H. McKee
C.N. Chinyama
W.F. Whimster †
W.V. Bogomoletz
G.S. Delides
C.J.M. de Wolf

Contributors

Arapantoni-Dadioti, P.M.   Metaxas Memorial Cancer Hospital, Department of Pathology, Piraeus, Greece.

Bogomoletz, W.V.   Formerly at Department of Pathology, Institut Jean Godinot, Reims, France.

Bonetti, F.   Università Degli Studi di Verona, Facoltà di Medicina e Chirurgia, Istituto di Anatomia Patologica, Verona, Italy.

Buckley, C.H.   Department of Reproductive Pathology, St Mary's Hospital, Whitworth Park, Manchester, United Kingdom.

Carneiro, F.   Institute of Molecular Pathology and Immunology of the University of Porto (IPATIMUP) and Faculty of Medicine, Porto, Portugal.

Chinyama, C.N.   Department of Histopathology, St. Thomas' Hospital, London, United Kingdom.

Colombari, R.   Università Degli Studi di Verona, Facoltà di Medicina e Chirurgia, Istituto di Anatomia Patologica, Verona, Italy.

David, L.   Institute of Molecular Pathology and Immunology of the University of Porto (IPATIMUP) and Faculty of Medicine, Porto, Portugal.

De Nictolis, M.   Istituto di Anatomia ed Istologia Patologica, Facoltà di Medicina e Chirurgia, Nuovo Ospedale Regionale, Torette Ancona, Italy.

Delides, G.S.   Department of Pathology, Faculty of Medicine, University of Crete, Greece.

Falkmer, S.   Pathology Unit, Institute of Laboratory Medicine, University Hospital, Norwegian University of Science and Technology, Trondheim, Norway.

Fletcher, C.D.M.   Department of Pathology, Brigham and Women's Hospital, Boston, U.S.A.

Hughes, D.E.   Department of Histopathology, Chesterfield and North Derbyshire Royal Hospital, United Kingdom.

Iakovidou, J.   Metaxas Memorial Cancer Hospital, Department of Pathology, Piraeus, Greece.

Iuzzolino, P.   Università Degli Studi di Verona, Facoltà di Medicina e Chirurgia, Istituto di Anatomia Patologica, Verona, Italy.

Kalmanti, M.   Department of Pediatric Haematology-Oncology, Faculty of Medicine, University of Crete, Greece.

Kanavaros, P.   Department of Histology, Faculty of Medicine, University of Thessaly, Larissa, Greece.

Lekka, J.   Metaxas Memorial Cancer Hospital, Department of Pathology, Piraeus, Greece.

Mariuzzi, G.M.   Università Degli Studi di Verona, Facoltà di Medicina e Chirurgia, Istituto di Anatomia Patologica, Verona, Italy.

Martignono, G.   Università Degli Studi di Verona, Facoltà di Medicina e Chirurgia, Istituto di Anatomia Patologica, Verona, Italy.

Matsouka, Ch.   Department of Pediatric Haematology-Oncology, Faculty of Medicine, University of Crete, Greece.

McKee, P.H.   Division of Dermatopathology, Brigham and Women's Hospital, Boston, USA.

Montironi, R.   Istituto di Anatomia ed Istologia Patologica, Facoltà di Medicina e Chirurgia, Nuovo Ospedale Regionale, Torette Ancona, Italy.

Morgan, P.R.   Department of Oral Medicine & Pathology, Guy's, King's College & St. Thomas' Hospitals (GKT) Dental Institute, Guy's Tower, Guy's Hospital, London, United Kingdom.

Parkinson, C.   UCL Hospitals NHS Trust, Institute of Urology, Department of Histopathology, London, United Kingdom.

Pea, M.

Università Degli Studi di Verona, Facoltà di Medicina e Chirurgia, Istituto di Anatomia Patologica, Verona, Italy.

Prete, E.

Istituto di Anatomia ed Istologia Patologica, Facoltà di Medicina e Chirurgia, Nuovo Ospedale Regionale, Torette Ancona, Italy.

Salisbury, J.R.

Department of Histopathology, Guy's King's and St. Thomas' School of Medicine, King's Denmark Hill Campus, London, United Kingdom.

Seopela, S.S.

Lancet Laboratories, Department of Anatomical Pathology, Sandton, Johannesburg, South Africa.

Sheppard, M.N.

Department of Cardiothoracic Histopathology, Royal Brompton Hospital, London, United Kingdom.

Sobrinho-Simões, M.

Institute of Molecular Pathology and Immunology of the University of Porto (IPATIMUP) and Faculty of Medicine, Porto, Portugal.

Sugar, J.

Nyirö Gyula and MÁV Hospital, Department of Pathology, Budapest, Hungary.

Tilakaratne, W.M.

Department of Oral Pathology, University of Peradeniya, Dental Sciences, Sri Lanka.

Wells, M.

Department of Pathology, University of Sheffield Medical School, Sheffield, United Kingdom.

Zamboni, G.

Università Degli Studi di Verona, Facoltà di Medicina e Chirurgia, Istituto di Anatomia Patologica, Verona, Italy.

Glossary

Adenocarcinoma	A malignant tumour arising from glandular epithelium or one showing glandular differentiation or mucin secretion.
Adenoma	A benign tumour of glandular epithelium.
Anaplastic neoplasm	A synonym for an undifferentiated neoplasm which by definition is malignant.
Atypia	An abnormal cytological appearance which may represent a reactive or a neoplastic process.
Benign	A tumour which is devoid of metastatic potential.
Cancer	A general term indicating a malignant neoplasm irrespective of its cell of origin.
Carcinoma	A malignant tumour of epithelial origin.
Carcinoma in situ	A carcinoma limited to the epithelium of origin and showing no evidence of invasion of the stroma. Glandular and squamous variants are recognised. By definition carcinoma in situ has no metastatic potential.
Choristoma	A tumour composed of tissues not normally present at that site.
Differentiation	An expression of the degree to which a tumour resembles its cell or tissue of origin.
Dysplasia	The combination of cytological and architectural abnormalities that indicate a pre-malignant state. When severe, the term "carcinoma in situ" is sometimes used.
Grade	A measurement of malignant potential based upon an estimation of a range of histological parameters including number of mitoses, pleomorphism, degree, differentiation, etc.
Intraepithelial carcinoma	A synonym for carcinoma in situ.

Intraepithelial neoplasia   A synonym for carcinoma in situ.

Malignant lymphoma   A malignant tumour of lymphocytic tissue.

Melanoma   A malignant tumour of melanin-producing cells of neuroectodermal derivation.

Metaplastic carcinoma   A carcinoma showing malignant mesenchymal differentiation.

Metastasis   A deposit of malignant tumour in an organ or tissue not in continuity with the primary lesion. Metastases may follow lymphatic or blood vessel involvement.

Neoplasm   A cellular proliferation which may be either benign or malignant.

Papilloma   An exophytic epithelial proliferation growing in a frond-like pattern.

Polyp   A benign, dysplastic or malignant intraluminal protrusion, usually but not invariably consisting of an epithelial proliferation covering a connective tissue core and joined to the tissue of origin by a stalk.

Recurrence   Reappearance of a tumour at the site of origin following excision.

Sarcoma   A malignant tumour of mesenchymal elements. The term is usually used in combination with the tissue of origin, e.g., leiomyosarcoma.

Squamous carcinoma   A malignant tumour of squamous epithelium or one showing squamous differentiation.

Teratoma   A tumour consisting of tissues arising from one or more germ cell layers.

Tumour   A general term for any abnormal mass or growth. Often it is used as a synonym for a neoplasm.

Undifferentiated neoplasm   A malignant neoplasm showing no evidence of differentiation; most are high grade.

Section 1

Tumours of the Eye and Adnexa

S. Falkmer

Tumour terminology Recommended terms are in **bold**	Synonyms	Comments
Actinic keratosis	Solar keratosis	See Tumours of Skin (Non-Melanocytic) (Section 41).
Adenocarcinoma glandulae sebacei	See sebaceous carcinoma	
Adenoid cystic carcinoma	Cylindroma	Almost half of the epithelial tumours of lacrimal glands are of this type. See Tumours of the Salivary Glands (Section 9).
Adenoma of the tarsal gland	See tarsal gland adenoma	
Angiomatosis retinae	See haemangioblastoma	
Astrocytic hamartoma	See Drusen	
Basal cell carcinoma	Basal cell epithelioma Basalioma Rodent ulcer	See Tumours of Skin (Non-Melanocytic) (Section 41).
Basal cell epithelioma	See basal cell carcinoma	
Basalioma	See basal cell carcinoma	
Benign lymphoepithelial lesion	Inflammatory pseudotumour	A non-neoplastic, chronic inflammatory, lymphocytic lesion, often of autoimmune origin. When bilateral, it can be a manifestation of Sjögren's or Mikulicz's syndromes. See Tumours of the Salivary Glands (Section 9).
Bowen's disease	Intraepidermal squamous cell carcinoma	See Tumours of Skin (Non-Melanocytic) (Section 41).
Carcinoma of the glands of Meibomian	See sebaceous carcinoma	

1

Tumour terminology Recommended terms are in **bold**	Synonyms	Comments
Carcinoma of the glands of Zeis	See sebaceous carcinoma	
Chalazion	Lipogranuloma	An inflammatory tumour-like lesion of the tarsal (Meibomian) glands.
Chloroma	See leukaemic infiltrate	
Complex choristoma	See dermoid	
Congenital oculodermal melanocytosis	See naevus of Ota	
Cornu cutaneum	See cutaneous horn	
Cutaneous horn		See Tumours of Skin (Non-Melanocytic) (Section 41).
Cylindroma	See adenoid cystic carcinoma	
Dacryocanaliculitis	See dacryops	
Dacryops	Dacryocanaliculitis	A non-neoplastic dilatation of the major excretory ducts of the lacrimal gland.
Dermofibrolipoma	See dermoid	
Dermoid	Complex choristoma Dermolipoma Dermofibrolipoma Epibulbar osseous choristoma Epibulbar osteoma	A hamartoma composed of skin and adnexa, cartilage, bone, and lacrimal gland parenchyma.
Dermolipoma	See dermoid	
Diktyoma	See medulloepithelioma	
Drusen	Astrocytic hamartoma	A tumour-like lesion composed of laminated calcified deposits within the optic nerve head. Affects mainly patients with tuberous sclerosis.
Embryonal neuroectodermal tumour	See medulloepithelioma	
Epibulbar osseous choristoma	See dermoid	
Epibulbar osteoma	See dermoid	

Tumour terminology Recommended terms are in **bold**	Synonyms	Comments
Epidermoid carcinoma	See squamous cell carcinoma	
Epithelial melanosis	See primary acquired melanosis	
Extraskeletal mesenchymal chondrosarcoma	Mesenchymal chondrosarcoma	See Tumours of Soft Tissue (Section 42).
Fibroepithelial polyp	Skin tag	See Tumours of Skin (Non-Melanocytic) (Section 41).
Fibrous histiocytoma	Fibroxanthoma	See Tumours of Skin (Non-Melanocytic) (Section 41).
Fibroxanthoma	See fibrous histiocytoma	
Haemangioblastoma	Angiomatosis retinae Hippel-Lindau syndrome (von) von Hippel-Lindau syndrome	A rare benign tumour. When it coexists with a haemangioblastoma in the cerebellum, it may form part of the von Hippel-Lindau syndrome. See Tumours of the Central Nervous System (Section 2).
Hippel-Lindau syndrome (von)	See haemangioblastoma	
Inflammatory pseudotumour	See benign lymphoepithelial lesion	
Intraepidermal squamous cell carcinoma	See Bowen's disease	
Juvenile xanthogranuloma	Naevoxantho-endothelioma Xanthogranuloma	See Tumours of Soft Tissue (Section 42).
Leukaemic infiltrate	Chloroma Mycloid sarcoma	See Tumours of the Bone Marrow and Leukaemia (Section 23).
Lipogranuloma	See chalazion	
Lymphoid pseudotumour	See reactive lymphoid hyperplasia	
Magnocellular naevus	Melanocytoma	A benign melanocytic lesion of the uveal tract.
Malignant fibrous histiocytoma		See Tumours of Soft Tissue (Section 42).

Tumour terminology Recommended terms are in **bold**	Synonyms	Comments
Malignant melanoma	Melanosarcoma Melanocarcinoma	See Tumours of Skin (Melanocytic) (Section 40).
Medulloepithelioma	Diktyoma Embryonal neuroectodermal tumour Teratoid medulloepithelioma	A rare childhood embryonal neoplasm of the non-pigmented part of the retina. The result of the histopathological assessment predicts its biological behaviour.
Melanocarcinoma	See malignant melanoma	
Melanocytoma	See magnocellular naevus	
Melanocytosis of Ota	See naevus of Ota	
Melanosarcoma	See malignant melanoma	
Melanosis oculi	See ocular melanocytosis	
Mesenchymal chondrosarcoma	See extraskeletal mesenchymal chondrosarcoma	
Mixed tumour of the lacrimal gland	See pleomorphic adenoma of the lacrimal gland	
Mucoepidermoid carcinoma		Rare lacrimal gland tumour. Highly malignant.
Myeloid sarcoma	See leukaemic infiltrate	
Naevoxantho- endothelioma	See juvenile xanthogranuloma	
Naevus of Ota	Congenital oculodermal melanocytosis Melanosis of Ota Oculodermal melanocytosis	See Tumours of Skin (Melanocytic) (Section 40).
Neurofibromatosis		See Tumours of Soft Tissue (Section 42).
Ocular melanocytosis	Melanosis oculi	Rarely benign unilateral congenital hyperpigmentation of the uveal tract.
Oculodermal melanocytosis	See naevus of Ota	

Tumour terminology Recommended terms are in **bold**	Synonyms	Comments
Oncocytoma	See oxyphil cell adenoma	
Orbital chemodectoma	See paraganglioma	
Oxyphil cell adenoma	Oncocytoma Oxyphilic adenoma	Extremely rare. Arises from an aberrant lacrimal gland. Benign tumour.
Oxyphilic adenoma	See oxyphil cell adenoma	
Paraganglioma	Orbital chemodectoma	Can occur in the orbit but only rarely. See tumours of the Adrenal Cortex, Adrenal Medulla, and Paraganglia (Section 6).
Pinguecula	See pterygium	
Pleomorphic adenoma of the lacrimal gland	Mixed tumour of the lacrimal gland Pleomorphic tumour of the lacrimal gland	This common lacrimal gland tumour is identical to the salivary gland variant. See Tumours of the Salivary Glands (Section 9).
Pleomorphic tumour of the lacrimal gland	See pleomorphic adenoma of the lacrimal gland	
Primary acquired melanosis	Epithelial melanosis	Unilateral, naevocellular hyperpigmentation. Benign but can rarely progress to a malignant melanoma.
Pterygium	Pinguecula	A tumour-like lesion of the conjunctiva due to elastotic degeneration of collagen in the bulbar conjunctiva, located nasally (pinguecula), or at the limbus, extending on to the cornea (pterygium).
Reactive lymphoid hyperplasia	Lymphoid pseudotumour	A tumour-like lesion of the orbit resulting from lymphoid tissue hyperplasia. Its differentiation from follicular lymphoma can be difficult.
Retinoblastoma		Highly malignant. The most frequent intraocular neoplasm of childhood. About one third are genetically determined, often bilateral.
Retinocytoma		A variant of retinoblastoma with a better prognosis.

Tumour terminology Recommended terms are in **bold**	Synonyms	Comments
Rodent ulcer	See basal cell carcinoma	
Sebaceous carcinoma	Adenocarcinoma glandulae sebacei Carcinoma of the gland of Zeis Carcinoma of the Meibomian gland	See Tumours of Skin (Non-Melanocytic) (Section 41).
Skin tag	See fibroepithelial polyp	
Solar keratosis	See actinic keratosis	
Squamous cell carcinoma	Epidermoid carcinoma	See Tumours of Skin (Non-Melanocytic) (Section 41).
Tarsal gland adenoma	Adenoma of the tarsal glands	Rare, benign tumour, arising from the tarsal glands of the eyelids, the ciliary sweat glands, and the accessory lacrimal glands (Krause's glands).
Teratoid medullo-epithelioma	See medulloepithelioma	
von-Hippel-Lindau syndrome	See haemangioblastoma	
Xanthelasma		A variant of plain xanthoma affecting the eyelids. See Tumours of Skin (Non-Melanocytic) (Section 41).
Xanthogranuloma	See juvenile xanthogranuloma	See Tumours of Soft Tissue (Section 42).
Xanthoma		See Tumours of Skin (Non-Melanocytic) (Section 41).

Section 2

Tumours of the Central Nervous System

P. Iuzzolino
G.M. Mariuzzi

Tumour terminology Recommended terms are in **bold**	Synonyms	Comments
Abrikossoff's tumour	See granular cell tumour	Obsolete term.
Adamantinous craniopharyngioma		Histopathological variant of craniopharyngioma.
Anaplastic astrocytoma	Grade 3 astrocytoma Malignant astrocytoma	Highly malignant tumour; median survival 2–3 years.
Anaplastic ependymoma	Grade 3 ependymoma Malignant ependymoma	Malignant tumour; seeding by cerebrospinal fluid pathway may occur.
Anaplastic ganglioglioma		A malignant variant of ganglioglioma.
Anaplastic meningioma		Meningioma with histological features of frank malignancy; high rate of recurrence.
Anaplastic neurofibroma	See malignant peripheral nerve sheath tumour	
Anaplastic oligo-astrocytoma	Malignant oligo-astrocytoma	A malignant oligo-astrocytoma.
Anaplastic oligodendroglioma	Grade 3 oligodendroglioma Malignant oligodendroglioma	A malignant oligodendroglioma.
Angioblastoma	See haemangioblastoma	
Angioendotheliomatosis		See Tumours of the Lymph Nodes and Spleen (Section 24).

Tumour terminology Recommended terms are in **bold**	Synonyms	Comments
Angiolipoma		See Tumours of Soft Tissue (Section 42).
Angiomatous meningioma		Histological variant of meningioma.
Angioreticuloma	See haemangioblastoma	Obsolete term.
Astroblastoma		Rare glial neoplasm; biological behaviour unpredictable.
Astrocytoma	Fibrillary astrocytoma Grade1-2 astrocytoma Low grade astrocytoma	Well differentiated neoplasm of fibrillary astrocytes, which grows slowly, but almost always recurs; median survival 7–8 years.
Astrocytoma of "juvenile type"	See pilocytic astrocytoma	
Atypical choroid plexus papilloma		Histological variant of choroid plexus papilloma showing cytologic atypia and mitotic activity not amounting to carcinoma.
Atypical meningioma		Meningioma with histological features that fall short of frank malignancy; biological behaviour intermediate between benign and malignant meningioma.
Atypical teratoid-rhabdoid tumour		Rare childhood malignant tumour of uncertain origin frequently involving the cerebellum.
Capillary haemangioblastoma	See haemangioblastoma	
Cellular ependymoma		Histological variant of ependymoma.
Cellular schwannoma		See Tumours of Soft Tissue (Section 42).
Central neurocytoma	Neurocytoma	Benign neuronal tumour.
Cerebellar neuroblastoma		Histological variant of medulloblastoma.
Cholesteatoma	See epidermoid cyst	
Chondrosarcoma		See Tumours of the Bone (Section 43).
Chordoid meningioma		Histological variant of meningioma.

Tumour terminology Recommended terms are in **bold**	Synonyms	Comments
Choriocarcinoma	Chorionepithelioma	Highly malignant germ cell tumour principally occurring in the pineal and suprasellar region.
Chorionepithelioma	See choriocarcinoma	
Choristoma	See granular cell tumour	
Choroid plexus carcinoma		Malignant choroid plexus tumour.
Choroid plexus papilloma	Plexus papilloma	Benign tumour of choroid plexus.
Circumscribed sarcoma of the arachnoid of the cerebellum	See desmoplastic medulloblastoma	
Clear cell ependymoma		Histological variant of ependymoma.
Clear cell meningioma		Histological variant of meningioma; potentially aggressive.
Colloid cyst of the third ventricle	Ependymal cyst	Benign lesion of endodermal origin.
Craniopharyngioma	Erdheim's tumour	Benign tumour of the sellar region or third ventricle.
Dermoid cyst		Benign lesion frequently occurring in the midline.
Desmoplastic infantile ganglioglioma	Desmoplastic supratentorial neuroepithelial tumour of infancy	Benign tumour of infancy.
Desmoplastic medulloblastoma	Circumscribed sarcoma of the arachnoid of cerebellum	Histological variant of medulloblastoma.
Desmoplastic supratentorial neuroepithelial tumour of infancy	See desmoplastic infantile ganglioglioma	
Diffuse meningeal melanosis		Benign diffuse melanocytic lesion involving the meninges with sparing of the brain.
Dysembryoblastic neuroepithelial tumour		Benign supratentorial tumour.
Dysgerminoma	See germinoma	

Tumour terminology Recommended terms are in **bold**	Synonyms	Comments
Dysplastic gangliocytoma of cerebellum	Lhermitte-Duclos disease	Very rare tumour-like neuronal lesion of cerebellum.
Embryonal carcinoma		Malignant germ cell tumour principally occurring in the pineal and suprasellar regions.
Endodermal cyst	See enterogenous cyst	
Endodermal sinus tumour	See yolk sac tumour	
Enterogenous cyst	Endodermal cyst	Benign cyst line by ciliated columnar or mucus-secreting epithelium.
Ependymal cyst	See colloid cyst of the third ventricle	
Ependymoblastoma		Rare malignant embryonal tumour.
Ependymoma	Grade 1–2 ependymoma	Slowly growing ependymal tumour of low malignant potential.
Epidermoid cyst	Cholesteatoma	Benign lesion frequently lying within the cerebellopontine angle.
Epithelioid malignant peripheral nerve sheath tumour		See Tumours of Soft Tissue (Section 42).
Erdheim's tumour	See craniopharyngioma	
Esthesioneuroblastoma	See olfactory neuroblastoma	
Fibrillary astrocytoma	See astrocytoma	
Fibrous (fibroblastic) meningioma		Histological variant of meningioma with a prominent fibrous component.
Fibrous histiocytoma		See Tumours of Soft Tissue (Section 42).
Gangliocytoma		Benign neuronal tumour.
Ganglioglioma		Benign mixed astrocytic-neuronal tumour.
Gemistocytic astrocytoma		Histological variant of astrocytoma.

Tumour terminology Recommended terms are in **bold**	Synonyms	Comments
Germinoma ˙	Dysgerminoma	Malignant germ cell tumour principally occurring in the pineal and suprasellar region.
Giant cell glioblastoma	Monstrocellular sarcoma	Histological variant of glioblastoma composed of glial and mesenchymal components.
Glioblastoma	Glioblastoma multiforme Grade 4 astrocytoma	Highly malignant glioma most closely related to fibrillary astrocytic tumours.
Glioblastoma multiforme	See glioblastoma	
Gliofibroma		Extremely rare benign tumour.
Gliomatosis cerebri		Diffuse malignant glioma.
Gliosarcoma		Histological variant of glioblastoma.
Grade 1–2 astrocytoma	See astrocytoma	
Grade 1–2 ependymoma	See ependymoma	
Grade 1–2 oligodendroglioma	See oligodendroglioma	
Grade 3 astrocytoma	See anaplastic astrocytoma	
Grade 3 ependymoma	See anaplastic ependymoma	
Grade 3 oligodendroglioma	See anaplastic oligodendroglioma	
Grade 4 astrocytoma	See glioblastoma	
Granular cell astrocytoma		Histological variant of astrocytoma.
Granular cell glioblastoma		Histological variant of glioblastoma.
Granular cell myoblastoma	See granular cell tumour	
Granular cell tumour	Granular cell myoblastoma Abrikossoff's tumour (obsolete)	Benign intra- or suprasellar tumour of the neurohypophysis. See Tumours of Soft Tissue (Section 42).

Tumour terminology Recommended terms are in **bold**	Synonyms	Comments
Granulocytic sarcoma		See Tumours of the Bone Marrow and Leukaemia (Section 23).
Haemangioblastoma	Angioblastoma Angioreticuloma (obsolete) Capillary haemangioblastoma von-Hippel-Lindau syndrome	Benign tumour most often involving cerebellum. Can form part of the von-Hippel-Lindau syndrome, i.e., comprising also angiomatosis retinae and cysts of the cerebellum, pancreas, and the kidneys.
Haemangiopericytic meningioma	See haemangiopericytoma	
Haemangiopericytoma	Haemangiopericytic meningioma	See Tumours of Soft Tissue (Section 42).
Hippel-Lindau syndrome (von)	See haemangioblastoma	
Hypothalamic neuronal hamartoma		Tumour-like lesion of the hypothalamus.
Immature teratoma		Malignant germ-cell tumour occurring principally in the pineal and suprasellar region.
Infantile desmoplastic astrocytoma		Benign astrocytic tumour of infancy.
Juvenile pilocytic astrocytoma	See pilocytic astrocytoma	
Large cell medulloblastoma		Histological variant of medulloblastoma with highly aggressive behaviour.
Lhermitte-Duclos disease	See dysplastic gangliocytoma of cerebellum	
Lipoma		See Tumours of Soft Tissue (Section 42).
Low grade astrocytoma	See astrocytoma	
Lymphoplasmacyte-rich meningioma		Histological variant of meningioma.
Malignant astrocytoma	See anaplastic astrocytoma	
Malignant ependymoma	See anaplastic ependymoma	

Tumour terminology Recommended terms are in **bold**	Synonyms	Comments
Malignant fibrous histiocytoma		See Tumours of Soft Tissue (Section 42).
Malignant lymphoma		See Tumours of the Lymph Nodes and Spleen (Section 24).
Malignant melanoma		See Tumours of Skin (Melanocytic) (Section 40).
Malignant oligo-astrocytoma	See anaplastic oligo-astrocytoma	
Malignant oligodendroglioma	See anaplastic oligodendroglioma	
Malignant peripheral nerve sheath tumour	Anaplastic neurofibroma Malignant schwannoma Neurogenic sarcoma	See Tumours of Soft Tissue (Section 42).
Malignant schwannoma	See malignant peripheral nerve sheath tumour	
Mature teratoma		Benign germ cell tumour usually involving the pineal and suprasellar regions.
Medulloblastoma		Malignant embryonal childhood tumour located in the cerebellum.
Medullocytoma		Histological variant of medulloblastoma.
Medulloepithelioma		Very rare malignant embryonal tumour.
Medullomyoblastoma		Histopathological variant of medulloblastoma.
Melanocytoma		Benign melanocytic tumour usually involving the meninges.
Melanotic medulloblastoma		Rare histological variant of medulloblastoma.
Melanotic neuroectodermal tumour of infancy		A rare, highly pigmented tumour presenting in infants usually in the maxilla. Benign although sometimes locally invasive.
Melanotic schwannoma		See Tumours of Soft Tissue (Section 42).
Meningeal gliomatosis		Rare astrocytic or oligodendroglial tumour arising primarily in the meninges.

Tumour terminology Recommended terms are in **bold**	Synonyms	Comments
Meningeal melanomatosis		Malignant diffuse tumour of leptomeninges.
Meningeal sarcomatosis		Malignant mesenchymal tumour arising from and diffusely infiltrating the meninges.
Meningioangiomatosis		Rare tumour-like lesion of meningothelial cells, fibroblasts, and blood vessels.
Meningioma		Benign meningeal tumour; the 5-year recurrence rate is less than 5%.
Meningothelial meningioma		Histological variant of meningioma.
Mesenchymal chondrosarcoma		See Tumours of Soft Tissue (Section 42).
Metaplastic meningioma		Histological variant of meningioma.
Microcystic meningioma		Histological variant of meningioma.
Microglioma		Obsolete term.
Mixed germ cell tumour		Malignant germ cell tumour usually involving the pineal and suprasellar regions.
Mixed glioma (other than oligoastrocytoma)		Extremely rare histological variant of glioma.
Monstrocellular sarcoma	See giant cell glioblastoma	
Myxopapillary ependymoma		Benign variant of ependymoma that occurs almost exclusively in the region of the cauda equina.
Nasal glial heterotopia	Nasal glioma	Benign nasal or paranasal tumour-like lesion.
Nasal glioma	See nasal glial heterotopia	
Neurilemmoma	See schwannoma	
Neurinoma	See schwannoma	
Neuroblastoma		Rare malignant embryonal tumour of infancy.
Neurocytoma	See central neurocytoma	

Tumour terminology Recommended terms are in **bold**	Synonyms	Comments
Neurofibroma		See Tumours of Soft Tissue (Section 42).
Neurogenic sarcoma	See malignant peripheral nerve sheath tumour	
Neuroglial cyst		Benign lesion.
Olfactory neuroblastoma	Esthesioneuroblastoma	Malignant but slowly progressive neuronal tumour involving the vault of the nose.
Olfactory neuroepithelioma		Rare histological variant of olfactory neuroblastoma.
Oligo-astrocytoma		Infiltrative tumour of low malignant potential.
Oligodendrocytoma	See oligodendroglioma	Obsolete term.
Oligodendroglioma	Grade 1–2 oligodendroglioma Oligodendrocytoma (obsolete)	Infiltrative tumour of low malignant potential.
Osteocartilaginous tumour		Benign tumour usually involving the meninges.
Papillary craniopharyngioma		Histological variant of craniopharyngioma occurring in adults.
Papillary ependymoma		Rare histological variant of ependymoma.
Papillary meningioma		Rare aggressive histological variant of meningioma.
Paraganglioma of the filum terminale		Benign neuroendocrine tumour.
Pilocytic astrocytoma	Astrocytoma of "juvenile type" Juvenile pilocytic astrocytoma	Circumscribed astrocytic tumour of young people; the prognosis is excellent.
Pituicytoma	See granular cell tumour	
Plasma cell granuloma		Tumour-like lesion usually involving the meninges.
Plasmacytoma		See Tumours of the Lymph Nodes and Spleen (Section 24).

Tumour terminology Recommended terms are in **bold**	Synonyms	Comments
Pleomorphic xanthoastrocytoma		Well demarcated astrocytic tumour characterised by a generally favourable prognosis.
Plexiform neurofibroma		See Tumours of Soft Tissue (Section 42).
Plexiform schwannoma		See Tumours of Soft Tissue (Section 42).
Plexus papilloma	See choroid plexus papilloma	
Polar spongioblastoma	Primitive polar spongioblastoma	Very rare childhood tumour with a variable biological behaviour.
Primitive neuroectodermal tumour		See Tumours of Soft Tissue (Section 42).
Primitive polar spongioblastoma	See polar spongioblastoma	
Protoplasmic astrocytoma		Rare histological variant of astrocytoma.
Psammomatous meningioma		Histological variant of meningioma.
Rathke's cleft cyst		Rare developmental abnormality of Rathke's cleft presenting as a benign intra- or suprasellar lesion.
Reticulum cell sarcoma		Obsolete term.
Rhabdomyosarcoma		See Tumours of Soft Tissue (Section 42).
Schwannoma	Neurilemmoma Neurinoma	See Tumours of Soft Tissue (Section 42).
Secretory meningioma		Histological variant of meningioma.
Subependymal giant cell astrocytoma		Benign intraventricular tumour typically occurring as part of the tuberous sclerosis complex.
Subependymoma		Benign intra- or periventricular tumour composed of ependymal and astrocyte-like cells.
Teratoma with malignant transformation		Rare malignant variant of teratoma principally occurring in the pineal and suprasellar regions.
Transitional (mixed) meningioma		Histological variant of meningioma.

Tumour terminology Recommended terms are in **bold**	Synonyms	Comments
von-Hippel-Lindau syndrome	See haemangioblastoma	
Yolk sac tumour	Endodermal sinus tumour	Malignant germ cell tumour principally occurring in the pineal and suprasellar regions.

Section 3

Tumours of the Pituitary Gland and Pineal Gland

S. Falkmer

Section 3a. Tumours of the Pituitary Gland

Tumour terminology Recommended terms are in **bold**	Synonyms	Comments
Abrikossoff's tumour	See granular cell tumour	
Acidophil adenoma	Acidophil cell adenoma Eosinophil adenoma	Histological variant of adenoma.
Acidophil cell adenoma	See acidophil adenoma	
Acidophil stem cell adenoma		Histological variant of adenoma.
Adenocarcinoma	See carcinoma	
Adenoma		Practically all pituitary adenomas are histopathologically benign. Multiple types. Classification may be based on tinctorial properties (e.g., acidophil adenoma) or on hormone production, (e.g., growth hormone). The resulting endocrine syndromes are related to the latter.
Basophil adenoma	Basophil cell adenoma Mucoid cell adenoma	Histological variant of adenoma.
Basophil cell adenoma	See basophil adenoma	
Carcinoma	Adenocarcinoma Chromophobe carcinoma Chromophobe cell carcinoma	Extremely rare. The diagnosis should only be made in the presence of known metastases.

18

Tumour terminology Recommended terms are in **bold**	Synonyms	Comments
Choristoma	See gangliocytoma	
Chromophobe adenoma	Chromophobe cell adenoma	Histological variant of adenoma.
Chromophobe carcinoma	See carcinoma	
Chromophobe cell adenoma	See chromophobe adenoma	
Chromophobe cell carcinoma	See carcinoma	
Corticotrophin adenoma	See corticotrophin-producing adenoma	
Corticotrophin cell adenoma	See corticotrophin-producing adenoma	
Corticotrophin-producing adenoma	Corticotrophin adenoma Corticotrophin cell adenoma	ACTH-producing tumour, which may be associated with Cushing's or Nelson's syndromes.
Craniopharyngioma		Benign tumour of childhood derived from vestigial remnants of Rathke's pouch.
Dermoid cyst		Tumour-like lesion. The cyst wall is composed of stratified squamous epithelium and includes hairs, sebaceous glands, and sweat glands.
Eosinophil adenoma	See acidophil adenoma	
Epidermoid cyst	Squamous cyst	Tumour-like lesion. The cyst wall is composed of stratified squamous epithelium.
Gangliocytoma	Choristoma	Extremely rare, benign tumour in the neurohypophysis. It may be associated with a growth-hormone-secreting pituitary adenoma causing acromegaly.
Glandular cyst		Tumour-like lesion. The wall is lined by cuboidal epithelium. It is believed to be derived from remnants of Rathke's pouch.
Gonadotroph adenoma	See gonadotrophin-producing adenoma	

Tumour terminology Recommended terms are in **bold**	Synonyms	Comments
Gonadotroph cell adenoma	See gonadotrophin-producing adenoma	
Gonadotrophin-producing adenoma	Gonadotroph adenoma Gonadotroph cell adenoma	In women, it may be associated with amenorrhoea and galactorrhoea. In males, the main symptom is loss of libido.
Granular cell myoblastoma	See granular cell tumour	
Granular cell tumour	Granular-cell myoblastoma Myoblastoma Abrikossoff's tumour	A benign tumour of possible Schwann cell derivation. It may, very rarely, be associated with diabetes insipidus.
Growth-hormone adenoma	See growth hormone-producing adenoma	
Growth-hormone cell adenoma	See growth hormone-producing adenoma	
Growth-hormone-producing adenoma	Growth-hormone adenoma Growth-hormone cell adenoma	May be associated with acromegaly, gigantism, galactorrhoea, and amenorrhoea.
Hyperplastic nodule	See nodular hyperplasia	
Mixed adenoma	Mixed cell adenoma	Histological variant of adenoma containing a mixture of growth hormone and prolactin-producing cells.
Mixed cell adenoma	See mixed adenoma	
Mucoid cell adenoma	See basophil adenoma	
Myoblastoma	See granular cell tumour	
Nodular hyperplasia	Hyperplastic nodule	Common, tumour-like, non-functioning hyperplastic nodules in the adenohypophysis.
Non-oncocytic adenoma	See null cell adenoma	
Null cell adenoma	Non-oncocytic adenoma	Non-functioning adenoma, presenting local symptoms only.
Oncocytic adenoma	See oncocytoma	

Tumour terminology Recommended terms are in **bold**	Synonyms	Comments
Oncocytoma	Oncocytic adenoma	Histological variant of adenoma characterised by the presence of eosinophilic granular cytoplasm due to excessive content of mitochondria.
Prolactin adenoma	See prolactin-producing adenoma	
Prolactin cell adenoma	See prolactin-producing adenoma	
Prolactin-producing adenoma	Prolactin adenoma Prolactin cell adenoma	May be associated with galactorrhoea and amenorrhoea.
Silent adenoma	See silent corticotroph adenoma	
Silent corticotroph adenoma	Silent adenoma	Histological variant of adenoma not associated with clinical evidence of hormone overproduction.
Squamous cyst	See epidermoid cyst	
Thyrotroph adenoma	See thyrotrophin-producing adenoma	
Thyrotroph cell adenoma	See thyrotrophin-producing adenoma	
Thyrotrophin-producing adenoma	Thyrotroph adenoma Thyrotroph cell adenoma	May be associated with hyperthyroidism.
Undifferentiated cell adenoma		Histological variant of adenoma.

Section 3b. Tumours of the Pineal Gland

Tumour terminology Recommended terms are in **bold**	Synonyms	Comments
Adult teratoma	See germ cell tumour	
Astroblastoma	See pineocytoma	
Choriocarcinoma	See germ cell tumour	
Dysgerminoma	See germ cell tumour	

Tumour terminology Recommended terms are in **bold**	Synonyms	Comments
Embryonal carcinoma	See germ cell tumour	
Ependymoma	See pineocytoma	
Germ cell tumour	Adult teratoma Choriocarcinoma Dysgerminoma Embryonal carcinoma Germinoma Seminoma Yolk-sac tumour	This represents the predominant primary tumour arising within the pineal gland.
Germinoma	See germ cell tumour	
Medulloblastoma	See pineoblastoma	
Malignant pineocytoma	See mixed pineocytoma-pineoblastoma	
Mixed pineocytoma-pineoblastoma	Malignant pineocytoma Pineocytoma without neuronal differentiation	This extremely rare tumour occupies a position in between pineocytoma and pineoblastoma in terms of structure and biological behaviour.
Neuroblastoma	See pineoblastoma	
Paraganglioma		Obsolete term.
Pineoblastoma	Medulloblastoma Neuroblastoma	This is an extremely rare malignant neuroepithelial tumour, which predominantly affects children. Infiltration of the adjacent brain and spread via the cerebrospinal fluid are common.
Pineocytoma	Astroblastoma Ependymoma	This is an extremely rare benign tumour of pineocytes, which tends to present in adults. In contrast to pineoblastoma it is well circumscribed and does not infiltrate the surrounding brain. Histological distinction from astroblastomas and ependymomas may be difficult.
Pineocytoma without neuronal differentiation	See mixed pineocytoma-pineoblastoma	
Seminoma	See germ-cell tumour	
Yolk-sac tumour	See germ-cell tumour	

Section 4

Tumours of the Thyroid Gland

L. David
M. Sobrinho-Simões

Tumour terminology Recommended terms are in **bold**	Synonyms	Comments
Adenoacanthoma		Obsolete term.
Adenocarcinoma	See follicular carcinoma and papillary carcinoma	
Adenochondroma		Extremely rare. Benign.
Adenolipoma		Extremely rare. Benign.
Adenoma	Embryonal adenoma (obsolete) Foetal adenoma (obsolete) Follicular adenoma	Several histological variants are recognised, including embryonal, foetal, macrofollicular, microfollicular, normofollicular, solid, and trabecular.
Adenoma with bizarre nuclei	See atypical adenoma	
Adenoma with papillary hyperplasia	Hyperplastic papillary adenoma	Benign. May occur in a setting of multi-nodular goitre. May be hyperfunctioning.
Adenomatous goitre	See nodular goitre	
Adenosquamous carcinoma		A variant of squamous cell carcinoma associated with mucin production.
Amphicrine carcinoma	See medullary carcinoma	Obsolete term.
Amyloid goitre		Tumour-like lesion.
Anaplastic carcinoma	See undifferentiated carcinoma	
Angioma	See haemangioma	
Angiosarcoma	Haemangioendothelioma Haemangiosarcoma	See Tumours of Soft Tissue (Section 42).

Tumour terminology Recommended terms are in **bold**	Synonyms	Comments
Askanazy adenoma	See oxyphilic adenoma	
Atypical adenoma	Adenoma with bizarre nuclei	A benign follicular tumour showing nuclear atypia but lacking unequivocal signs of capsular or vascular invasion.
Benign metastasising goitre		Obsolete term.
Carcinoma showing thymus-like differentiation	CASTLE	Extremely rare, low grade tumour characterised by late local recurrence.
Carcinosarcoma	See metaplastic carcinoma	
CASTLE	See carcinoma showing thymus-like differentiation	
C-cell carcinoma	See medullary carcinoma	
C-cell hyperplasia		Rare condition thought to precede familial medullary carcinoma.
Clear cell carcinoma		Descriptive term encompassing any variant of thyroid carcinoma showing clear cell change.
Colloid goitre	See nodular goitre	
Columnar cell carcinoma	See poorly differentiated carcinoma	This term may also be applied to a variant of papillary carcinoma, which carries a guarded prognosis.
Cystic variant of papillary carcinoma	See papillary carcinoma	
De Quervain's thyroiditis	See granulomatous thyroiditis	
Diffuse follicular variant of papillary carcinoma		A rare histological variant of papillary carcinoma occurring in young adults. It is associated with aggressive behaviour and metastasises to lymph nodes, lungs, and bones.
Diffuse sclerosing variant of papillary carcinoma		A rare histological variant of papillary carcinoma, which occurs in children and young adults. It commonly metastasises to lymph nodes and the lung. The prognosis is guarded.

Tumour terminology Recommended terms are in **bold**	Synonyms	Comments
Embryonal adenoma	See adenoma	Obsolete term.
Encapsulated follicular carcinoma	See minimally invasive follicular carcinoma	
Encapsulated medullary carcinoma	See medullary carcinoma	Obsolete term.
Encapsulated papillary carcinoma		Rare histological variant of papillary carcinoma. Despite the presence of lymph node metastases the prognosis is excellent.
Fibrosing thyroiditis	See Riedel's thyroiditis	
Foetal adenoma	See adenoma	Obsolete term.
Follicular adenoma	See adenoma	
Follicular carcinoma		The prognosis depends mainly on the extent of invasion. Minimally invasive and widely invasive variants are recognised. The former is a histological term and refers to focal capsular or vascular invasion. The latter relates to a tumour in which there is extensive invasion of the adjacent thyroid and widespread involvement of blood vessels.
Follicular variant of medullary carcinoma		Histological variant of medullary carcinoma.
Follicular variant of papillary carcinoma		Histological variant of papillary carcinoma with variable prognosis. It appears to be more prone to give bloodborne metastasis.
Giant cell carcinoma		A histological variant of undifferentiated follicular carcinoma in which in addition to recognisable epithelial elements, highly pleomorphic spindle cell areas containing numerous multinucleate giant cells are seen.
Giant cell variant of medullary carcinoma		Histological variant of medullary carcinoma characterised by striking pleomorphism and giant cells. The prognosis is uncertain.
Goitre		Tumour-like lesion, which may present in a variety of clinical settings, e.g., Grave's disease.

Tumour terminology Recommended terms are in **bold**	Synonyms	Comments
Granulomatous thyroiditis	De Quervain's thyroiditis	Tumour-like inflammatory lesion.
Haemangioendothelioma	See angiosarcoma	
Haemangioma	Angioma	See Tumours of Soft Tissue (Section 42).
Haemangiosarcoma	See angiosarcoma	
Hashimoto's thyroiditis		Tumour-like inflammatory lesion. Autoimmune disorder.
Hürthle cell adenoma	See oxyphilic adenoma	
Hürthle cell carcinoma	See oxyphilic carcinoma	
Hyalinising trabecular adenoma	Hyalinising trabecular tumour (obsolete) Paraganglioma-like adenoma (obsolete)	This histological variant of adenoma shares morphological features with papillary carcinoma. Diagnosis is often problematical.
Hyalinising trabecular carcinoma	Hyalinising trabecular tumour (obsolete)	This is an extremely rare tumour, which may be related to the trabecular variant of papillary carcinoma.
Hyalinising trabecular tumour	See hyalinising trabecular adenoma and carcinoma	Obsolete term.
Hyperfunctioning adenoma	Plummer adenoma (obsolete) Toxic adenoma	Adenoma associated with hyperthyroidism.
Hyperplastic papillary adenoma	See adenoma with papillary hyperplasia	
Insular carcinoma	See poorly differentiated carcinoma	
Intrathyroid epithelial thymoma	See carcinoma showing thymus-like differentiation	
Latent papillary carcinoma	See papillary microcarcinoma	
Leiomyoma		See Tumours of Soft Tissue (Section 42).
Leiomyosarcoma		See Tumours of Soft Tissue (Section 42).
Lymphangioma		See Tumours of Soft Tissue (Section 42).
Lymphocytic thyroiditis		Tumour-like inflammatory lesion.

Tumour terminology Recommended terms are in **bold**	Synonyms	Comments
Macrofollicular adenoma	See adenoma	
Macrofollicular variant of papillary carcinoma		Histological variant of papillary carcinoma with low malignant potential.
Malakoplakia		Tumour-like inflammatory lesion.
Malignant lymphoma		See Tumours of the Lymph Nodes and Spleen (Section 24).
Malignant peripheral nerve sheath tumour	Neurofibrosarcoma	See Tumours of Soft Tissue (Section 42).
Malignant schwannoma		See Tumours of Soft Tissue (Section 42).
Malignant teratoma	See spindle epithelial tumour with thymus-like differentiation	
Medullary carcinoma	Amphicrine carcinoma (obsolete) C-cell carcinoma Encapsulated medullary carcinoma (obsolete) Solid amyloidotic carcinoma (obsolete)	This rare neuroendocrine tumour may be sporadic or familial (alone or in the settings of MEN IIA and MEN IIB syndromes). A number of histological variants are recognised including glandular, oxyphilic, giant cell, clear cell, spindle cell, pigmented, squamous, papillary, small cell, hyalinising trabecular adenoma-like, and medullary microcarcinoma.
Medullary carcinoma with thyroglobulin immunoreactivity	See mixed thyroid carcinoma	
Melanotic (pigmented) carcinoma		Histological variant of medullary carcinoma containing melanin–pigment.
Metaplastic carcinoma	Carcinosarcoma	This is a highly pleomorphic rare variant of thyroid undifferentiated carcinoma showing mesenchymal differentiation and therefore may contain skeletal muscle, bone, or cartilage. See also undifferentiated carcinoma.
Microcarcinoma	See papillary microcarcinoma	
Microfollicular adenoma	See adenoma	
Minimally invasive follicular carcinoma	Encapsulated follicular carcinoma	Histological variant of follicular carcinoma with low malignant potential.

Tumour terminology Recommended terms are in **bold**	Synonyms	Comments
Mixed follicular-parafollicular carcinoma	See mixed thyroid carcinoma	
Mixed medullary-follicular carcinoma	See mixed thyroid carcinoma	
Mixed medullary-papillary carcinoma	See mixed thyroid carcinoma	
Mixed thyroid carcinoma	Medullary carcinoma with thyroglobulin immunoreactivity Mixed follicular-parafollicular carcinoma Mixed medullary-follicular carcinoma Mixed medullary-papillary carcinoma	This is a rare tumour characterised by dual follicular and parafollicular differentiation. Whenever one is not certain about the dual origin of the neoplastic cells, the term "medullary" with thyroglobulin immunoreactivity may be used.
Mucinous carcinoma		Rare histological variant of thyroid carcinoma characterised by marked epithelial mucin production.
Mucoepidermoid carcinoma		Rare histological variant combining a mucus-secreting glandular component with areas of squamous differentiation. May be related to papillary carcinoma.
Multinodular goitre	See nodular goitre	
Neurilemmoma	See Schwannoma	
Neurofibrosarcoma	See malignant peripheral nerve sheath tumour	
Nodular goitre	Adenomatous goitre Colloid goitre Multinodular goitre Nodular hyperplasia	This common condition may represent either a hyperplastic or a benign neoplastic lesion.
Nodular hyperplasia	See nodular goitre	
Non-encapsulated sclerosing carcinoma	See papillary microcarcinoma	
Normofollicular adenoma	See adenoma	Histological variant of follicular adenoma.
Occult papillary carcinoma	See papillary microcarcinoma	

Tumour terminology Recommended terms are in **bold**	Synonyms	Comments
Occult sclerosing papillary carcinoma		Histological variant of papillary microcarcinoma.
Oncocytic adenoma	See oxyphilic adenoma	
Oncocytic carcinoma	See oxyphilic carcinoma	
Oxyphilic adenoma	Askanazy adenoma Hürthle cell adenoma Oncocytic adenoma	This variant of follicular adenoma is composed of intensely eosinophilic oxyphilic (Hürthle, oncocytic) cells.
Oxyphilic carcinoma	Hürthle cell carcinoma Oncocytic carcinoma	This tumour is sometimes subdivided into follicular and papillary types. Other authors classify them as a single entity.
Oxyphilic tumour	Papillary oncocytic neoplasm Papillary oxyphilic neoplasm	This term encompasses oxyphilic adenoma and oxyphilic carcinoma regardless of their papillary or follicular nature. Behaviour in this group is unpredictable.
Papillary carcinoma	Microcarcinoma Non-encapsulated sclerosing carcinoma Papillary cystadenocarcinoma (obsolete)	The most frequent form of thyroid carcinoma. It is commonly associated with nodal metastases despite being very slowly growing. A number of histological variants including follicular, solid, encapsulated, diffuse sclerosing, diffuse follicular, tall cell, macrofollicular, oxyphilic, and trabecular are recognised. In addition papillary carcinoma may be associated with a nodular fasciitis-like stroma. Tumours with a favourable prognosis include the micro-carcinomatous, cystic, macrofollicular, and encapsulated subtypes. Histological variants with a guarded prognosis include the diffuse follicular, diffuse sclerosing, and tall cell variants.
Papillary carcinoma with nodular fasciitis-like stroma		Histological variant of papillary carcinoma. The spindle cell element may obscure the underlying carcinoma.
Papillary cystadenocarcinoma	See papillary carcinoma	Obsolete term.

Tumour terminology Recommended terms are in **bold**	Synonyms	Comments
Papillary microcarcinoma		Variant of papillary carcinoma implying a tumour less than 1 cm in diameter, which may represent either an occult papillary carcinoma (one that is identified following the discovery of metastatic disease) or a latent papillary carcinoma (an incidental finding following surgical resection). Such a tumour has a very low malignant potential and a very favourable prognosis. Histologically, the tumour is often densely fibrotic (hence the term "occult sclerosing papillary carcinoma").
Papillary oncocytic neoplasm	See oxyphilic tumour	
Papillary oxyphilic neoplasm	See oxyphilic tumour	
Papillary variant of medullary carcinoma	See medullary carcinoma	
Paraganglioma		Extremely rare in the thyroid. See Tumours of the Adrenal Cortex, Adrenal Medulla, and Paraganglia (Section 6).
Paraganglioma-like adenoma	See hyalinising trabecular adenoma	Obsolete term. This term was sometimes abbreviated to the acronym PLAT.
Plummer adenoma	See hyperfunctioning adenoma	Obsolete term.
Poorly differentiated carcinoma	Columnar cell carcinoma Insular carcinoma Trabecular carcinoma	This group has been delineated to identify tumours occupying an intermediate position in terms of histological features and biological potential between well differentiated and undifferentiated variants. They are prone to give nodal and bloodborne metastases. Several histological variants are recognised.
Riedel's thyroiditis	Fibrosing thyroiditis	Tumour-like inflammatory lesion.
Salivary gland type tumour		Extremely rare. Benign. Looks like a pleomorphic adenoma.
Sarcomatoid carcinoma	See undifferentiated carcinoma	
Schwannoma		See Tumours of Soft Tissue (Section 42).

Tumour terminology Recommended terms are in **bold**	Synonyms	Comments
Sclerosing mucoepidermoid carcinoma with eosinophilia		This rare tumour of low malignant potential is associated with Hashimoto's thyroiditis.
SETTLE	See spindle epithelial tumour with thymus-like differentiation	
Small cell carcinoma	See undifferentiated carcinoma	
Solid adenoma	See adenoma	
Solid amyloidotic carcinoma	See medullary carcinoma	Obsolete term.
Solitary fibrous tumour		See Tumours of Soft Tissue (Section 42).
Spindle cell carcinoma	See undifferentiated carcinoma	
Spindle epithelial tumour with mucous cysts	See spindle epithelial tumour with thymus-like differentiation	
Spindle epithelial tumour with thymus-like differentiation	Malignant teratoma SETTLE Spindle epithelial tumour with mucous cysts	An extremely rare tumour occurring in children and young adults.
Squamoid carcinoma	See undifferentiated carcinoma	
Squamous cell carcinoma		Rare; differential diagnosis includes metastasis from a squamous cell carcinoma elsewhere in the body.
Tall cell variant of papillary carcinoma		Histological variant of papillary carcinoma with a guarded prognosis particularly when it arises in the elderly. It may coexist with foci or columnar cell carcinoma.
Teratoma		This germ cell tumour is usually benign in neonates and infants. In adults, it is extremely rare and usually malignant.
Thyroglossal duct cyst		Tumour-like developmental anomaly.

Tumour terminology Recommended terms are in **bold**	Synonyms	Comments
Toxic adenoma	See hyperfunctioning adenoma	
Trabecular adenoma	See adenoma	
Trabecular carcinoma	See poorly differentiated carcinoma	
Trabecular variant of papillary carcinoma	See papillary carcinoma	Histological variant of papillary carcinoma with variable prognosis.
Undifferentiated carcinoma	Anaplastic carcinoma Sarcomatoid carcinoma Small cell carcinoma Spindle cell carcinoma Squamoid carcinoma	This is a high grade type of carcinoma with extremely poor prognosis, which includes the following variants: giant cell carcinoma (in which the tumour cells may resemble osteoclasts), metaplastic (a tumour in which, in addition to an epithelial component, shows mesenchymal differentiation, e.g., smooth muscle, bone, or cartilage. This lesion is also sometimes referred to as spindle cell or sarcomatoid carcinoma and carcinosarcoma), small cell carcinoma (which is a heterogeneous group of tumours including variants of medullary carcinoma, poorly differentiated, and neuroendocrine carcinoma), and squamoid carcinoma (which represents an undifferentiated carcinoma in which a hint of squamous differentiation is apparent).
Well differentiated carcinoma, NOS		Descriptive term encompassing rare partly encapsulated tumours that share features of follicular and papillary carcinoma.
Widely invasive follicular carcinoma		Histological variant of follicular carcinoma.

Section 5

Tumours of the Parathyroid Gland

L. David
M. Sobrinho-Simões

Tumour terminology Recommended terms are in **bold**	Synonyms	Comments
Adenocarcinoma	See carcinoma	
Adenoma		A number of subtypes are recognised based on histological appearances. These include chief cell adenoma, water-clear cell adenoma, mixed cell adenoma, and oxyphil cell adenoma. The last type owes its name to the presence of abundant granular eosinophilic cytoplasm. An adenoma may be non-functioning or functioning, i.e., associated with hyperparathyroidism.
Atypical adenoma		Benign or unpredictable behaviour. An imprecise term designating tumours that show cytological features usually associated with carcinoma but lack unequivocal signs of malignancy.
Carcinoma	Adenocarcinoma	The diagnosis is based on the presence of invasion of adjacent structures and/or metastases. It is usually but not invariably associated with hyperparathyroidism. Rarely it may be seen in association with familial hyperparathyroidism.
Chief cell adenoma		Histological variant of adenoma.
Clear cell adenoma	See water-clear cell adenoma	

Tumour terminology Recommended terms are in **bold**	Synonyms	Comments
Cyst		Rare tumour-like lesion, which most often presents in the neck and represents a developmental abnormality.
Hamartoma	See lipoadenoma	
Hyperplasia	See primary nodular hyperplasia See primary water-clear cell hyperplasia	
Lipoadenoma	Hamartoma	A rare benign pseudotumour composed of an admixture of adipose and parathyroid tissue. It may be associated with hyperparathyroidism.
Mixed cell adenoma		Histological variant of adenoma.
Nodular hyperplasia	See primary nodular hyperplasia	
Oncocytic adenoma	Oxyphilic cell adenoma	Histological variant of adenoma. The cells exhibit eosinophilic cytoplasm. Usually non-functional.
Oncocytic parathyroid carcinoma		Histological variant of carcinoma.
Oxyphilic cell adenoma	See oncocytic adenoma	
Parathyroidomatosis		A rare condition characterised by the presence of hyperplastic and/or supernumerary glands in the neck and/or mediastinum. It is usually associated with hyperparathyroidism.
Primary chief cell hyperplasia	See primary nodular hyperplasia	
Primary clear cell hyperplasia	See primary water-clear cell hyperplasia	
Primary nodular hyperplasia	Hyperplasia Nodular hyperplasia Primary chief cell hyperplasia	Tumour-like lesion usually involving all four glands and associated with hyperparathyroidism. Frequently familial within the frame of multiple endocrine neoplasia, type I (MEN I) or multiple endocrine neoplasia, type II (MEN IIA).

Tumour terminology Recommended terms are in **bold**	Synonyms	Comments
Primary water-clear cell hyperplasia	Hyperplasia Primary clear cell hyperplasia	This is a rare tumour-like lesion, which usually involves all four glands and is associated with hyperparathyroidism. There is no apparent familial incidence or evidence of any of the multiple endocrine neoplasia syndromes.
Secondary hyperparathyroidism		This term refers to hyperplasia involving all glands as a consequence of a sustained stimulus for parathormone secretion.
Tertiary hyperparathyroidism		This term refers to the development of autonomous (hyperplastic or neoplastic) parathyroid hyperfunction in patients with previously documented secondary hyperparathyroidism.
Third pharyngeal pouch cyst		Tumour-like lesion. Contains both thymus and parathyroid tissue.
Water-clear cell adenoma	Clear cell adenoma	Histological variant of adenoma.

Section 6

Tumours of the Adrenal Cortex, Adrenal Medulla, and Paraganglia

S. Falkmer

Tumour terminology Recommended terms are in **bold**	Synonyms	Comments
Adenocarcinoma of the adrenal cortex	See adrenal cortical carcinoma	
Adenoma of the adrenal cortex	See adrenal cortical adenoma	
Adrenal carcinoma	See adrenal cortical carcinoma	
Adrenal cortical adenocarcinoma	See adrenal cortical carcinoma	
Adrenal cortical adenoma	Adenoma of the adrenal cortex Aldosteronoma Black adenoma Clear cell adenoma Compact cell adenoma Glomerulosa cell adenoma Mixed cell adenoma Single nodule of the adrenal cortex Spongiocytic adenoma	These tumours are most often non-functional. The rare functioning variants may be classified according to their function, e.g., adenoma associated with hyperaldosteronism may be referred to as an aldosteronoma. In black adenoma the pigmentation is due to the presence of lipofuscin and/or neuromelanin. Clear cell adenoma contains abundant lipid. Mixed cell adenoma may be associated with aldosterone secretion (Conn's syndrome).
Adrenal cortical carcinoma	Adenocarcinoma of the adrenal cortex Adrenal carcinoma Adrenal cortical adenocarcinoma Adrenocortical carcinoma	This rare tumour is highly malignant. On occasions differentiation from a large adenoma can be difficult. Reliable factors indicating malignancy include tumour weight >100 g, large necrotic areas, poor encapsulation, vascular invasion, high mitotic activity, and overproduction of feminising corticosteroids.

Tumour terminology Recommended terms are in **bold**	Synonyms	Comments
Adrenal cyst	See cyst of the adrenal glands	
Adrenal incidentaloma	Incidentaloma	This term refers to the incidental discovery of a nodular enlargement of one or both adrenal glands.
Adrenergic tumour	See phaeochromocytoma	
Adrenocortical angioma	See haemangioma	
Adrenocortical carcinoma	See adrenal cortical carcinoma	
Aldosteronoma	See adrenal cortical adenoma	
Angioma	See haemangioma	
Angioma of the adrenal cortex	See haemangioma	
Black adenoma	See adrenal cortical adenoma	
Bone marrow heterotopia	See myelolipoma	
Carotid body tumour	See paraganglioma	
Chemoblastomatosis	See paraganglioma	
Chemodectoma	See paraganglioma	
Chromaffin cell tumour	See phaeochromocytoma	
Chromaffinoma	See phaeochromocytoma	
Chromophil tumour	See phaeochromocytoma	
Clear cell adenoma	See adrenal cortical adenoma	
Compact cell adenoma	See adrenal cortical adenoma	
Composite paraganglioma	Paraganglioma of the cauda equina	An extremely rare, benign tumour of the filum terminale of the spinal cord.
Composite phaeochromocytoma	Gangliocytoma	This rare, usually benign tumour is composed of an admixture of a phaeochromocytoma and collections of mature ganglion cells, which sometimes aggregate to form small ganglioneuromata.

Tumour terminology Recommended terms are in **bold**	Synonyms	Comments
Cyst of the adrenal gland	Adrenal cyst	This is a rare lesion and most often represents a pseudocyst developing after haemorrhage. Occasionally lymphangiectatic variants are encountered.
Cystic medullary struma of the adrenal	See phaeochromocytoma	
Extra-adrenal phaeochromocytoma	See paraganglioma	
Functional pigmented adenoma	See black adenoma	
Gangliocytic paraganglioma of duodenum		Extremely rare, benign polypoid lesion in the second portion of duodenum.
Gangliocytoma	See composite phaeochromocytoma	The term is sometimes also used as synonym for a ganglioneuroblastoma; this should be avoided.
Gangliocytoneuroma	See ganglioneuroma	
Ganglioma	See ganglioneuroma	
Ganglion cell tumour	See ganglioneuroma	
Ganglioneuroblastoma	See neuroblastoma	Obsolete term.
Ganglioneuroma	Gangliocytoneuroma Ganglioma Ganglion cell tumour Neuroganglioneuroma Sympaticocytoma	This benign tumour is usually an incidental finding in the sympathetic ganglia of the retroperitoneum or in the adrenal medulla. Most often it is small and completely asymptomatic. It consists of an admixture of ganglion cells and neurofibromatous tissue.
Ganglioneurosarcoma	See neuroblastoma	
Glomerulosa cell adenoma	See adrenal cortical adenoma	
Glomus caroticum tumour	See paraganglioma	
Glomus jugulare tumour	See paraganglioma	
Glomus tumour	See paraganglioma	

Tumour terminology Recommended terms are in **bold**	Synonyms	Comments
Haemangioma	Adrenocortical angioma Angioma Angioma of the adrenal cortex	See Tumours of Soft Tissue (Section 42).
Immature ganglioneuroma	See neuroblastoma	
Incidentaloma	See adrenal incidentaloma	
Intra-adrenal paraganglioma	See phaeochromocytoma	
Jugularis tumour	See paraganglioma	
Jugulotympanic tumour	See paraganglioma	
Leiomyoma	Myoma	See Tumours of Soft Tissue (Section 42).
Malignant ganglioneuroma	See neuroblastoma	A synonym for the ganglioneuroblastoma variant of neuroblastoma.
Medullary adenoma of adrenal	See phaeochromocytoma	
Microadenomatous adrenal	See micronodular adrenal disease	
Micronodular adrenal disease	Microadenomatous adrenal Micronodular cortical adenomatosis Polymicroadenomatosis Primary nodular hyperplasia	This is a rare benign lesion, which occurs in children. By definition the adrenal gland is of normal size.
Micronodular cortical adenomatosis	See micronodular adrenal disease	
Mixed cell adenoma	See adrenal cortical adenoma	
Multinodular adrenal	Nodular adrenal Nodular hyperplasia	This is the most frequently encountered lesion in the adrenal cortex. It is not a genuine neoplasm and is usually discovered incidentally at autopsy. Functional effects do not occur.

Tumour terminology Recommended terms are in **bold**	Synonyms	Comments
Multinodular hyperplasia	Multiple nodular hyperplasia Pseudoadenomatous hyperplasia	This is a rare condition characterised by enlargement of the adrenal glands. It is not a true neoplasm.
Multiple endocrine adenopathy (MEA)	See multiple endocrine neoplasia (MEN)	
Multiple endocrine neoplasia (MEN)	Multiple endocrine adenopathy (MEA) Neuroectodermal syndromes Polyendocrine syndromes	*MEN-1* (MEN-I; Wermer's syndrome) Parathyroid adenoma, giving rise to hyperparathyroidism. Pituitary adenoma, giving rise to acromegaly or to Morbus Cushing. Islet cell tumour ("insuloma") of the pancreas, giving rise to hyperinsulinism ("insulinoma"), or to the "glucagonoma syndrome", or to the Verner-Morrison (watery diarrhoea)-syndrome. "Gastrinoma" in pancreas or duodenum is giving rise to hypergastrinaemia and the Zollinger-Ellison syndrome. ECL cell carcinoid of the stomach which develops as a consequence of hypergastrinaemia *MEN-2* (MEN-IIa; Sipple's syndrome) Medullary thyroid carcinoma, giving rise to hypercalcinaemia. Phaeochromocytoma, giving rise to paroxysmal hypertension. Parathyroid adenoma, giving rise to hyperparathyroidism. *MEN-3* (MEN-IIb; Gorlin syndrome) Same components as in MEN-2. Gastrointestinal mucosal neuromas. Marfanoid habitus.
Multiple nodular hyperplasia	See multinodular hyperplasia	
Myeloid metaplasia	See myelolipoma	
Myelolipoma	Bone marrow heterotopia Myeloid metaplasia	This not uncommon lesion represents heterotopic bone marrow in the adrenal medulla. It is often an incidental finding at autopsy.
Myoma	See leiomyoma	

Tumour terminology Recommended terms are in **bold**	Synonyms	Comments
Neuroblastoma	Ganglioneuroblastoma (obsolete) Ganglioneurosarcoma Immature ganglioneuroma Malignant ganglioneuroma Neurocytoma Neurosarcoma Sympatheticoblastoma (obsolete) Sympatheticogonioma (obsolete)	A group of usually highly malignant, neuroendocrine neoplasms in infants and children, arising not only from the adrenal medulla, but also from the sympathetic ganglia. Marked variations in differentiation can occur. Sympatheticogonioma, ganglioneuroblastoma, and sympatheticoblastoma are obsolete terms that were used to imply varying degrees of differentiation.
Neurocytoma	See neuroblastoma	
Neuroectodermal syndromes	See multiple endocrine neoplasia (MEN)	
Neuroganglioneuroma	See ganglioneuroma	
Neurosarcoma	See neuroblastoma	
Nodular adrenal	See multinodular adrenal	
Nodular hyperplasia	See multinodular adrenal	
Non-chromaffin paraganglioma	See paraganglioma	
Orbital chemodectoma	See paraganglioma	
Paraganglioma	Carotic body tumour Chemoblastomatosis Chemodectoma Composite paraganglioma Extra-adrenal phaeochromocytoma Glomus caroticum tumour Glomus jugulare tumour Glomus tumour Jugularis tumour Jugulotympanic tumour Non-chromaffin paraganglioma Orbital chemodectoma Pulmonary chemodectoma Stromal mesothelioma Vagal body tumour	This tumour is analogous to the phaeochromocytoma of the adrenal medulla. It is difficult to predict its biological behaviour. Most are benign although occasional non-encapsulated variants with a tendency to local recurrence are encountered. Although the two most common sites are the carotid body and the jugulotympanic paraganglia, paragangliomas can appear as primary tumours in several additional organs including the urinary bladder, larynx, heart, and remnants of the organ of Zuckerkandl.

Tumour terminology Recommended terms are in **bold**	Synonyms	Comments
Paraganglioma of the cauda equina	See composite paraganglioma	
Phaeochromoblastoma	See phaeochromocytoma	
Phaeochromocytoma	Adrenergic tumour Chromaffin cell tumour Chromaffinoma Chromophil tumour Cystic medullary struma of the adrenal Intra-adrenal paraganglioma Medullary adenoma of the adrenal Phaeochromoblastoma	This neuroendocrine tumour arises in the adrenal medulla. It is difficult to predict the biological behaviour but metastases may be seen in up to 10% of patients. It may be a feature of multiple endocrine neoplasia (MEN) syndrome type 2. It is often called "the 10% tumour", due to the fact that roughly 10% of them are bilateral, 10% occur in children, 10% are extra-adrenal, 10% are familial (MEN-2), and 10% are malignant (see above).
Polyendocrine syndromes	See Multiple endocrine neoplasia (MEN)	
Polymicroadenomatosis	See micronodular adrenal disease	
Primary nodular hyperplasia	See micronodular adrenal disease	
Pseudoadenomatous hyperplasia	See multinodular hyperplasia	
Pulmonary chemodectoma	See paraganglioma	
Single nodule of the adrenal cortex	See adrenal cortical adenoma	
Spongiocytic adenoma	See adrenal cortical adenoma	
Stromal mesothelioma	See paraganglioma	
Sympatheticoblastoma	See neuroblastoma	Obsolete term.
Sympatheticocytoma	See ganglioneuroma	
Sympatheticogonioma	See neuroblastoma	Obsolete term.
Vagal body tumour	See paraganglioma	

Section 7

Tumours of the Exocrine and Endocrine Pancreas

G. Zamboni
G.M. Mariuzzi

Tumour terminology Recommended terms are in **bold**	Synonyms	Comments
Acinar cell adenoma		Entity of doubtful existence.
Acinar cell carcinoma		Rare form of pancreatic carcinoma, which accounts for about 1% of all exocrine tumours.
Acinar cell cystadenocarcinoma		A predominantly cystic variant of acinar carcinoma.
ACTHoma	ACTH-secreting tumour	Low grade malignant neuroendocrine tumour.
ACTH-secreting tumour	See ACTHoma	
Adenoacanthoma	See adenosquamous carcinoma	
Adenocarcinoma	See ductal adenocarcinoma	
Adenosquamous (spindle cell) carcinoma	See adenosquamous carcinoma	
Adenosquamous carcinoma	Adenoacanthoma Adenosquamous (spindle cell) carcinoma Mucoepidermoid carcinoma	Rare histological variant of ductal adenocarcinoma.
Anaplastic carcinoma	See undifferentiated carcinoma	
Angiosarcoma	Haemangiosarcoma	See Tumours of Soft Tissue (Section 42).

Tumour terminology Recommended terms are in **bold**	Synonyms	Comments
Calcitonin-secreting tumour		Low grade malignant neuroendocrine tumour.
Carcinoid tumour	See neuroendocrine tumour	
Clear cell "sugar" tumour		An extremely rare, benign tumour.
Clear cell carcinoma		Rare form of pancreatic carcinoma, which must be differentiated from metastatic renal carcinoma.
Colloid carcinoma	See mucinous non-cystic carcinoma	
Cyst	See pancreatic cyst	
Cystadenocarcinoma		Malignant serous or mucinous tumour with cystic differentiation.
Cystadenoma		Benign serous or mucinous cystic tumour.
Dermoid cyst	See mature cystic teratoma	
Diffuse intraductal papillary adenocarcinoma	See intraductal papillary-mucinous tumour	
Duct cell carcinoma	See ductal adenocarcinoma	
Ductal adenocarcinoma	Adenocarcinoma Duct cell carcinoma	This tumour represents the most frequent variant of exocrine carcinoma (90% of all cases). It is graded into well, moderate, and poorly differentiated types. Histological variants include adenosquamous carcinoma, mucinous non-cystic carcinoma, and signet ring cell carcinoma.
Ductectatic mucinous cystadenocarcinoma	See intraductal papillary-mucinous tumour	
Ductectatic mucinous cystadenoma	See intraductal papillary-mucinous tumour	
Ductectatic mucinous cystic neoplasm	See intraductal papillary-mucinous tumour	
Endocrine pancreatic tumour	See neuroendocrine tumour	

Tumour terminology Recommended terms are in **bold**	Synonyms	Comments
Focal lymphoid hyperplasia		Pseudolymphomatous tumour-like lesion.
Functioning neuroendocrine tumour		This is characterised by the presence of a clinical syndrome resulting from the secretion of one or more hormones.
Gastrinoma		This is a low grade malignant neuroendocrine tumour. It is frequently associated with the sporadic form of Zollinger-Ellison syndrome and sometimes with MEN1.
Gelatinous carcinoma	See mucinous non-cystic carcinoma	
Giant cell carcinoma	See undifferentiated carcinoma	
Giant cell tumour of the osteoclastoid type	See osteoclast-like giant cell tumour	
Glucagonoma		Low grade malignant neuroendocrine tumour associated with diabetes mellitus and skin rash.
Glycogen-rich cystadenoma	See serous cystadenoma	
GRFoma	Growth hormone releasing-factor tumour	Low grade malignant neuroendocrine tumour.
Growth hormone releasing-factor tumour	See GRFoma	
Haemangiosarcoma	See angiosarcoma	
Infantile carcinoma	See pancreatoblastoma	
Inflammatory fibroblastic tumour	See Inflammatory pseudotumour	
Inflammatory myofibroblastic tumour	See Inflammatory pseudotumour	
Inflammatory pseudotumour	Inflammatory fibroblastic tumour Inflammatory myofibroblastic tumour Plasma cell granuloma	Tumour-like lesion characterised by vascular and fibroblastic proliferation and inflammatory cell infiltration.
Insular adenoma	See neuroendocrine tumour	

Tumour terminology Recommended terms are in **bold**	Synonyms	Comments
Insular adenomatosis	See neuroendocrine tumour	Most often a focal lesion (cf. "Nesidioblastosis").
Insular carcinoma	See neuroendocrine tumour	
Insulinoma		Neuroendocrine tumour. Benign in about 90% of cases associated with episodes of hypoglycaemia.
Insuloma	See neuroendocrine tumour	
Intraductal mucin-hypersecreting tumour	See intraductal papillary-mucinous tumour	
Intraductal oncocytic papillary neoplasm		Rare histological variant of intraductal papillary-mucinous tumour.
Intraductal papillary tumour	See intraductal papillary-mucinous tumour	
Intraductal papillary-mucinous adenoma	See intraductal papillary-mucinous tumour	
Intraductal papillary-mucinous carcinoma	See intraductal papillary-mucinous tumour	
Intraductal papillary-mucinous tumour	Diffuse intraductal papillary adenocarcinoma Ductectatic mucinous cystadenocarcinoma Ductectatic mucinous cystadenoma Ductectatic mucinous cystic neoplasm Intraductal mucin-hypersecreting tumour Intraductal papillary tumour Intraductal papillary-mucinous adenoma Intraductal papillary-mucinous carcinoma Intraductal papilloma IPMT Mucin-producing tumour Mucinous duct ectasia Papillary carcinoma Villous adenoma	This term encompasses a wide range of intraductal tumours with variable papillary proliferation, mucin secretion, and cystic change. Behaviour is variable, the following subtypes are recognised: adenoma, atypically proliferating (borderline malignant), and malignant.

Tumour terminology Recommended terms are in **bold**	Synonyms	Comments
Intraductal papilloma	See intraductal papillary-mucinous tumour	
IPMT	See intraductal papillary-mucinous tumour	
Islet cell adenoma	See neuroendocrine tumour	
Islet cell adenomatosis	See neuroendocrine tumour	Most often a focal lesion (cf. "Nesidioblastosis").
Islet cell carcinoma	See neuroendocrine tumour	
Lymphoepithelial cyst		Tumour-like lesion.
Malignant fibrous histiocytoma of the giant cell type	See osteoclast-like giant cell tumour	
Mature cystic teratoma	Dermoid cyst	A benign, mature extragonadal germ cell tumour, rare in the pancreas.
Microadenocarcinoma	Microglandular adenocarcinoma Solid microglandular carcinoma	Heterogeneous group of tumours including ductal, acinar, neuroendocrine, and mixed.
Microcystic serous adenocarcinoma	See serous cystadenocarcinoma	
Microcystic serous adenoma	See serous cystadenoma	
Microglandular adenocarcinoma	See microadenocarcinoma	
Mixed acinar-endocrine carcinoma	Mixed acinar-islet cell carcinoma	An extremely rare tumour with mixed acinar and neuroendocrine components.
Mixed acinar-islet cell carcinoma	See mixed acinar-endocrine carcinoma	
Mixed ductal-endocrine carcinoma	Mixed duct-islet cell carcinoma	An extremely rare tumour with mixed ductal and neuroendocrine differentiation.
Mixed duct-islet cell carcinoma	See mixed ductal-endocrine carcinoma	

Tumour terminology Recommended terms are in **bold**	Synonyms	Comments
Mixed duct-islet-acinar cell carcinoma		An extremely rare tumour with mixed ductal, acinar, and neuroendocrine differentiation.
Mucinous carcinoma	See mucinous non-cystic carcinoma	
Mucinous cystadenocarcinoma	See mucinous cystic tumour	
Mucinous cystadenoma	See mucinous cystic tumour	
Mucinous cystic tumour	Mucinous cystadenocarcinoma Mucinous cystadenoma Mucinous cystic tumours with moderate dysplasia	A generic name for a group of mucus-secreting cystic neoplasms of variable malignant potential including adenomatous, borderline malignant (mucinous cystic tumour with moderate dysplasia), and carcinoma (invasive and non-invasive variants).
Mucinous cystic tumour with moderate dysplasia	See mucinous cystic tumour	
Mucinous duct ectasia	See intraductal papillary-mucinous tumour	
Mucinous non-cystic carcinoma	Colloid carcinoma Gelatinous carcinoma Mucinous carcinoma	A histological variant of ductal adenocarcinoma composed of well differentiated neoplastic glands dispersed within mucinous lakes (comprising more than 50% of the neoplasm). The prognosis is better than with conventional ductal carcinoma and signet ring cell carcinoma.
Mucin-producing tumour	See intraductal papillary-mucinous tumour	
Mucoepidermoid carcinoma	See adenosquamous carcinoma	
Multihormonal endocrine tumour		A low grade malignant tumour characterised by multiple hormone production.
Nesidioblastosis	See neuroendocrine tumour	A controversial term, indicating a diffusely hyperplastic lesion of the islets of Langerhans, usually in infants, associated with persistent hypoglycaemia with hyperinsulinism.

Tumour terminology Recommended terms are in **bold**	Synonyms	Comments
Neuroendocrine tumour	Carcinoid tumour Endocrine pancreatic tumour Functioning neuroendocrine tumour Insular adenoma Insular adenomatosis Insular carcinoma Insuloma Islet cell adenoma Islet cell adenomatosis Islet cell carcinoma Mixed acinar-islet cell carcinoma Mixed ductal-endocrine carcinoma Nesidioblastosis Non-functioning endocrine tumour Pancreatic endocrine tumour PET	From the omnipotent cells of the epithelium of the ends of the ductuli, and from the parenchyma of the islets of Langerhans, a multitude of focally ("adenomatosis") or diffusely ("nesidioblastosis") hyperplastic or genuinely neoplastic ("insuloma") lesions can arise. As in most other neuroendocrine neoplasms, their degree of malignancy can be difficult to assess histopathologically. As a rule of thumb, it can be said that about $\frac{1}{3}$ of them are functionally inactive, $\frac{1}{3}$ secrete proinsulin/insulin, and $\frac{1}{3}$ secrete other peptide hormones and/or biogenic amines. Those causing clinical syndromes are often known by terms formed from the name of the hormone with addition of the letters "-oma" (e.g., "insulinoma").
Neurotensinoma		A low grade malignant neuroendocrine tumour.
Non-functioning endocrine tumour		This is a low grade malignant tumour in which clinical symptoms are absent and hormonal production variably demonstrable within tumour cells by immunohistochemistry.
Oat cell carcinoma	See small cell carcinoma	
Oncocytic carcinoma		An extremely rare histological variant.
Osteoclast-like giant cell tumour	Giant cell carcinoma (osteoclastoid type) Giant cell tumour of the osteoclastic type Malignant fibrous histiocytoma of the giant cell type Osteoclastoma Osteoclast-type giant cell tumour Pleomorphic carcinoma of giant or large cell type Pleomorphic carcinoma with osteoclast-like cells Pleomorphic large cell carcinoma	An extremely rare malignant histological variant of ductal adenocarcinoma rich in osteoclast-like giant cells. Should be distinguished from undifferentiated carcinoma because of the favourable prognosis.

Tumour terminology Recommended terms are in **bold**	Synonyms	Comments
Osteoclastoma	See osteoclast-like giant cell tumour	
Osteoclast-type giant cell tumour	See osteoclast-like giant cell tumour	
Pancreatic cyst	Cyst	Tumour-like cystic lesion formed by non-neoplastic epithelial or mesenchymal cells. Variants include pseudocyst, retention cyst, parasitic cyst, and congenital cyst.
Pancreatic endocrine tumour	See neuroendocrine tumour	"PET".
Pancreatic polypeptide-producing tumour	See PPoma	
Pancreatoblastoma	Infantile carcinoma	A rare malignant tumour, which typically occurs in children. Rare examples have been described in adults.
Papillary carcinoma	See intraductal papillary mucinous tumour	
Papillary cystic tumour	See solid-pseudopapillary tumour	
Parathyroid hormone-secreting tumour	See PTHoma	
PET	See neuroendocrine tumour	Pancreatic endocrine tumour.
Plasma cell granuloma	See inflammatory pseudotumour	
Pleomorphic carcinoma of giant cell type	See osteoclast-like giant cell tumour	
Pleomorphic carcinoma of giant or large cell type	See osteoclast-like giant cell tumour	
Pleomorphic carcinoma small cell type	See undifferentiated carcinoma	
Pleomorphic carcinoma with osteoclast-like cells	See osteoclast-like giant cell carcinoma	
Pleomorphic large cell carcinoma	See undifferentiated carcinoma	

Tumour terminology Recommended terms are in **bold**	Synonyms	Comments
PPoma	Pancreatic polypeptide-producing tumour	Low grade malignant neuroendocrine tumour.
PTHoma	Parathyroid hormone-secreting tumour	Low grade malignant neuroendocrine tumour.
Sarcomatoid carcinoma	See undifferentiated carcinoma	
Serotonin-secreting tumour		Neuroendocrine tumour.
Serous cystadenocarcinoma	Microcystic serous adenocarcinoma	This is an extremely rare tumour.
Serous cystadenoma	Glycogen-rich cystadenoma Microcystic serous adenoma	This tumour most often presents in elderly females.
Signet ring cell carcinoma		This is an extremely rare histological variant.
Small cell carcinoma	Oat cell carcinoma	In the past this tumour was believed to represent a variant of undifferentiated carcinoma. It is now recognised as a poorly differentiated neuroendocrine tumour.
Solid and cystic tumour	See solid-pseudopapillary tumour	
Solid microglandular carcinoma	See microadenocarcinoma	
Solid-pseudopapillary tumour	Papillary cystic tumour Solid and cystic tumour	Most tumours are of borderline malignant (atypically proliferating) potential. Frankly malignant variants are extremely rare.
Somatostatinoma		Low grade malignant neuroendocrine tumour.
Spindle cell carcinoma	See undifferentiated carcinoma	
Squamous cell carcinoma		An excessively rare histological variant.

Tumour terminology Recommended terms are in **bold**	Synonyms	Comments
Undifferentiated carcinoma	Anaplastic carcinoma Giant cell carcinoma Pleomorphic carcinoma giant cell type Pleomorphic carcinoma small cell type Pleomorphic large cell carcinoma Sarcomatoid carcinoma Spindle cell carcinoma	This term encompasses a heterogeneous group of tumours, all of which are characterised by aggressive behaviour.
Villous adenoma	See intraductal papillary-mucinous tumour	
VIPoma	VIP-producing tumour	Low grade malignant neuroendocrine tumour associated with watery diarrhoea, hypokalaemia achlorhydria (WDHA)— Verner-Morrison syndrome.
VIP-producing tumour	See VIPoma	

Section 8

Tumours of the Oral Cavity, Pharynx, and Tongue

F. Bonetti
W.M. Tilakaratne
P.R. Morgan
G.M. Mariuzzi

Tumour terminology Recommended terms are in **bold**	Synonyms	Comments
Abrikossoff's tumour	See granular cell tumour	Obsolete term.
Acantholytic squamous cell carcinoma	Adenoid squamous cell carcinoma Pseudoglandular squamous cell carcinoma	See Tumours of Skin (Non-Melanocytic) (Section 41).
Adenoid squamous cell carcinoma	See acantholytic squamous cell carcinoma	
Adenosquamous carcinoma		A rare tumour composed of both glandular and squamous malignant elements.
Angiosarcoma		See Tumours of Soft Tissue (Section 42).
Basal cell carcinoma	Rodent ulcer	See Tumours of Skin (Non-Melanocytic) (Section 41).
Basaloid squamous cell carcinoma		See Tumours of Skin (Non-Melanocytic) (Section 41).
Carcinoma with sarcoma-like (spindle cell) stroma	See spindle cell squamous carcinoma	
Carcinosarcoma	See metaplastic carcinoma	

Tumour terminology Recommended terms are in **bold**	Synonyms	Comments
Congenital epulis	Congenital gingival granular cell tumour Congenital myoblastoma (obsolete) Gingival granular cell tumour Granular cell epulis	This rare tumour is found in neonates. Although it is histologically similar to granular cell tumour, it is currently believed to be of pericyte or myofibroblastic differentiation rather than of Schwann cell derivation.
Congenital gingival granular cell tumour	See congenital epulis	
Congenital myoblastoma	See congenital epulis	Obsolete term.
Denture granuloma	See fibroepithelial polyp	
Denture injury tumour	See fibroepithelial polyp	Obsolete term.
Eosinophilic granuloma	See Langerhans cell histiocytosis	
Epidermoid carcinoma	See squamous cell carcinoma	
Epulis		A general description for a localised swelling of the gum.
Epulis fissuratum	See fibroepithelial polyp	Obsolete term.
Erythroplakia	Erythroplasia	This is a clinical descriptive term for a red mucosal plaque. The underlying pathology is invariably dysplastic.
Erythroplasia	See erythroplakia	
Fibroepithelial polyp	Denture granuloma Denture injury tumour (obsolete) Epulis fissuratum (obsolete) Fibroma	A pseudotumour consisting of squamous epithelium covering a fibrous connective tissue core. It most often is associated with chronic trauma.
Fibroma	See fibroepithelial polyp	
Fibrous epulis		A reactive fibroepithelial swelling of the gingiva.
Florid oral papillomatosis		A rare lesion characterised by numerous papilloma-like nodules clinically similar to verrucous carcinoma.

Tumour terminology Recommended terms are in **bold**	Synonyms	Comments
Focal epithelial hyperplasia	Heck's disease	Rare condition characterised by multiple flat mucosal nodules occurring mainly in children. It has a viral aetiology.
Giant cell fibroma		Histological variant of fibroepithelial polyp characterised by atypical stellate and multinucleate myofibroblasts.
Giant cell epulis	Peripheral giant cell reparative granuloma	This benign pseudotumour is composed of multinucleate osteoclast-like giant cells. It must be distinguished from osteoclastoma of the jaw and hyperparathyroidism.
Gingival epithelial hamartoma		Rare hamartomatous condition composed of odontogenic epithelium.
Gingival granular cell tumour	See congenital epulis	
Granular cell epulis	See congenital epulis	
Granular cell myoblastoma	See granular cell tumour	
Granular cell Schwannoma	See granular cell tumour	
Granular cell tumour	Abrikossoff's tumour (obsolete) Granular cell myoblastoma Granular cell Schwannoma Myoblastic myoma	See Tumours of Soft Tissue (Section 42).
Hairy leukoplakia		A hyperplastic virus-induced proliferation of oral epithelium often observed in AIDS patients.
Heck's disease	See focal epithelial hyperplasia	
Hereditary benign intraepithelial dyskeratosis		A very rare inherited condition characterised by soft spongy white lesions. It is not associated with any risk of malignancy.
Keratoacanthoma		See Tumours of Skin (Non-Melanocytic) (Section 41).

Tumour terminology Recommended terms are in **bold**	Synonyms	Comments
Lethal midline granuloma	Midline lethal granulomatosis (obsolete) Midline malignant reticulosis (obsolete) Midline necrotising lesion (obsolete) Polymorphic reticulosis	This clinical term is used to refer to a destructive condition of the nose and related sinuses due to a variety of diseases including Wegener's granulomatosis, angiocentric T-cell lymphoma (lymphomatoid granulomatosis), and other lymphomas.
Leukoplakia		This is a clinical term referring to a white adherent plaque on the oral mucosa. It has a variety of causes including dysplastic lesions, in situ and invasive squamous cell carcinoma.
Lipoma		See Tumours of Soft Tissue (Section 42).
Lymphoepithelial carcinoma	See nasopharyngeal carcinoma	
Lymphoepithelioma	See nasopharyngeal carcinoma	
Lymphoepithelioma-like carcinoma	See nasopharyngeal carcinoma	
Lymphomatoid granulomatosis		Obsolete term. This condition is now believed to represent an angiocentric T-cell lymphoma.
Malignant melanoma	See melanoma	
Malignant mixed tumour	See metaplastic carcinoma	
Melanocytic nevi		See Tumours of Skin (Melanocytic) (Section 40).
Melanoma	Malignant melanoma	See Tumours of Skin (Melanocytic) (Section 40).
Metaplastic carcinoma	Carcinocarcinoma Malignant mixed tumour	This is a very rare high grade tumour showing both malignant epithelial and mesenchymal differentiation.
Midline lethal granulomatosis	See lethal midline granuloma	Obsolete term.
Midline malignant reticulosis	See lethal midline granuloma	Obsolete term.

Tumour terminology Recommended terms are in **bold**	Synonyms	Comments
Midline necrotising lesion	See lethal midline granuloma	Obsolete term.
Mucosal neuroma		This is most often plexiform in type and when multiple is often associated with multiple endocrine neoplasia syndrome type III.
Myoblastic myoma	See granular cell tumour	
Myofibroma(tosis) infantile		See Tumours of Soft Tissue (Section 42).
Nasopharyngeal carcinoma	Lymphoepithelial carcinoma Lymphoepithelioma Lymphoepithelioma-like carcinoma	This high grade tumour is aetiologically related to Epstein-Barr virus. Metastasis to lymph nodes is common.
Neurilemmoma		See Tumours of Soft Tissue (Section 42).
Neurofibroma		See Tumours of Soft Tissue (Section 42).
Oral focal mucinosis		Tumour-like lesion presenting as one or more mucosal nodules. The gingiva is most often affected.
Papillary hyperplasia of palate		Tumour-like lesion presenting as multiple soft nodules.
Papilloma	See squamous cell papilloma	
Peripheral ameloblastoma		See Tumours of Jaws and Teeth (Section 44).
Peripheral giant cell reparative granuloma	See giant cell epulis	
Peripheral odontogenic fibroma		Tumour-like lesion originally thought to represent the peripheral counterpart of central odontogenic fibroma.
Peripheral ossifying fibroma		A tumour-like reactive gingival nodule. It is unrelated to fibro-osseous lesions of the jaw.
Polymorphic reticulosis	See lethal midline granuloma	
Pregnancy epulis		A clinical variant of pyogenic granuloma.

Tumour terminology Recommended terms are in **bold**	Synonyms	Comments
Pseudoglandular squamous cell carcinoma	See acantholytic squamous cell carcinoma	
Pyogenic granuloma	Vascular epulis	See Tumours of Soft Tissue (Section 42).
Rodent ulcer	See basal cell carcinoma	
Sarcomatoid Carcinoma	See spindle cell squamous carcinoma	
Spindle cell squamous carcinoma	Carcinoma with sarcoma-like (spindle cell) stroma Sarcomatoid carcinoma	See Tumours of Skin (Non-Melanocytic) (Section 41).
Squamous cell carcinoma	Epidermoid carcinoma	This is the most common malignant tumour of the oral cavity and tongue, accounting for about 80% of all malignant tumours in this location. Prognostic parameters include: stage, site, size, growth pattern, and cell differentiation.
Squamous cell papilloma	Papilloma	This common lesion is composed of squamous epithelium overlying a connective tissue core. It is not pre-malignant.
Vascular epulis	See pyogenic granuloma	
Verruciform xanthoma		A rare exophytic lesion of unknown aetiology. It most commonly occurs on the gingiva and may be clinically mistaken for an early squamous or verrucous carcinoma.
Verrucoid squamous cell carcinoma	See verrucous carcinoma	
Verrucous carcinoma	Verrucoid squamous cell carcinoma	This is a rare variant of squamous cell carcinoma, which is often associated with human papilloma virus infection. Although recurrence may occur metastases are very rare.
White sponge naevus		This is an inherited disease characterised by the presence of bilateral white plaques on the oral mucosal epithelium.

Section 9

Tumours of the Salivary Glands

P. Arapantoni-Dadioti
W.M. Tilakaratne
P.R. Morgan

Tumour terminology Recommended terms are in **bold**	Synonyms	Comments
Acinic cell adenocarcinoma	See acinic cell carcinoma	
Acinic cell carcinoma	Acinic cell adenocarcinoma Acinic cell tumour	A malignant tumour of variable behaviour. Over 80% occur in the parotid gland.
Acinic cell tumour	See acinic cell carcinoma	
Adenocarcinoma (NOS)		A salivary gland carcinoma, which does not fit into any of the described categories. Prognosis depends on histological grade and high grade tumours have the poorest outcome among all salivary gland tumours.
Adenoid cystic carcinoma	Basalioma (obsolete) Basaloid mixed tumour (obsolete) Cylindroma (obsolete)	This is an aggressive tumour, which frequently shows perineural spread and therefore has a high recurrence rate.
Adenolymphoma	See Warthin's tumour	
Adenomatoid hyperplasia of mucous salivary glands		A pseudotumour which most often occurs on the palate and which may represent a hyperplastic or a hamartomatous process.
Adenomyoepithelioma	See myoepithelioma	Obsolete term.
Adenosquamous carcinoma		A rare and highly aggressive tumour associated with a poor prognosis.

Tumour terminology Recommended terms are in **bold**	Synonyms	Comments
Basal cell adenocarcinoma		A low grade malignancy. Over 90% occur in parotid.
Basal cell adenoma	Dermal anlage tumour	A benign tumour, which may sometimes resemble cylindroma of the skin.
Basalioma	See adenoid cystic carcinoma	Obsolete term.
Basaloid mixed tumour	See adenoid cystic carcinoma	Obsolete term.
Benign lymphoepithelial lesion	Mikulicz disease Myoepithelial sialadenitis	Tumour-like lesion, which is frequently associated with Sjögren's syndrome. Malignant transformation occasionally develops.
Benign metastasising pleomorphic adenoma	See metastasising pleomorphic adenoma	
Benign mixed tumour	See pleomorphic adenoma	
Canalicular adenoma		Benign tumour, which most often occurs in the upper lip.
Carcinoma arising in lymphoepithelial lesion	See lymphoepithelial carcinoma	
Carcinoma arising in mixed tumour	See carcinoma arising in pleomorphic adenoma	
Carcinoma arising in pleomorphic adenoma	Carcinoma arising in mixed tumour Malignant mixed tumour	This rare lesion represents carcinoma arising in a background of pleomorphic adenoma. It is an aggressive tumour, which shows a recurrence rate of up to 50%.
Carcinoma in Warthin's tumour		Malignancy arising in an underlying Warthin's tumour is extremely rare. Squamous cell carcinoma most commonly occurs but occasionally lymphomatous transformation occurs.
Carcinosarcoma	See metaplastic carcinoma	
Chronic sclerosing sialadenitis	Kuttner tumour	Tumour-like inflammatory lesion in submandibular salivary gland.
Cylindroma	See adenoid cystic carcinoma	Obsolete term.

Tumour terminology Recommended terms are in **bold**	Synonyms	Comments
Cystic lymphoid hyperplasia in AIDS		Tumour-like lesion consisting of lymphoid tissue containing multiple cystic cavities filled with mucin.
Dermal anlage tumour	See basal cell adenoma	
Dysgenetic disease of parotid gland	Polycystic salivary gland disease	Development malformation presenting as a tumour-like lesion.
Embryonal carcinoma		A very rare malignant tumour showing variable differentiation.
Epithelial myoepithelial carcinoma		Intermediate grade malignancy, which usually presents in old age. Local recurrence sometimes occurs.
Extrapulmonary oat cell carcinoma	See small cell carcinoma	
Haemangioma		See Tumours of Soft Tissue (Section 42).
Inflammatory pseudotumour		See Tumours of Soft Tissue (Section 42).
Intraductal papilloma		A very rare benign tumour of the excretory ducts of the minor salivary glands.
Inverted duct papilloma		An extremely rare benign tumour of the salivary duct.
Kuttner tumour	See chronic sclerosing sialadenitis	
Large cell undifferentiated carcinoma		High grade aggressive tumour that frequently metastasises and is associated with a poor prognosis.
Lipoma		See Tumours of Soft Tissue (Section 42).
Lobular carcinoma	See polymorphous low grade adenocarcinoma	Obsolete term.
Lymphadenoma		Extremely rare benign tumour.
Lymphoepithelial carcinoma	Carcinoma arising in lymphoepithelial lesion Malignant lymphoepithelial lesion Undifferentiated carcinoma with lymphoid stroma	Uncommon variant of undifferentiated carcinoma associated with a relatively good prognosis.

Tumour terminology Recommended terms are in **bold**	Synonyms	Comments
Malignant lymphoepithelial lesion	See lymphoepithelial carcinoma	
Malignant lymphoma		See Tumours of the Lymph Nodes and Spleen (Section 24).
Malignant mixed tumour	See carcinoma arising in pleomorphic adenoma	
Malignant myoepithelioma	See myoepithelial carcinoma	
Malignant oncocytoma	See oncocytic carcinoma	
Malignant oxyphilic granular cell tumour	See oncocytic carcinoma	
MALT Lymphoma	MALToma	Low grade B cell lymphoma frequently associated with Sjögren's syndrome.
MALToma	See MALT lymphoma	
Metaplastic carcinoma	Carcinosarcoma	High grade tumour with both carcinomatous and sarcomatous features. The five-year survival rate is poor.
Metastasising mixed tumour	See metastasising pleomorphic adenoma	
Metastasising pleomorphic adenoma	Benign metastasising pleomorphic adenoma Metastasising mixed tumour	This is an extremely rare histologically benign tumour, which behaves in a malignant fashion. Metastases to local lymph nodes may follow multiple recurrences.
Mikulicz disease	See benign lymphoepithelial lesion	
Mixed epidermoid and mucous-secreting carcinoma	See mucoepidermoid carcinoma	Obsolete term.
Mixed tumour	See pleomorphic adenoma	
Monomorphic adenoma		Obsolete term. This is used to designate a group of benign tumours
Mucinous adenocarcinoma		Rare low grade malignancy with a good prognosis. The majority of the tumour contains mucin.

Tumour terminology Recommended terms are in **bold**	Synonyms	Comments
Mucinous cystadenoma		Benign tumour. Histological appearances are much similar to malignant counterpart.
Mucoepidermoid carcinoma	Mixed epidermoid and mucous-secreting carcinoma (obsolete)	Most common malignant salivary gland tumour. Prognosis depends on the grade.
Multifocal oncocytic adenomatous hyperplasia		Rare tumour-like growth in the parotid gland, which can histologically mimic malignancy due to the presence of satellite foci.
Myoepithelial adenoma	See myoepithelioma	
Myoepithelial carcinoma	Malignant myoepithelioma	A very rare locally destructive tumour, which predominantly occurs in the parotid gland. Metastasis is infrequent.
Myoepithelial sialadenitis	See benign lymphoepithclial lesion	
Myoepithelioma	Adenomyoepithelioma (obsolete) Myoepithelial adenoma	Benign neoplasm closely related to pleomorphic adenoma and with similar potential for recurrence.
Necrotising sialometaplasia	Salivary gland infarction	Pseudotumour, which usually affects the minor salivary glands of the palate.
Oncocytic adenoma	See oncocytoma	
Oncocytic carcinoma	Malignant oncocytoma Malignant oxyphilic granular cell tumour	High grade malignant tumour, which frequently metastasises.
Oncocytoma	Oncocytic adenoma Oxyphilic adenoma (obsolete) Oxyphilic granular cell adenoma (obsolete)	Benign tumour.
Oncocytosis		A very rare non-neoplastic condition of the parotid gland.
Oxyphilic adenoma	See oncocytoma	Obsolete term.
Oxyphilic granular cell adenoma	See oncocytoma	Obsolete term.
Papillary cystadenocarcinoma		Rare low grade malignant tumour.

Tumour terminology Recommended terms are in **bold**	Synonyms	Comments
Papillary cystadenoma		Benign tumour, which closely resembles Warthin's tumour.
Papillary cystadenoma lymphomatosum	See Warthin's tumour	
Pleomorphic adenoma	Benign mixed tumour Mixed tumour	This is the most common benign salivary gland tumour. Malignant transformation may rarely occur particularly in long-standing lesions.
Polycystic salivary gland disease	See dysgenetic salivary gland disease	
Polymorphous low grade adenocarcinoma	Lobular carcinoma (obsolete) Terminal duct carcinoma	Low grade malignant tumour that appears to arise only in the minor salivary glands.
Salivary duct carcinoma		Extremely rare aggressive neoplasm with poor prognosis, which occurs almost exclusively in the parotid gland.
Salivary gland infarction	See necrotising sialometaplasia	
Sebaceous adenoma		Rare benign tumour composed of cells resembling sebaceous glands of skin.
Sebaceous carcinoma		Rare intermediate grade malignant tumour, which occurs exclusively in the parotid gland.
Sebaceous lymphadenocarcinoma		Extremely rare intermediate grade malignant tumour.
Sebaceous lymphadenoma		Rare benign tumour showing an admixture of sebaceous tissue and lymphoid cells.
Sialadenoma papilliferum		Rare benign tumour of ductal origin.
Sialadenosis	See sialosis	
Sialoblastoma		Extremely rare low grade malignant congenital or perinatal tumour.
Sialosis	Sialadenosis	Non-neoplastic and non-inflammatory swelling of major salivary glands, which may be associated with systemic disease.

Tumour terminology Recommended terms are in **bold**	Synonyms	Comments
Sjögren's syndrome		An autoimmune disorder. The risk of developing malignant lymphoma is forty times higher than in the normal population.
Small cell carcinoma	Extrapulmonary oat cell carcinoma	Extremely rare tumour. The possibility of a bronchial metastasis must always be excluded.
Squamous cell carcinoma		Primary squamous cell carcinoma of the salivary gland is very rare.
Terminal duct carcinoma	See polymorphous low grade adenocarcinoma	
Undifferentiated carcinoma		Rare malignant tumour.
Undifferentiated carcinoma with lymphoid stroma	See lymphoepithelial carcinoma	
Unilocular cystic sebaceous lymphadenoma		Rare benign tumour, which usually occurs in the parotid gland.
Warthin's tumour	Adenolymphoma Papillary cystadenoma lymphomatosum	Usually benign tumour that occurs almost exclusively in the parotid gland. This consists of oncocytic cells surrounded by lymphoid stroma.

Section 10

Tumours of the Oesophagus

W.V. Bogomoletz

Tumour terminology Recommended terms are in **bold**	Synonyms	Comments
Abrikossoff's tumour	See granular cell tumour	
Adenocarcinoma		Most cases arise in distal oesophagus in conjunction with Barrett's oesophagus. Histological variants include tubular and papillary (both common), mucinous, and signet ring cell (both rare).
Adenoid cystic carcinoma		Rare histological variant, which may be associated with squamous or undifferentiated carcinoma. Associated with aggressive behaviour.
Adenoma	Adenomatous polyp	Rare at this site. It is composed of dysplastic columnar epithelium and usually develops in association with Barrett's oesophagus.
Adenomatous polyp	See adenoma	
Adenosquamous carcinoma		Rare high grade histological variant of carcinoma showing both glandular and squamous differentiation. It should be treated as conventional squamous cell carcinoma. Most cases occur in the lower oesophagus, associated with Barrett's oesophagus.
Amyloid tumour		Vary rare tumour-like amyloid deposit.
Anaplastic carcinoma	See undifferentiated carcinoma	
Barrett's metaplasia	See Barrett's oesophagus	

Tumour terminology Recommended terms are in **bold**	Synonyms	Comments
Barrett's oesophagus	Barrett's metaplasia CELLO Columnar lined lower oesophagus	This is a condition in which oesophageal ulceration, as a consequence of reflux of gastric contents, is followed by re-epithelialisation by gastric and/or intestinal-type mucosa. This is associated with an increased risk of developing glandular epithelial dysplasia and adenocarcinoma.
Basaloid-squamous carcinoma		Histological variant of squamous carcinoma associated with aggressive behaviour and frequent metastases.
Carcinosarcoma	See metaplastic carcinoma	
CELLO	See Barrett's ocsophagus	Abbreviation of columnar lined lower oesophagus.
Columnar lined lower oesophagus	See Barrett's oesophagus	
Diffuse leiomyomatosis		Rare tumour-like condition of unknown aetiology in which there is hyperplasia involving the whole muscularis propria of the oesophagus. Sporadic autosomal dominant inherited forms have been described.
Early adenocarcinoma	See superficial adenocarcinoma	
Early squamous carcinoma	See superficial squamous carcinoma	
Endocrine tumour	See small cell carcinoma	
Epidermoid carcinoma	See squamous carcinoma	
Fibrous polyp	See fibrovascular polyp	
Fibrovascular polyp	Fibrous polyp	A polyp composed of fibrous or adipose connective tissue and blood vessels covered by normal squamous epithelium. Most common in the upper oesophagus.
Focal lymphoid hyperplasia	Pseudolymphoma	A rare reactive condition of the lymphoid tissue.
Glycogenic acanthosis		Multiple white elevations of the squamous epithelium due to increased cytoplasmic glycogen.

Tumour terminology Recommended terms are in **bold**	Synonyms	Comments
Granular cell myoblastoma	See granular cell tumour	
Granular cell tumour	Abrikossoff's tumour Granular cell myoblastoma	See Tumours of Soft Tissue (Section 42).
Haemangioma		See Tumours of Soft Tissue (Section 42).
Inflammatory fibroid polyp	Inflammatory pseudotumour	This is a tumour-like lesion probably of inflammatory origin and most common in middle and distal oesophagus. It is composed of oedematous fibrovascular tissue.
Inflammatory pseudotumour	See inflammatory fibroid polyp	
Kaposi's sarcoma		Oesophageal involvement is usually associated with AIDS. See Tumours of Soft Tissue (Section 42).
Leiomyoma		Most common benign non-epithelial tumour composed of smooth muscle. See Tumours of Soft Tissue (Section 42).
Leiomyosarcoma		A malignant smooth muscle tumour, which is rarely encountered in the oesophagus. Well differentiated variants may be difficult to distinguish from leiomyoma. Metastases are uncommon. See Tumours of Soft Tissue (Section 42).
Leukoplakia		A gross descriptive term for any mucosal white or whitish plaque. Obsolete term.
Malignant lymphoma		Involvement of the oesophagus by primary malignant lymphoma is very uncommon. See Tumours of the Lymph Nodes and Spleen (Section 24).
Malignant melanoma		This rarely occurs in the oesophagus and is usually associated with a poor prognosis. Metastatic melanoma is more common.
Metaplastic carcinoma	Carcinosarcoma Polypoid carcinoma Pseudosarcoma Spindle cell carcinoma Squamous cell carcinoma with spindle cell stroma	A high grade tumour characterised by both malignant epithelial and mesenchymal components.

Tumour terminology Recommended terms are in **bold**	Synonyms	Comments
Microinvasive adenocarcinoma	See superficial adenocarcinoma	
Microinvasive squamous carcinoma	See superficial squamous carcinoma	
Mucoepidermoid carcinoma		A rare form of carcinoma composed of squamous and mucous-secreting glands. Some are small, low grade, and arise from salivary-type submucosal oesophageal gland. Others are large, more aggressive, and may metastasise.
Neuroendocrine tumour	See small cell carcinoma	
Oat cell carcinoma	See small cell carcinoma	
Papilloma	See squamous cell papilloma	
Papillomatosis		Multiple squamous cell papillomas, which may be related to HPV infection.
Pleomorphic adenoma		A rare tumour, which arises from the submucosal mucous glands and resembles that which arises in the salivary glands.
Polypoid carcinoma		A gross descriptive term for a tumour protruding into the lumen. It is often used as a synonym for metaplastic carcinoma.
Pseudolymphoma	See focal lymphoid hyperplasia	
Pseudosarcoma	See metaplastic carcinoma	
Small cell carcinoma	Apudocarcinoma APUD-oma Neuroendocrine tumour Oat cell carcinoma	This is a high grade tumour, which resembles the bronchial equivalent. It is very rarely associated with hormone production.
Spindle cell carcinoma	See metaplastic carcinoma	
Squamous carcinoma	Epidermoid carcinoma	The most common malignant epithelial tumour of oesophagus.
Squamous cell carcinoma with spindle cell stroma	See metaplastic carcinoma	
Squamous cell papilloma	Papilloma	An uncommon benign tumour, which may be related to chronic irritation or HPV infection.

Tumour terminology Recommended terms are in **bold**	Synonyms	Comments
Superficial adenocarcinoma	Early adenocarcinoma Microinvasive adenocarcinoma	Adenocarcinoma confined to mucosa or submucosa, regardless of lymph node status.
Superficial squamous carcinoma	Early squamous carcinoma Microinvasive squamous carcinoma	Squamous cell carcinoma confined to mucosa or submucosa, regardless of lymph node status.
Undifferentiated carcinoma	Anaplastic carcinoma	High grade malignant epithelial tumour without any glandular or squamous differentiation.
Verrucous carcinoma		A rare variant of squamous cell carcinoma with an indolent course.

Section 11

Tumours of the Stomach

F. Carneiro

Tumour terminology Recommended terms are in **bold**	Synonyms	Comments
Abrikossoff's tumour	See granular cell tumour	
ACAG carcinoid	See carcinoid	ACAG: Type A of Chronic Atrophic Gastritis.
Adenocarcinoid tumour	See mixed carcinoid-adenocarcinoma	
Adenocarcinoma		This is the most common malignant epithelial tumour in the stomach. It may be graded into well, moderate, or poorly differentiated variants or else into low grade (well/moderately differentiated) and high grade (poorly differentiated). Histological variants include papillary, tubular, mucinous, signet ring cell, and adenosquamous. Prognosis is mainly dependent on the staging of the tumour.
Adenocarcinoma in situ	See carcinoma in situ	
Adeno-endocrine cell carcinoma	See mixed carcinoid-adenocarcinoma	
Adenoma	Adenomatous polyp	A pre-malignant tumour, which is relatively rare in the stomach. It is composed of dysplastic epithelium. Histological variants include tubular, tubulovillous, and villous. The epithelial atypia is classified as mild, moderate, or severe dysplasia. It may be associated with familial adenomatous polyposis.
Adenomatous polyp	See adenoma	
Adenomyoma	See pancreatic heterotopia	

Tumour terminology Recommended terms are in **bold**	Synonyms	Comments
Adeno-small cell carcinoma		A rare malignant tumour with similar biological behaviour as neuroendocrine small cell carcinoma. A term to be avoided.
Adenosquamous carcinoma		A rare histological variant of adenocarcinoma showing both malignant glandular and squamous differentiation. The overall prognosis tends to be worse than that of pure adenocarcinoma.
Anaplastic carcinoma	See undifferentiated carcinoma	
APUD carcinoma	See carcinoid tumour	Obsolete term.
APUD-oma	See carcinoid tumour	Obsolete term.
Atypical carcinoid	See carcinoid tumour	
Benign lymphoid hyperplasia	Lymphoid hyperplasia	Tumour-like lesion composed of reactive polyclonal lymphoid tissue.
Blue cell carcinoma	See lymphoepithelioma-like carcinoma	
Brunner gland heterotopia	See gastric gland heterotopia	
Carcinoid tumour	ACAG carcinoid APUD carcinoma (obsolete) APUD-oma (obsolete) Atypical carcinoid ECL cell carcinoid ECL-oma Endocrine tumour Neuroendocrine tumour Non-ACAG carcinoid	Two major types exist. One, the (atypical) "Non-ACAG" carcinoid, is rare; it is essentially the homologue in the gastric mucosa of the common small gut carcinoid. The markedly predominating type is the "ACAG" carcinoid, usually occurring in patients with the A-type of chronic atrophic gastritis and hypergastrinaemia (also in Zollinger-Ellison's syndrome). Its neoplastic parenchyma is formed by the histamine-producing Entero-Chromaffin-Like (ECL) cells ("ECL-oma"). It often appears as multiple polyps. When large, it can recur and metastasise (to the regional lymph nodes and liver). Neoplastic ECL cells can form the major part of the mixed carcinoid/adenocarcinomas.
Carcinoma in situ	Adenocarcinoma in situ	The term "dysplasia" is preferred for this early neoplastic proliferation. Not to be confused with intramucosal carcinoma.

Tumour terminology Recommended terms are in **bold**	Synonyms	Comments
Carcinoma with lymphoid stroma	See lymphoepithelioma-like carcinoma	
Carcinosarcoma	See metaplastic carcinoma	
Choriocarcinoma		Rare, but can occur in pure form or associated with adenocarcinoma. Associated with raised human chorionic-gonadotrophin.
Colloid adenocarcinoma	See mucinous adenocarcinoma	
Composite tumour	See mixed carcinoid-adenocarcinoma	
Cronkhite-Canada polyposis		This is a rare tumour-like lesion, which also affects other segments of gastro-intestinal tract. The polyps are benign but there is an increased risk of malignancy. It is associated with protein-losing enteropathy, alopecia, nail atrophy, and skin pigmentation. Exceptionally, disease is limited to the stomach.
Desmoplastic carcinoma	See signet ring cell carcinoma	
Diffuse carcinoma	See signet ring cell carcinoma	
Early carcinoma	Early gastric cancer Intramucosal adenocarcinoma Intramucosal carcinoma Microinvasive gastric cancer Submucosal carcinoma Superficial gastric cancer Surface gastric cancer	This term is used to describe adenocarcinoma confined to the mucosa (intramucosal carcinoma) or submucosa (submucosal carcinoma), regardless of histological type and the presence of lymph node and/or distant metastases.
Early gastric cancer	See early carcinoma	
ECL cell carcinoid	See carcinoid tumour	
ECL-oma	See carcinoid tumour	
Endocrine tumour	See carcinoid tumour	

Tumour terminology Recommended terms are in **bold**	Synonyms	Comments
Eosinophilic granuloma	See inflammatory fibroid polyp	
Epithelioid leiomyoma	Leiomyoblastoma (benign variant)	See Tumours of Soft Tissue (Section 42).
Epithelioid leiomyosarcoma	Leiomyoblastoma (malignant variant)	See Tumours of Soft Tissue (Section 42).
Expanding carcinoma		A term included in Ming's classification of gastric cancer and used to describe relatively circumscribed tumours with pushing growth margin, regardless of histological type.
Fibroid polyp	See inflammatory fibroid polyp	
Fundic gland hyperplasia	See Zollinger-Ellison syndrome	
Fundic gland polyp	Fundic gland polyposis Hamartomatous cystic polyp Polyp with fundic glandular cysts	Tumour-like hamartomatous condition characterised by microcysts lined by fundic epithelium. Can be multiple. Strong association with familial adenomatous polyposis (FAP).
Fundic gland polyposis	See fundic gland polyp	
GANT	See gastrointestinal autonomic nerve tumour	
Gastric gland heterotopia	Brunner gland heterotopia Submucosal cyst	Tumour-like lesion consisting of heterotopic Brunner's glands located in the submucosa. Other constituents include large ducts and smooth muscle.
Gastrinoma		This is a rare variant of neuroendocrine tumour (not classified under the term "carcinoid tumour"), which is associated with the production of gastrin. It may be associated with Zollinger-Ellison syndrome.
Gastritis cystica polyposa	Stomal polypoid hypertrophic gastritis	This tumour-like lesion occurs at or near to a gastrojejunal or gastroduodenal anastomosis.
Gastritis cystica profunda		Submucosal cyst. On occasions represents a heterotopic condition.

Tumour terminology Recommended terms are in **bold**	Synonyms	Comments
Gastrointestinal Autonomic Nerve Tumour	GANT Plexosarcoma	These tumours may be classified into malignant or borderline malignant variants. Some cases occur in the context of Carney syndrome (associated with pulmonary chondroma and extra-adrenal paragangliomas).
Gastrointestinal Stromal Tumour	GIST Stromal tumour	Generic term for benign, borderline, or malignant spindle tumours of mostly neurogenic or myogenic origin. Some tumours are of indeterminate histogenesis.
Giant fold hyperplasia	See hypertrophic/hyperplastic gastropathy	
Giant hypertrophic gastritis	See hypertrophic/hyperplastic gastropathy	
Giant rugal hypertrophy	See Ménétrier's disease	
GIST	See gastrointestinal stromal tumour	
Glandular carcinoma		This term is used in some classifications to describe tumours with a predominantly glandular structure. It may be used as a synonym for intestinal, tubular, and papillary carcinomas.
Granular cell myoblastoma	See granular cell tumour	
Granular cell tumour	Abrikossoff's tumour Granular cell myoblastoma	See Tumours of Soft Tissue (Section 42).
Granuloblastoma	See inflammatory fibroid polyp	
Hamartomatous cystic polyp	See fundic gland polyp	
Hepatoid carcinoma		Very rare, high grade, histological variant of gastric adenocarcinoma combining conventional glandular components with hepatoma-like areas.
Hyperplasiogenic polyp	See hyperplastic polyp	
Hyperplastic gastropathy	See hypertrophic/hyperplastic gastropathy	

Tumour terminology Recommended terms are in **bold**	Synonyms	Comments
Hyperplastic polyp	Hyperplasiogenic polyp Inflammatory polyp Regenerative polyp	The most common benign gastric polyp, which exhibits elongation of the foveolar glands with some cystic change. Low risk of malignancy. Can be multiple.
Hypertrophic gastropathy	See hypertrophic/ hyperplastic gastropathy	
Hypertrophic hypersecretory gastropathy		Variant of hypertrophic/hyperplastic gastropathy in which there is a strong association with peptic ulcer. Hypergastrinaemia is typically absent.
Hypertrophic hypersecretory gastropathy with protein loss		Very rare variant of hypertrophic/ hyperplastic gastropathy associated with acid hypersecretion and protein loss.
Hypertrophic rugal lesion	See hypertrophic/ hyperplastic gastropathy	
Hypertrophic/ hyperplastic gastropathy	Giant fold hyperplasia Giant hypertrophic gastritis Hyperplastic gastropathy Hypertrophic gastropathy Hypertrophic rugal lesion Ménétrier's disease	Tumour-like lesion consisting of markedly enlarged mucosal folds in the body and fundus of the stomach. The antrum is spared. Prominent foveolar hyperplasia is associated with hypo/ achlorhydria and protein loosing enteropathy. Variants include Zollinger-Ellison syndrome, hypertrophic hypersecretory gastropathy, and hypertrophic hypersecretory gastropathy with protein loss.
Infiltrating carcinoma		A term used in Ming's classification of gastric cancer to describe tumours with a widely infiltrative growth pattern irrespective of histological type.
Inflammatory fibroid polyp	Eosinophilic granuloma Fibroid polyp Granuloblastoma	A pseudotumour characterised by oedematous fibro-vascular proliferation and inflammatory cells with prominent eosinophils.
Inflammatory polyp	See hyperplastic polyp	
Intestinal carcinoma	Intestinal cell type carcinoma	A term used in Laurén's classification to describe tumours with a glandular structure (papillary and/or tubular), usually occurring in a background of chronic atrophic gastritis with intestinal metaplasia.

Tumour terminology Recommended terms are in **bold**	Synonyms	Comments
Intestinal cell type carcinoma	See intestinal carcinoma	
Intramucosal adenocarcinoma	See early carcinoma	
Intramucosal carcinoma	See early carcinoma	
Isolated-cell type carcinoma	See signet ring cell carcinoma	
Juvenile polyp/polyposis	Retention polyp	A hamartomatous polyp, which occurs most frequently in the colon, but can also arise in the stomach. Oedematous stroma surrounds cystically dilated benign glands. Can be multiple (polyposis).
Leiomyoblastoma (benign variant)	See epithelioid leiomyoma	See Tumours of Soft Tissue (Section 42).
Leiomyoblastoma (malignant variant)	See epithelioid leiomyosarcoma	See Tumours of Soft Tissue (Section 42).
Leiomyoma		This is the most common benign non-epithelial tumour of the stomach. See Tumours of Soft Tissue (Section 42).
Leiomyosarcoma		This is the most common malignant non-epithelial tumour of the stomach. See Tumours of Soft Tissue (Section 42).
Linitis plastica	See signet ring cell carcinoma	Obsolete term.
Lymphoepithelial carcinoma	See lymphoepithelioma-like carcinoma	
Lymphoepithelioma-like carcinoma	Blue cell carcinoma Carcinoma with lymphoid stroma Lymphoepithelial carcinoma Medullary carcinoma with lymphoid stroma	A histological variant of adenocarcinoma characterised by an undifferentiated epithelial cell population surrounded by a dense, diffuse lymphocytic infiltrate. It may be associated with Epstein-Barr virus infection. The prognosis is favourable when compared with typical gastric adenocarcinoma.
Lymphoid hyperplasia	See benign lymphoid hyperplasia	
Malignant lymphoma	MALT lymphoma MALToma	Most gastric lymphomas are of the MALToma type. (Mucosa associated lymphoma). See Tumours of the Lymph Nodes and Spleen (Section 24).

Tumour terminology Recommended terms are in **bold**	Synonyms	Comments
MALT lymphoma	See malignant lymphoma	
MALToma	See malignant lymphoma	
Medullary carcinoma	See undifferentiated carcinoma	
Medullary carcinoma with lymphoid stroma	See lymphoepithelioma-like carcinoma	
Melanoma		Primary melanoma is extremely rare. Metastasis should always be excluded.
Ménétrier's disease	Giant rugal hypertrophy	This tumour-like lesion is a variant of hypertrophic/hyperplastic gastropathy and is associated with hypochlorhydria/achlorhydria and protein loss.
Metaplastic carcinoma	Carcinosarcoma Sarcomatoid carcinoma	A rare high grade histological variant of gastric adenocarcinoma, which is composed of an admixture of glandular and spindle cells commonly associated with heterologous differentiation such as smooth muscle, cartilage etc.
Microcarcinoid		Microscopic proliferation of neuroendocrine ECL cells against the background of the A-type of Chronic Atrophic Gastritis (ACAG).
Microinvasive gastric cancer	See early carcinoma	
Mixed carcinoid-adenocarcinoma	Adenocarcinoid tumour Adeno-endocrine cell carcinoma Composite tumour	This histological variant of carcinoid tumour is rare in the stomach. It is composed of an admixture of neuroendocrine elements, usually ECL cells, and adenocarcinomatous parenchyma.
Mixed carcinoma		A term used in some classifications to encompass tumours with more than one histological type. Prognosis is usually worse than that of carcinoma of pure histological type.
Mixed hyperplastic and adenomatous polyp		This pre-malignant condition encompasses both hyperplastic and dysplastic areas.

Tumour terminology Recommended terms are in **bold**	Synonyms	Comments
Mucinous adenocarcinoma	Colloid adenocarcinoma Mucoid adenocarcinoma Muconodular adenocarcinoma	Histological variant of adenocarcinoma characterised by the presence of abundant extracellular mucin.
Mucocellular carcinoma	See signet ring cell carcinoma	
Mucoid adenocarcinoma	See mucinous adenocarcinoma	
Muconodular adenocarcinoma	See mucinous adenocarcinoma	
Mucous cell carcinoma	See signet ring cell carcinoma	
Myoepithelial hamartoma	See pancreatic heterotopia	
Neuroendocrine cell hyperplasia		This pre-neoplastic condition is associated with A-type Chronic Atrophic Gastritis (ACAG), hyper-gastrinemia, with or without pernicious anaemia.
Neuroendocrine tumour	See carcinoid tumour	
Non-ACAG carcinoid	See carcinoid tumour	ACAG: Type A of Chronic Atrophic Gastritis
Pancreatic heterotopia		Submucosal collection of normal pancreatic tissue, which may clinically present as a mass.
Papillary adenocarcinoma		Histological variant of adenocarcinoma characterised by a papillary architecture.
Parietal cell carcinoma		A rare variant of gastric carcinoma with eosinophilic cells rich in mitochondria.
Peutz-Jeghers' polyp		Hamartomatous polyp, which consists of arborescent smooth muscle fibres, lined by benign epithelial cells. Malignant change is rare. Can be multiple.
Plasmacytoma		This lesion is rare in the stomach. See Tumours of the Lymph Nodes and Spleen (Section 24).
Plexosarcoma	See gastrointestinal autonomic nerve tumour	

Tumour terminology Recommended terms are in **bold**	Synonyms	Comments
Polyp with fundic glandular cysts	See fundic gland polyp	
Regenerative polyp	See hyperplastic polyp	
Retention polyp	See juvenile polyp / polyposis	
Sarcomatoid carcinoma	See metaplastic carcinoma	
Scirrhous carcinoma	See signet ring cell carcinoma	
Signet ring cell carcinoma	Desmoplastic carcinoma Diffuse carcinoma Isolated-cell type carcinoma Linitis plastica (obsolete) Mucocellular carcinoma Mucous cell carcinoma	This histological variant of adenocarcinoma consists of signet ring cells containing abundant intracytoplasmic mucin. It is characterised by a tendency for widespread peritoneal dissemination and nodal metastases. Tumours may be associated with an abundant fibrous stroma (desmoplastic or scirrhous carcinoma). When the entire stomach is involved, the term "linitis plastica" is sometimes applied. Some have hereditary conditioning.
Simplex carcinoma	See undifferentiated carcinoma	
Small cell carcinoma		High grade neuroendocrine tumour morphologically and prognostically similar to the pulmonary counterpart.
Solid carcinoma	See undifferentiated carcinoma	
Solid medullary carcinoma	See undifferentiated carcinoma	
Squamous cell carcinoma		Most tumours present in the cardia as a result of spread from an oesophageal primary lesion.
Stomal polypoid hypertrophic gastritis	See gastritis cystica polyposa	
Stromal tumour	See gastrointestinal stromal tumour	
Submucosal carcinoma	See early carcinoma	

Tumour terminology Recommended terms are in **bold**	Synonyms	Comments
Submucosal cyst	See gastric gland heterotopia	
Superficial gastric cancer	See early carcinoma	
Surface gastric cancer	See early carcinoma	
Tubular adenocarcinoma		Histological variant of adenocarcinoma characterised by a tubular architecture. Most intestinal carcinomas are tubular.
Tubular adenoma		Histological variant of adenoma characterised by a tubular architecture.
Tubulovillous adenoma		Histological variant of adenoma characterised by a tubulovillous architecture.
Undifferentiated carcinoma	Anaplastic carcinoma Medullary carcinoma Simplex carcinoma Solid carcinoma Solid medullary carcinoma	High grade histological variant of carcinoma devoid of glandular or squamous cell differentiation.
Villous adenoma		Histological variant of adenoma characterised by a villous (papillary) structure.
Zollinger-Ellison syndrome	Fundic gland hyperplasia See also carcinoid tumour See also gastrinoma	This syndrome is the result of a tumour-like lesion and a variant of hypertrophic/hyperplastic gastropathy. It is characterised by peptic ulceration and increased gastrin secretion complicating a gastrinoma or neuroendocrine cell hyperplasia/tumour. It may be associated with multiple endocrine neoplasia (MEN I).

Section 12

Tumours of the Small Intestine Including Duodenum and Ampulla of Vater

W.V. Bogomoletz

Tumour terminology Recommended terms are in **bold**	Synonyms	Comments
Abrikossoff's tumour	See granular cell tumour	
Adenocarcinoma		Adenocarcinoma is rare at this site. Most tumours occur in the ampullary or periampullary region and many arise in pre-existent adenomas. Subtypes: adenocarcinoma NOS, mucinous, and signet ring.
Adenocarcinoma NOS	.	Histological variant of adenocarcinoma in which there are no specific distinguishing features, i.e., not otherwise specified.
Adenoma	Adenomatous polyp	This tumour most often occurs in the ampullary and periampullary regions. May be classified as villous, tubular, and tubulovillous with low or high grade dysplasia.
Adenomatosis		Multiple adenomas are often associated with familial adenomatous polyposis of the colon.
Adenomatous polyp	See adenoma	
Adenosquamous carcinoma		Extremely rare variant of adenocarcinoma showing foci of squamous differentiation.
Anaplastic carcinoma	See undifferentiated carcinoma	
APUD carcinoma	See carcinoid tumour	Obsolete term.

Tumour terminology Recommended terms are in **bold**	Synonyms	Comments
APUD-oma	See carcinoid tumour	Obsolete term.
Benign lymphoid polyp	See lymphoid hyperplasia	
Brunner's gland adenoma	Brunneroma Brunner's gland hyperplasia Polypoid hamartoma	This tumour-like proliferation of Brunner's glands probably represents a hyperplasia or hamartoma.
Brunner's gland hyperplasia	See Brunner's gland adenoma	
Brunneroma	See Brunner's gland adenoma	
Carcinoid tumour	APUD carcinoma (obsolete) APUD-oma (obsolete) Endocrine tumour Neuroendocrine cell tumour	Low grade malignant tumour arising in the diffuse neuroendocrine system. Metastases to the liver may be associated with the carcinoid syndrome.
Colloid carcinoma	See mucinous adenocarcinoma	
Cronkhite-Canada polyposis		This non-inherited syndrome is characterised by the presence of tumour-like hamartomatous lesions in the gastro-intestinal tract associated with alopecia, nail atrophy, skin hyperpigmentation, and protein loss.
Diffuse ganglioneuromatosis		Intestinal ganglioneuromatosis may occur in association with multiple endocrine neoplasia type IIB (MEN-3) See Tumours of the Adrenal Cortex, Adrenal Medulla, and Paraganglia (Section 6).
Diffuse nodular lymphoid hyperplasia	Lymphoid polyposis	This hyperplastic condition may develop in association with adult primary hypogammaglobulinaemia.
Endocrine tumour	See carcinoid tumour	
Endometriosis		Tumour-like condition due to the presence of endometrial glands and stroma, which may be confused with a carcinoma or sarcoma.

Tumour terminology Recommended terms are in **bold**	Synonyms	Comments
Enteropathy associated T-cell lymphoma	See T-cell malignant lymphoma	
Eosinophilic granulomatous polyp	See inflammatory fibroid polyp	
Gangliocytic paraganglioma	Nonchromaffin paraganglioma Paraganglioma	This is an extremely rare, benign tumour of endocrine and ganglion cells, which presents as a polypoid lesion in the second part of duodenum. See Tumours of the Adrenal Cortex, Adrenal Medulla, and Paraganglia (Section 6).
Ganglioneuroma		This very rare benign tumour consists of an admixture of ganglion cells and neurofibromatous tissue.
GANT	See gastrointestinal autonomic nerve tumour	
Gastric heterotopia	Heterotopic tumour	Tumour-like lesion composed of ectopic gastric mucosa.
Gastrointestinal autonomic nerve tumour	GANT Plexosarcoma	Malignant tumour of variable grade derived from autonomic nervous tissue.
Gastrointestinal stromal tumour	GIST	Generic name for benign or malignant stromal spindle cell tumours of uncertain histogenesis. In particular they do not usually express smooth muscle or neural markers.
GIST	See gastrointestinal stromal tumour	
Granular cell myoblastoma	See granular cell tumour	
Granular cell tumour	Abrikossoff's tumour Granular cell myoblastoma	See Tumours of Soft Tissue (Section 42).
Heterotopic tumour	See gastric heterotopia See pancreatic heterotopia	Tumour-like lesion consisting of ectopic pancreatic or gastric tissue most commonly found in the duodenum or Meckel's diverticulum.
Immunoproliferative small intestinal disease	IPSID Mediterranean lymphoma Malignant lymphoma	B-cell lymphoma distinct in the small intestine associated with malabsorbtion and occurring in patients of Mediterranean origin. See Tumours of the Lymph Nodes and Spleen (Section 24).

Tumour terminology Recommended terms are in **bold**	Synonyms	Comments
Inflammatory fibroid polyp	Eosinophilic granulomatous polyp Inflammatory pseudotumour	The small intestine is the most common site for this inflammatory tumour-like lesion composed of oedematous fibrovascular tissue with prominent eosinophils.
Inflammatory pseudotumour	See inflammatory fibroid polyp	
IPSID	See immunoproliferative small intestinal disease	
Juvenile polyp		This hamartomatous lesion may occasionally occur in the small intestine. See Tumours of the Large Intestine and Appendix (Section 13).
Juvenile polyposis		Multiple juvenile polyps. See Tumours of the Large Intestine and Appendix (Section 13).
Kaposi's sarcoma		Small intestinal lesions are usually associated with AIDS. See Tumours of Soft Tissue (Section 42).
Leiomyoma		See Tumours of Soft Tissue (Section 42).
Leiomyosarcoma		Most frequently encountered malignant non-epithelial tumour in the small intestine. See Tumours of Soft Tissue (Section 42).
Lipohyperplasia of ileocaecal valve		A benign tumour-like lesion composed of fat.
Lipoma		See Tumours of Soft Tissue (Section 42).
Lymphangioma		See Tumours of Soft Tissue (Section 42).
Lymphoid hyperplasia	Benign lymphoid polyp Pseudolymphoma	Tumour-like benign lesion usually occurring in terminal ileum of children.
Lymphoid polyposis	See diffuse nodular lymphoid hyperplasia	
Malignant lymphoma	See immunoproliferative small intestinal disease See mucosa associated lymphoid tissue lymphoma	

Tumour terminology Recommended terms are in **bold**	Synonyms	Comments
MALToma	See mucosa associated lymphoid tissue lymphoma	
Mediterranean lymphoma	See immunoproliferative small intestinal disease	
Mucinous adenocarcinoma	Colloid carcinoma Mucoid carcinoma	Histological variant of adenocarcinoma characterised by abundant mucin production.
Mucoid carcinoma	See mucinous adenocarcinoma	
Mucosa associated lymphoid tissue lymphoma	MALToma Malignant lymphoma	See Tumours of the Lymph Nodes and Spleen (Section 24).
Neurilemmoma	Schwannoma	See Tumours of Soft Tissue (Section 42).
Neuroendocrine cell tumour	See carcinoid tumour	
Neurofibroma		See Tumours of Soft Tissue (Section 42).
Nonchromaffin paraganglioma	See gangliocytic paraganglioma	
Oat cell carcinoma	See small cell carcinoma	
Pancreatic heteropia	Heterotopic tumour	Tumour-like lesion consisting of ectopic pancreatic tissue.
Paraganglioma	See gangliocytic paraganglioma	See Tumours of the Adrenal Cortex, Adrenal Medulla, and Paraganglia (Section 6).
Peutz-Jeghers' polyp		Hamartomatous lesion most often arising in a background of Peutz-Jeghers' syndrome (see below). It may rarely present as an isolated lesion.
Peutz-Jeghers' polyposis	See Peutz-Jeghers' syndrome	
Peutz-Jeghers' syndrome	Peutz-Jeghers' polyposis	Hamartomatous polyps are a feature of this autosomal dominant inherited condition. Multiple lentigines are also characteristic. The development of malignancy is a very rare complication.
Plexosarcoma	See gastrointestinal autonomic nerve tumour	

Tumour terminology Recommended terms are in **bold**	Synonyms	Comments
Polypoid ganglioneuromatosis		Small intestinal involvement may occur in association with juvenile polyposis and Cowden's syndrome.
Polypoid hamartoma	See Brunner's gland adenoma	
Pseudolymphoma	See lymphoid hyperplasia	
Schwannoma	See neurilemmoma	
Signet ring cell carcinoma		Histological variant of adenocarcinoma characterised by the presence of intracellular mucin.
Small cell carcinoma	Oat cell carcinoma	This rare variant of neuroendocrine carcinoma is associated with a poor prognosis and is similar to the bronchial counterpart.
T-cell malignant lymphoma	Enteropathy associated T-cell lymphoma	T-cell lymphoma associated with coeliac disease. See Tumours of the Lymph Nodes and Spleen (Section 24).
Undifferentiated carcinoma	Anaplastic carcinoma	High grade malignant epithelial tumour without any recognisable glandular differentiation.

Section 13

Tumours of the Large Intestine and Appendix

W.V. Bogomoletz

Tumour terminology Recommended terms are in **bold**	Synonyms	Comments
Abrikossoff's tumour	See granular cell tumour	
Adenocarcinoid	See goblet cell carcinoid	
Adenocarcinoma		Most common malignant epithelial tumour of the large intestine. Appendiceal lesions are very rare. Histological variants include adenosquamous, mucinous, signet ring, and metaplastic squamous tumours.
Adenoma	Adenomatous polyp	A common pre-malignant lesion, which may present as solitary or multiple tumours, is classified into tubular, tubulovillous, or villous subtypes.
Adenomatosis	Polyposis	The term implies multiple adenomas, which may present in a non-familial or familial setting (see also familial adenomatous polyposis).
Adenomatous polyp	See adenoma	
Adenosquamous carcinoma		Histological variant of adenocarcinoma showing foci of squamous differentiation.
Anaplastic carcinoma	See undifferentiated carcinoma	
APUD carcinoma	See carcinoid tumour	Obsolete term.
APUD-oma	See carcinoid tumour	Obsolete term.
Basaloid carcinoma	Cloacogenic carcinoma	Exceptionally rarely this tumour may present in the rectum.

Tumour terminology Recommended terms are in **bold**	Synonyms	Comments
Benign lymphoid polyp	Lymphoid hyperplasia Pseudolymphoma	Reactive condition composed of hyperplastic lymphoid tissue; may be single or present as multiple lesions (polyposis). The rectum is the most frequent site. It must be distinguished from true malignant lymphoma.
Cap polyp	See inflammatory polyp	
Carcinoid tumour	APUD carcinoma, APUD-oma Endocrine tumour Neuroendocrine tumour	Most common primary tumour of the appendix. In the large intestine carcinoid tumours are uncommon—the rectum being the most frequently affected site. Appendiceal tumours are usually incidental findings and very rarely behave aggressively (see goblet cell carcinoid). Metastasis from a rectal primary is rare.
Cloacogenic carcinoma	See basaloid carcinoma	
Colloid carcinoma	See mucinous adenocarcinoma	
Cowden's syndrome	Multiple hamartoma syndrome	Rare syndrome combining the presence of juvenile polyposis with tricholemomas and acral keratosis.
Cronkhite-Canada polyposis		A non-inherited syndrome characterised by the presence of tumour-like hamartomatous polyps in the gastro-intestinal tract associated with alopecia, nail atrophy, skin pigmentation, and protein loss.
Crypt cell carcinoma	See goblet cell carcinoid	
Cystadenoma	See mucinous cystadenoma	
Diffuse ganglioneuromatosis		This condition may develop in association with multiple endocrine neoplasia type IIB (MEN-3). It may also arise in a background of von Recklinghausen's disease.
Endocrine tumour	See carcinoid tumour	
Familial adenomatous polyposis	Adenomatosis Familial polyposis FAP	This hereditary autosomal dominant condition is characterised by the presence of innumerable adenomatous polyps and usually presents in the second decade. Malignant transformation is almost inevitable.

Tumour terminology Recommended terms are in **bold**	Synonyms	Comments
Familial polyposis	See familial adenomatous polyposis	
FAP	See familial adenomatous polyposis	
Ganglioneuroma		This rare tumour may present as a solitary lesion or as part of diffuse ganglioneuromatosis. See above and Tumours of the Adrenal Cortex, Adrenal Medulla, and Paraganglia (Section 6).
GANT	See gastrointestinal autonomic nerve tumour	
Gardner's syndrome		This rare syndrome combines the features of familial adenomatous polyposis with soft tissue fibromatosis, skull/mandibular osteomas, and multiple epidermoid cysts.
Gastric heterotopia		Tumour-like lesion composed of ectopic gastric mucosa.
Gastrointestinal autonomic nerve tumour	GANT Plexosarcoma	These tumours may be classified into malignant or borderline malignant variants. Some cases occur in the context of Carney syndrome (associated with pulmonary chondroma and extra-adrenal paragangliomas).
Gastrointestinal stromal tumour	GIST	Generic name for benign or malignant neurogenic or smooth muscle tumours.
GIST	See gastrointestinal stromal tumour	
Goblet cell carcinoid	Adenocarcinoid Crypt cell carcinoma Goblet cell type adenocarcinoid Microglandular carcinoma Mixed carcinoid-adenocarcinoma Mucinous carcinoid Mucinous carcinoid tumour	This variant occurs only in the appendix and is believed to behave in a more aggressive fashion than classical carcinoid tumour. It is composed of an admixture of mucus containing signet ring/goblet cells and neuroendocrine cells. It must be distinguished from signet ring cell carcinoma.

Tumour terminology Recommended terms are in **bold**	Synonyms	Comments
Goblet cell type adenocarcinoid	See goblet cell carcinoid	
Granular cell myoblastoma	See granular cell tumour	
Granular cell neurofibroma	See granular cell tumour	
Granular cell tumour	Abrikossoff's tumour Granular cell myoblastoma Granular cell neurofibroma	See Tumours of Soft Tissue (Section 42).
Haemangioma		See Tumours of Soft Tissue (Section 42).
Hyperplastic polyp	Metaplastic polyp	Tumour-like lesion mainly found in the sigmoid colon and rectum. It has no malignant potential.
Hyperplastic polyposis	Metaplastic polyposis	Multiple hyperplastic polyps, which affect the entire colon and rectum and may additionally show coexisting adenomas or mixed adenoma-hyperplastic polyps.
Inflammatory myoglandular polyp		Tumour-like lesion composed of hyperplastic epithelium, granulation tissue, and smooth muscle.
Inflammatory polyp	Cap polyp	This inflammatory pseudotumour may complicate ulcerative colitis or ureterosigmoidostomy.
Juvenile polyp	Retention polyp	This common hamartomatous lesion may be single or multiple. Malignant change is exceptionally rare.
Juvenile polyposis		This rare condition may present in young children with intussusception and protein-losing enteropathy or as rectal bleeding. Dysplastic changes are not uncommon.
Kaposi's sarcoma		At this site it is mainly associated with AIDS. See Tumours of Soft Tissue (Section 42).
Leiomyoma		See Tumours of Soft Tissue (Section 42).
Leiomyosarcoma		See Tumours of Soft Tissue (Section 42).

Tumour terminology Recommended terms are in **bold**	Synonyms	Comments
Lipoma		See Tumours of Soft Tissue (Section 42).
Lymphangioma		See Tumours of Soft Tissue (Section 42).
Lymphoid hyperplasia	See benign lymphoid polyp	
Malignant lymphoma		Rare in the large intestine. May complicate chronic ulcerative colitis and AIDS. The great majority of these tumours are of the MALToma type. See Tumours of the Small Intestine (Section 12).
Metaplastic polyp	See hyperplastic polyp	
Metaplastic polyposis	See hyperplastic polyposis	
Microglandular carcinoma	See goblet cell carcinoid	
Mixed carcinoid-adenocarcinoma		Variant of goblet cell carcinoid tumour characterised by an infiltrating growth pattern and associated with a poorer prognosis than the common appendiceal carcinoid. It only occurs in the appendix.
Mucinous adenocarcinoma	Colloid carcinoma Mucoid carcinoma	Histological variant of adenocarcinoma in which by definition at least 50% of the tumour is composed of extracellular mucin.
Mucinous carcinoid	See goblet cell carcinoid	
Mucinous carcinoid tumour	See goblet cell carcinoid	
Mucinous cystadenocarcinoma		Malignant variant of mucinous cystadenoma, which only occurs in the appendix and may be associated with the development of pseudomyxoma peritoneii.
Mucinous cystadenoma	Cystadenoma	This tumour only occurs in the appendix and may predispose to the development of a mucocele.
Mucocele		The term refers to cystic dilatation of the appendix occurring as a consequence of mucus accumulation. It may result from an inflammatory or neoplastic process.

Tumour terminology Recommended terms are in **bold**	Synonyms	Comments
Mucoid carcinoma	See mucinous adenocarcinoma	
Multiple hamartoma syndrome	See Cowden's syndrome	
Neurilemmoma	Schwannoma	See Tumours of Soft Tissue (Section 42).
Neuroendocrine cell tumour	See carcinoid tumour See small cell carcinoma	
Neurofibroma		See Tumours of Soft Tissue (Section 42).
Neurofibromatosis		Large bowel involvement may occur in patients with von Recklinghausen's disease. See Tumours of Soft Tissue (Section 42).
Oat cell carcinoma	See small cell carcinoma	
Peutz-Jeghers' polyposis	See Peutz-Jeghers' syndrome	
Peutz-Jeghers' syndrome	Peutz-Jeghers' polyposis	These hamartomatous polyps may also affect the large intestine.
Plexosarcoma	See gastrointestinal autonomic nerve tumour	
Polypoid ganglioneuromatosis		This rare condition may present with multiple mucosal polyps. See Tumours of the Small Intestine (Section 12).
Polyposis	See adenomatosis	
Pseudolymphoma	See benign lymphoid polyp	
Pseudomyxoma peritoneii		Generic term for rupture of an appendiceal mucocele of neoplastic nature with shedding of malignant mucous-secreting epithelial cells into the peritoneal cavity.
Retention polyp	See juvenile polyp	
Schwannoma	See neurilemmoma	
Signet ring cell carcinoma		High grade histological variant of adenocarcinoma in which the presence of intracytoplasmic mucin gives rise to a signet ring cell appearance.

Tumour terminology Recommended terms are in **bold**	Synonyms	Comments
Small cell carcinoma	Neuroendocrine cell tumour Oat cell carcinoma	Histological variant of large bowel carcinoma showing neuroendocrine differentiation and associated with a very poor prognosis.
Solitary rectal ulcer		Tumour-like lesion, which presents as a polypoid or ulcerated lesion usually complicating mucosal prolapse.
Squamous cell carcinoma		A rare tumour resulting from almost complete squamous metaplasia of an adenocarcinoma.
Torre-Muir syndrome		The association of colonic carcinoma with cutaneous sebaceous tumours and keratoacanthoma.
Tubular adenoma	See adenoma	
Tubular type adenocarcinoid		This is a histological variant of carcinoid tumour characterised by a pure glandular morphology.
Tubulovillous adenoma	See adenoma	
Undifferentiated carcinoma	Anaplastic carcinoma	High grade malignant epithelial tumour without any glandular or squamous differentiation.
Villous adenoma	See adenoma	

Section 14

Tumours of the Anal Canal and Anus

W.V. Bogomoletz

Tumour terminology Recommended terms are in **bold**	Synonyms	Comments
Adenocarcinoma		Most of these tumours arise in the upper part of the anal canal and are morphologically identical to rectal tumours.
Anal papillae	See fibroepithelial polyp	
Anal tag	See fibroepithelial polyp	
Anaplastic carcinoma	See undifferentiated carcinoma	
Basaloid carcinoma	Cloacogenic carcinoma Transitional carcinoma	Rare form of poorly differentiated squamous cell carcinoma arising from the transitional zone (dentate line) of the anal canal.
Bowen's disease		See Tumours of Skin (Non-Melanocytic) (Section 41).
Bowenoid papulosis		See Tumours of Skin (Non-Melanocytic) (Section 41).
Buschke-Löwenstein tumour	See giant condyloma acuminatum	
Cloacogenic carcinoma	See basaloid carcinoma	
Condyloma acuminatum	Venereal wart Viral wart	Viral-induced squamous papillary lesion, often multiple. See Tumours of Skin (Non-Melanocytic) (Section 41).
Cystic hamartoma		Retrorectal tumour-like lesion.
Epidermotropic carcinoma	See extramammary Paget's disease	

Tumour terminology Recommended terms are in **bold**	Synonyms	Comments
Epidermotropic carcinoma	See extramammary Paget's disease	
Extramammary Paget's disease	Epidermotropic carcinoma Pagetoid dermatosis	See Tumours of Skin (Non-Melanocytic) (Section 41).
Fibroepithelial polyp	Anal papillae Anal tag	See Tumours of Skin (Non-Melanocytic) (Section 41).
Flat dysplastic lesion		"Flat" pre-cancerous lesion, often identified in high-risk populations (homosexuals, AIDS patients). Often viral induced.
Giant condyloma acuminatum	Buschke-Löwenstein tumour	Large viral-induced cauliflower-like lesion, histologically resembling condyloma acuminatum. Slow growing, prone to recurrences and associated with sinus and fistula formation. Does not metastasise.[1]
Inflammatory cloacogenic polyp		A tumour-like lesion of the anorectal junction, which develops as a complication of mucosal prolapse syndrome.
Leukoplakia		Clinical term meaning white plaque.
Melanoma		Rare at this site. It is usually high grade with a poor prognosis.
Mucinous adenocarcinoma		Rare variant of adenocarcinoma, which arises in association with a chronic anorectal fistula.
Oleogranuloma		Tumour-like lesion, which usually follows injection of haemorrhoids.
Pagetoid dermatosis	See extramammary Paget's disease	
Papilloma	See squamous cell papilloma	

[1] Other authors consider giant cell condyloma (synonym Buschke-Löwenstein tumour) and verrucous carcinoma as the same lesion: See Section 36 (Tumours of the Vagina), Section 37 (Tumours of the Vulva), and Section 41 (Tumours of the Skin, Non-Melanocytic)

Tumour terminology Recommended terms are in **bold**	Synonyms	Comments
Papillomatosis		Refers to multiple squamous cell papillomas.
Squamous cell carcinoma		Common in male homosexuals with AIDS. Most cases arise from the transitional zone (dentate line) of the anal canal. May be keratinising or non-keratinising, the latter often referred to as basaloid carcinoma. Preceded by dysplasia.
Squamous cell papilloma	Papilloma	Arises from squamous epithelium of anal canal. May be HPV-Induced and is then referred to as condyloma acuminatum. Frequently multiple.
Transitional carcinoma	See basaloid carcinoma	
Undifferentiated carcinoma	Anaplastic carcinoma	High grade malignant epithelial tumour without any glandular or squamous differentiation.
Venereal wart	See condyloma acuminatum	
Verrucous carcinoma		Well differentiated keratinising squamous cell carcinoma often resulting from the rare malignant transformation of condyloma acuminatum and giant condyloma acuminatum.
Viral wart	See condyloma acuminatum	

Section 15

Tumours of the Liver and Intrahepatic Bile Ducts

R. Colombari
G.M. Mariuzzi

Tumour terminology Recommended terms are in **bold**	Synonyms	Comments
Adenocarcinoma of the liver	See cholangiocarcinoma	
Adenomatoid hyperplasia	See dysplastic nodule	
Adenomatous hyperplasia	See dysplastic nodule	
Adenosquamous carcinoma	See cholangiocarcinoma	
Anaplastic carcinoma	See undifferentiated carcinoma	
Angioendothelioma	See infantile haemangioendothelioma	
Angiomatosis hepatis	See peliosis hepatis	
Angiomyolipoma		Benign tumour variably composed of smooth muscle, vessels, fat, and haemopoietic tissue. It may be associated with a similar tumour in the kidney and/or tuberous sclerosis.
Angiosarcoma	Haemangiosarcoma Kupffer cell sarcoma Malignant haemangioendothelioma	Most common mesenchymal malignant tumour of the liver. See Tumours of Soft Tissue (Section 42).
Atypical adenomatous hyperplasia	See dysplastic nodule	
Benign cholangioma	See bile duct adenoma	

98

Tumour terminology Recommended terms are in **bold**	Synonyms	Comments
Benign hepatoma	See hepatocellular adenoma	
Benign mesenchymoma	See mesenchymal hamartoma	
Bile duct adenoma	Benign cholangioma Cholangioadenoma Tubular adenoma	An incidental, usually solitary subcapsular nodule composed of small bile ducts.
Bile duct carcinoma	See cholangiocarcinoma	
Bile duct cystadenocarcinoma	Biliary cystadenocarcinoma Hepatic cystadenocarcinoma Hepatobiliary cystadenocarcinoma	Mucin-secreting and multilocular malignant counterpart of bile duct cystadenoma. "Borderline" variants are recognised.
Bile duct cystadenoma	See intrahepatic bile duct cystadenoma	
Bile duct fibroadenoma	See mesenchymal hamartoma	
Biliary adenofibroma	Biliary fibroadenoma	Rare, benign lesion, which may either represent a variant of biliary hamartoma or a true tumour in its own right. It should be distinguished from bile duct adenoma.
Biliary cystadenocarcinoma	See bile duct cystadenocarcinoma	
Biliary cystadenoma	See intrahepatic bile duct cystadenoma	
Biliary fibroadenoma	See biliary adenofibroma	
Biliary hamartoma	Biliary microhamartoma Von Meyenburg complex	Tumour-like lesion, which sometimes forms part of congenital hepatic fibrosis. It consists of numerous cystically dilated bile ducts surrounded by fibrous tissue.
Biliary microhamartoma	See biliary hamartoma	
Biliary papillomatosis	Intraductal papillary carcinoma Intraductal papillomatosis	Rare tumour of unpredictable biological behaviour best regarded as potentially malignant. It consists of multiple sessile papillary tumours, which may arise in either intrahepatic or extrahepatic bile ducts or even the gall bladder.

Tumour terminology Recommended terms are in **bold**	Synonyms	Comments
Botryoid rhabdomyosarcoma	See embryonal rhabdomyosarcoma	
Cavernous angioma	See infantile haemangioendothelioma	
Cavernous haemangioma	See haemangioma	
Cholangioadenoma	See bile duct adenoma	
Cholangiocarcinoma	Adenocarcinoma of the liver Bile duct carcinoma Cholangiocellular carcinoma (obsolete) Duct carcinoma Intrahepatic cholangiocarcinoma Malignant cholangioma Papillary adenocarcinoma Peripheral bile duct carcinoma	Malignant tumour of bile duct epithelium with prominent fibrosis. It can be differentiated from hepatocellular carcinoma by the presence of mucin secretion and lack of bile secretion. Peripheral, major duct, hilar, and intraductal papillary subtypes are recognized. Histological variants include acinar, adenosquamous, anaplastic, clear cell, giant cell, mucinous, mucoepidermoid, papillary, sarcomatoid, signet ring, squamous, and solid variants.
Cholangiocellular carcinoma	See cholangiocarcinoma	Obsolete term.
Cholangio-hepatocellular carcinoma	See combined hepatocellular and cholangiocarcinoma	
Clear cell carcinoma	See clear cell hepatocellular carcinoma	
Clear cell hepatocellular carcinoma	Clear cell carcinoma Fat cell hepatocellular carcinoma Fatty hepatocellular carcinoma	By definition in excess of 50% of cells must contain clear cytoplasm due to glycogen or lipid accumulation. This variant must be distinguished from metastatic renal cell carcinoma.
Combined hepatocellular and cholangiocarcinoma	Cholangio-hepatocellular carcinoma Combined hepato-cholangiocarcinoma Hepato-cholangio-carcinoma Malignant cholangio-hepatoma	This rare tumour combines liver cell carcinoma and cholangiocarcinoma.

Tumour terminology Recommended terms are in **bold**	Synonyms	Comments
Combined hepato-cholangiocarcinoma	See combined hepatocellular and cholangiocarcinoma	
Cystic mesenchymal hamartoma	See mesenchymal hamartoma	
Diffuse nodular hyperplasia of the liver	See nodular transformation of the liver	
Diffuse systemic haemangiomatosis		A rare disease of adults presenting with multiple haemangiomas affecting many organs including the liver.
Duct carcinoma	See cholangiocarcinoma	
Dysplastic nodule	Adenomatoid hyperplasia Adenomatous hyperplasia Atypical adenomatous hyperplasia Hepatocellular pseudotumour Macro-regenerative nodule	A well circumscribed nodule of hepatocytes arranged in typical cords containing portal tracts. It arises secondary to submassive hepatocellular necrosis or advanced cirrhosis of any cause. Large and small cell dysplasia has been described, but only small cell type dysplasia is nowadays regarded as a true pre-malignant lesion of the liver.
Embryonal rhabdomyosarcoma	Botryoid rhabdomyosarcoma Sarcoma botryoides	Extremely rare tumour of skeletal muscle encountered in children.
Embryonal sarcoma	See undifferentiated sarcoma	
Epidermoid carcinoma	See squamous carcinoma	
Epithelioid haemangioendothelioma		Rare vascular tumour of unpredictable malignant potential. See Tumours of Soft Tissue (Section 42).
Fat cell hepatocellular carcinoma	See clear cell hepatocellular carcinoma	
Fatty hepatocellular carcinoma	See clear cell hepatocellular carcinoma	

Tumour terminology Recommended terms are in **bold**	Synonyms	Comments
Fibrolamellar carcinoma	Fibrolamellar hepatoma Fibrolamellar oncocytic hepatoma Oncocytic hepatocellular carcinoma Polygonal cell type hepatocellular carcinoma with fibrous stroma	Morphologic and clinical variant of hepatocellular carcinoma. It usually arises in non-cirrhotic liver and affects adolescents or young adults. The prognosis is considered more favourable than usual hepatocellular carcinoma.
Fibrolamellar hepatoma	See fibrolamellar carcinoma	
Fibrolamellar oncocytic hepatoma	See fibrolamellar carcinoma	
Fibroma	See localized fibrous tumour	
Fibrosing hepatocellular carcinoma	See sclerosing hepatocellular carcinoma	
Focal cirrhosis	See focal nodular hyperplasia	
Focal nodular hyperplasia	Focal cirrhosis Hamartomatous cholangiohepatoma Hepatic hamartoma Mixed adenoma Solitary hyperplastic nodule	Well circumscribed, usually solitary tumour-like lesion characterised by a central fibrous scar. More common in women, but the association with oral contraceptive therapy has recently been denied: when present it has to be considered fortuitous. On needle biopsies the characteristic nodular pattern has to be differentiated from cirrhosis. Surgical excision is not necessary, unless the patient complains of symptoms due to compression.
Giant cell carcinoma	See giant cell hepatocellular carcinoma	
Giant cell hepatocellular carcinoma	Giant cell carcinoma	This is a poorly differentiated variant of hepatocellular carcinoma characterised by the presence of conspicuous multinucleate giant cells.
Haemangioma	Cavernous haemangioma Sclerosing haemangioma	Most common benign mesenchymal tumour of the liver. The cavernous variant is the most frequently encountered variant. See Tumours of Soft Tissue (Section 42).

Tumour terminology Recommended terms are in **bold**	Synonyms	Comments
Haemangiosarcoma	See angiosarcoma	
Haemolymphangioma	See lymphangioma	
Hamartomatous cholangiohepatoma	See focal nodular hyperplasia	
Hepatic adenoma	See hepatocellular adenoma	
Hepatic cystadenocarcinoma	See bile duct cystadenocarcinoma	
Hepatic hamartoma	See focal nodular hyperplasia	
Hepatic mixed tumour of childhood	See hepatoblastoma	
Hepatobiliary cystadenocarcinoma	See bile duct cystadenocarcinoma	
Hepatobiliary cystadenoma	See intrahepatic bile duct cystadenoma	
Hepatoblastoma	Hepatic mixed tumour of childhood Malignant hepatoblastoma Mesenchymal hepatoblastoma	Malignant tumour, which occurs mostly but not exclusively in children. It is composed of embryonal or foetal hepatocytes with or without heterologous elements.
Hepatocarcinoma	See hepatocellular carcinoma	
Hepatocellular adenoma	Benign hepatoma Hepatic adenoma Liver cell adenoma	Benign tumour occurring most often in women taking oral contraceptive steroids. It may also be seen in men and children of either sex taking anabolic or androgenic steroids. It may undergo spontaneous regression after drug discontinuation but may also rarely progress to malignancy.
Hepatocellular adenomatosis	Liver adenomatosis Liver cell adenomatosis Miliary hepatocellular adenomatosis Multiple hepatocellular adenomatosis	A rare condition characterised by the presence of ten or more hepatocellular adenomas. There is no sexual predominance or association with steroids.

Tumour terminology Recommended terms are in **bold**	Synonyms	Comments
Hepatocellular carcinoma	Hepatocarcinoma Hepatoma Liver cell carcinoma Malignant hepatoma Primary hepatic carcinoma Primary hepatocellular carcinoma	Most common primary malignant epithelial tumour of the liver. Usually but not exclusively arises in the background of cirrhosis due to any cause, more frequently nowadays hepatitis C. Subtypes include fibrolamellar, spindle cell, clear cell, giant cell, and sclerosing hepatocellular carcinoma.
Hepatocellular pseudotumour	See dysplastic nodule	
Hepato-cholangiocarcinoma	See combined hepatocellular and cholangiocarcinoma	
Hepatoma	See hepatocellular carcinoma	
Heterotopia		Tumour-like lesion composed of ectopic pancreatic, splenic, or adrenal tissue.
Infantile haemangioendothelioma	Angioendothelioma Cavernous angioma	A vascular tumour usually affecting children under 6 months of age. It may be multinodular and affect other organs. It usually follows an indolent course but metastases can occur. It is sometimes complicated by congestive cardiac failure.
Inflammatory myofibroblastic tumour	See inflammatory pseudotumour	
Inflammatory pseudotumour	Inflammatory myofibroblastic tumour Plasma cell granuloma Post-inflammatory tumour	A localised fibro-inflammatory mass consisting of spindle cells admixed with inflammatory cells. The aetiology is unclear.
Intraductal papillary carcinoma	See biliary papillomatosis	
Intraductal papillomatosis	See biliary papillomatosis	
Intrahepatic bile duct adenoma	See bile duct adenoma	
Intrahepatic bile duct cystadenoma	Bile duct cystadenoma Biliary cystadenoma Hepatobiliary cystadenoma Mucinous cystadenoma	A rare multilocular tumour, which resembles cystadenoma of the pancreas and ovary. Histological variants include mucinous, serous, and papillary cyst tumour. Malignant transformation may occur.

Tumour terminology Recommended terms are in **bold**	Synonyms	Comments
Intrahepatic cholangiocarcinoma	See cholangiocarcinoma	
Kupffer cell sarcoma	See angiosarcoma	
Liver adenomatosis	See hepatocellular adenomatosis	
Liver cell adenoma	See hepatocellular adenoma	
Liver cell adenomatosis	See hepatocellular adenomatosis	
Liver cell carcinoma	See hepatocellular carcinoma	
Localized fibrous mesothelioma	See localized fibrous tumour	
Localized fibrous tumour	Fibroma Localized fibrous mesothelioma	Benign spindle cell tumour, which resembles solitary fibrous tumour of the pleura.
Lymphangioma	Haemolymphangioma	Benign solitary or multiple collection of dilated lymphatics sometimes containing red blood cells.
Lymphangiomatosis		This rare condition is characterised by numerous lymphangiomas affecting the internal viscera including the liver.
Macro-regenerative nodule	See dysplastic nodule	
Malignant cholangio-hepatoma	See combined hepatocellular and cholangiocarcinoma	
Malignant cholangioma	See cholangiocarcinoma	
Malignant haemangioendothelioma	See angiosarcoma	
Malignant hepatoblastoma	See hepatoblastoma	
Malignant hepatoma	See hepatocellular carcinoma	
Malignant mesenchymoma	See undifferentiated sarcoma	

Tumour terminology Recommended terms are in **bold**	Synonyms	Comments
Mesenchymal hamartoma	Benign mesenchymoma Bile duct fibroadenoma Cystic mesenchymal hamartoma	A rare benign tumour-like lesion composed of sometimes cystically dilated bile ducts admixed with a mature stroma.
Mesenchymal hepatoblastoma	See hepatoblastoma	
Miliary hepatocellular adenomatosis	See hepatocellular adenomatosis	
Mixed adenoma	See focal nodular hyperplasia	
Mucinous adenocarcinoma	See mucinous carcinoma	
Mucinous carcinoma	Mucinous adenocarcinoma	Histological variant of cholangiocarcinoma.
Mucinous cystadenoma	See intrahepatic bile duct cystadenoma	
Mucoepidermoid carcinoma		Histological variant of cholangiocarcinoma.
Multiple hepatocellular adenomatosis	See hepatocellular adenomatosis	
Nodular non-cirrhotic liver	See nodular transformation of the liver	
Nodular regenerative hyperplasia	See nodular transformation of the liver	
Nodular transformation of the liver	Diffuse nodular hyperplasia of the liver Nodular non-cirrhotic liver Nodular regenerative hyperplasia Non-cirrhotic nodulation of the liver Partial nodular transformation	A tumour-like lesion in which the liver undergoes micronodular transformation usually as a consequence of vascular damage. By definition fibrous septa are absent.
Non-cirrhotic nodulation of the liver	See nodular transformation of the liver	

Tumour terminology Recommended terms are in **bold**	Synonyms	Comments
Oncocytic hepatocellular carcinoma	See fibrolamellar carcinoma	
Papillary adenocarcinoma	See cholangiocarcinoma	
Partial nodular transformation	See nodular transformation of the liver	
Peliosis hepatis	Angiomatosis hepatis	Tumour-like lesion consisting of multiple small, dilated, and blood-filled cavities devoid of endothelium.
Peripheral bile duct carcinoma	See cholangiocarcinoma	
Plasma cell granuloma	See inflammatory pseudotumour	
Polygonal cell type hepatocellular carcinoma with fibrous stroma	See fibrolamellar carcinoma	
Post-inflammatory tumour	See inflammatory pseudotumour	
Primary hepatic carcinoma	See hepatocellular carcinoma	
Primary hepatocellular carcinoma	See hepatocellular carcinoma	
Sarcoma botryoides	See embryonal rhabdomyosarcoma	
Sarcomatoid hepatocellular carcinoma	See spindle cell hepatocellular carcinoma	
Sclerosing haemangioma	See haemangioma	
Sclerosing hepatocellular carcinoma	Fibrosing hepatocellular carcinoma	Variant of hepatocellular carcinoma with abundant fibrous stroma and associated with hypercalcaemia.
Solitary hyperplastic nodule	See focal nodular hyperplasia	
Spindle cell hepatocellular carcinoma	Sarcomatoid hepatocellular carcinoma	This rare variant of hepatocellular carcinoma is most commonly seen in men. The clinical features are similar to classical hepatocellular carcinoma.

Tumour terminology Recommended terms are in **bold**	Synonyms	Comments
Squamous cell carcinoma	Adenoacanthoma Epidermoid carcinoma	Primary squamous cell carcinoma is extremely rare and may arise in a background of chronic inflammation. Metastases should be excluded.
Tubular adenoma	See bile duct adenoma	
Undifferentiated carcinoma	Anaplastic carcinoma	This term can be equally applied to undifferentiated variants of hepatocellular carcinoma and cholangiocarcinoma.
Undifferentiated mesenchymal sarcoma	See undifferentiated sarcoma	
Undifferentiated sarcoma	Embryonal sarcoma Malignant mesenchymoma Undifferentiated mesenchymal sarcoma	High grade tumour occurring primarily in children, consisting of primitive mesenchymal elements in a myxoid stroma. Heterologous components are absent.
Von Meyenburg complex	See biliary hamartoma	

Section 16

Tumours of the Gall Bladder and Extrahepatic Bile Ducts

R. Colombari
G.M. Mariuzzi

Tumour terminology Recommended terms are in **bold**	Synonyms	Comments
Adenoacanthoma	See adenocarcinoma	
Adenocarcinoma		The most common malignant tumour of the gall bladder and extrahepatic bile ducts often associated with gallstones. Histological variants include adenocarcinoma of intestinal type, adenoacanthoma, adenosquamous carcinoma, clear cell carcinoma, mucoepidermoid carcinoma, mucinous (colloid) adenocarcinoma, papillary adenocarcinoma, signet cell adenocarcinoma.
Adenocarcinoma of intestinal type	See adenocarcinoma	
Adenoma	Adenomatous polyp Papilloma	Pre-malignant lesion. Histological variants: tubular, papillary, tubulopapillary.
Adenomatosis	See papillomatosis	
Adenomatous polyp	See adenoma	
Adenomyoma	See adenomyomatous hyperplasia	
Adenomyomatosis	See adenomyomatous hyperplasia	
Adenomyomatous hyperplasia	Adenomyoma Adenomyomatosis	Tumour-like lesion.

Tumour terminology Recommended terms are in **bold**	Synonyms	Comments
Adenosquamous carcinoma	See adenocarcinoma	
Amputation neuroma	Traumatic neuroma	Tumour-like lesion. See Tumours of Soft Tissue (Section 42).
Anaplastic carcinoma	See undifferentiated carcinoma	
Angiosarcoma		See Tumours of Soft Tissue (Section 42).
Botryoid rhabdomyosarcoma	See rhabdomyosarcoma	
Carcinoid tumour	Neuroendocrine carcinoma	Gall bladder lesions are uncommon and predominantly affect the neck or cystic duct.
Carcinosarcoma	See metaplastic carcinoma	
Cholesterol polyp		Tumour-like lesion secondary to accumulation of lipid-laden macrophages in the submucosa.
Clear cell carcinoma		Histological variant of adenocarcinoma.
Colloid carcinoma		Histological variant of adenocarcinoma.
Composite glandular-endocrine cell carcinoma	See mixed carcinoid-adenocarcinoma	
Cystadenocarcinoma		Rare, malignant transformation of a cystadenoma.
Cystadenoma		Rare multiloculated tumour resembling cystadenoma of the pancreas or ovary.
Epidermoid carcinoma	See squamous cell carcinoma	
Granular cell myoblastoma	See granular cell tumour	
Granular cell tumour	Granular cell myoblastoma	See Tumours of Soft Tissue (Section 42).
Haemangioma		See Tumours of Soft Tissue (Section 42).
Heterotopia		Tumour-like lesion.
Inflammatory polyp		Tumour-like lesion.

Tumour terminology Recommended terms are in **bold**	Synonyms	Comments
Kaposi's sarcoma		Occurs within the context of AIDS. See Tumours of Soft Tissue (Section 42).
Leiomyoma		See Tumours of Soft Tissue (Section 42).
Leiomyosarcoma		See Tumours of Soft Tissue (Section 42).
Lipoma		See Tumours of Soft Tissue (Section 42).
Lymphangioma		See Tumours of Soft Tissue (Section 42).
Malignant mixed tumour	See metaplastic carcinoma	
Melanoma		Primary lesions in the gall bladder are exceptionally rare.
Metaplastic carcinoma	Carcinosarcoma Malignant mixed tumour Sarcomatoid carcinoma	This tumour, which is rare in the gall bladder, consists of adenocarcinomatous and spindle cell components with or without heterologous differentiation.
Mixed carcinoid-adenocarcinoma	Composite glandular-endocrine cell carcinoma	Rare. Not enough data available about the long-term survival.
Mucinous adenocarcinoma		Histological variant of adenocarcinoma.
Mucoepidermoid carcinoma		Histological variant of adenocarcinoma showing squamous differentiation.
Neuroendocrine carcinoma	See carcinoid tumour	
Neurofibroma		Exceedingly rare at this site. See Tumours of Soft Tissue (Section 42).
Oat cell carcinoma	See small cell carcinoma	
Papillary adenocarcinoma		Histological variant of adenocarcinoma.
Papillary adenoma	See adenoma	
Papillary hyperplasia		Tumour-like lesion.
Papilloma	See adenoma	
Papillomatosis	Adenomatosis	Histological variant of adenoma characterised by multiple recurring adenomas in the extrahepatic bile ducts, which may extend into the gall bladder and intrahepatic bile ducts.

Tumour terminology Recommended terms are in **bold**	Synonyms	Comments
Paraganglioma		This lesion is extremely rare in the gall bladder.
Pleomorphic carcinoma	See undifferentiated carcinoma	
Rhabdomyosarcoma	Botryoid rhabdomyosarcoma	This tumour is exceedingly rare in the gall bladder. See Tumours of Soft Tissue (Section 42).
Sarcomatoid carcinoma	See metaplastic carcinoma	
Signet cell adenocarcinoma		Histological variant of adenocarcinoma.
Small cell anaplastic carcinoma	See small cell carcinoma	
Small cell carcinoma	Oat cell carcinoma Small cell anaplastic carcinoma Small cell undifferentiated carcinoma	Resembling small cell carcinoma of the bronchus and lung. More common in the gall bladder than in the extrahepatic bile ducts.
Small cell undifferentiated carcinoma	See small cell carcinoma	
Squamous cell carcinoma	Epidermoid carcinoma	Probably arising from extensive squamous metaplasia of adenocarcinoma.
Traumatic neuroma	See amputation neuroma	
Tubular adenoma	See adenoma	
Tubulopapillary adenoma	See adenoma	
Undifferentiated carcinoma	Anaplastic carcinoma Pleomorphic carcinoma	More common in the gall bladder than in the extrahepatic bile ducts.

Section 17

Tumours of the Middle and Inner Ear

S. Falkmer

Primary cutaneous tumours of the external ear are dealt with in Skin Melanocytic and Non-Melanocytic Tumours, Sections 42 and 43.

Tumour terminology Recommended terms are in **bold**	Synonyms	Comments
Acoustic nerve tumour	See acoustic neuroma	
Acoustic neurilemmoma	See acoustic neuroma	
Acoustic neurinoma	See acoustic neuroma	
Acoustic neurofibroma	See acoustic neuroma	
Acoustic neuroma	Acoustic nerve tumour Acoustic neurilemmoma Acoustic neurinoma Acoustic neurofibroma Neurilemmoma of the vestibular-cochlear nerve Schwannoma of the VIIIth cranial nerve	This is the most common primary neurogenic tumour of the ear arising from the VIIIth cranial nerve. Although benign, it can cause considerable destruction of adjacent tissues due to local pressure. In addition it may give rise to seedling deposits in the inner ear.
Adenocarcinoma of the middle ear	See papillary adenocarcinoma	
Adenoid cystic carcinoma		Histological variant of ceruminous gland carcinoma. See Tumours of the Salivary Glands (Section 9).
Aggressive papillary middle ear tumour	See papillary adenocarcinoma	
APMET	See papillary adenocarcinoma	

Tumour terminology Recommended terms are in **bold**	Synonyms	Comments
Aural hidradenocarcinoma		Rare malignant tumour of the ceruminous gland. Variants include adenoid cystic carcinoma and mucoepidermoid carcinoma.
Aural hidradenoma	See ceruminoma	
Aural polyp	See inflammatory polyp	
Ceruminoma	Aural hidradenoma Ceruminous gland tumour Hidradenoma of the external acoustic meatus	This is a rare slowly growing tumour, which affects the external auditory meatus. It is sometimes locally invasive and may infiltrate the middle ear. Histologically it is composed of glands lined by a double layer of epithelium showing apocrine secretion. Spread from a parotid gland tumour should be excluded.
Ceruminous gland tumour	See ceruminoma	
Chemodectoma	See paraganglioma	
Cholesteatoma	Cholesteatosis Epidermoid cholesteatoma Epidermoidosis Keratinic cyst Squamous cholesteatosis Squamous epitheliosis	This common lesion represents a form of epidermoid cyst arising in the middle ear or temporal bone as an irreversible complication of chronic otitis media. Although not a true neoplasm, it is characterised by a high recurrence rate and is extremely difficult to eradicate. The term "cholesteatoma" is a misnomer.
Cholesteatosis	See cholesteatoma	
Epidermoid cholesteatoma	See cholesteatoma	
Epidermoidosis	See cholesteatoma	
Exostosis		Usually multiple and bilateral tumour-like masses composed of lamellar bone which present in the external auditory canal. Swimmers are most often affected.
Glomus tumour	See paraganglioma	
Granulation polyp	See inflammatory polyp	
Hidradenoma of the external acoustic meatus	See ceruminoma	

Tumour terminology Recommended terms are in **bold**	Synonyms	Comments
Inflammatory polyp	Aural polyp Granulation polyp Otic polyp Polyp	Tumour-like lesion composed of inflamed granulation tissue usually complicating otitis media.
Jugular glomus tumour	See paraganglioma	
Jugularis tumour	See paraganglioma	
Jugulotympanic body tumour	See paraganglioma	
Jugulotympanic paraganglioma	See paraganglioma	
Keratinic cyst	See cholesteatoma	
Keratosis obturans	Squamous cell papilloma of the external acoustic meatus	This rare lesion of the external auditory canal consists of hyperkeratotic and thickened skin. Its origin is uncertain. Occasionally it may be associated with development of squamous cell carcinoma.
Low grade adenocarcinoma of probable endolymphatic sac origin	See papillary adenocarcinoma	
Mucoepidermoid carcinoma		Histological variant of ceruminoma.
Neurilemmoma of the vestibular cochlear nerve	See acoustic neuroma	
Non-chromaffin paraganglioma	See paraganglioma	
Osteoma		Usually solitary tumour-like mass arising in the external auditory canal composed of lamellar bone and including a marrow component.
Otic polyp	See inflammatory polyp	
Papillary adenocarcinoma	Adenocarcinoma of the middle ear Aggressive papillary middle ear tumour APMET Low grade adeno-carcinoma of probably endolymphatic sac origin	Extremely rare tumour, which may mimic a metastasis from thyroid. The prognosis is poor.

Tumour terminology Recommended terms are in **bold**	Synonyms	Comments
Paraganglioma	Chemodectoma Glomus tumour Jugular glomus tumour Jugularis tumour Jugulotympanic body tumour Jugulotympanic paraganglioma Non-chromaffin paraganglioma Paraganglioma of the glomus jugulare Tympanic body tumour Tympanic tumour of carotic body type	Paraganglioma arising in the glomus jugulare is the most common tumour of the middle ear. It is a slowly growing, usually non-encapsulated, neuroendocrine tumour. It may invade the jugular fossa, extend into the tympanic cavity and perforate the tympanic membrane, thereby presenting as a haemorrhagic polyp in the external auditory meatus. Recurrences are common but metastasis is extremely rare.
Paraganglioma of the glomus jugulare	See paraganglioma	
Polyp	See inflammatory polyp	
Schwannoma of the VIIIth cranial nerve	See acoustic neuroma	
Squamous cell carcinoma		Rarely arises in the middle ear. Local invasion may be considerable, making treatment difficult.
Squamous cell papillomas of the external acoustic meatus	See keratosis obturans	
Squamous cholesteatosis	See cholesteatoma	
Squamous epitheliosis	See cholesteatoma	
Tympanic body tumour	See paraganglioma	
Tympanic body tumour of carotid body type	See paraganglioma	

Section 18

Tumours of the Nasal Cavity and Paranasal Sinuses

G. Martignoni

G.M. Mariuzzi

Tumour terminology Recommended terms are in **bold**	Synonyms	Comments
Acinic cell carcinoma	Acinic cell tumour	Rare. Low grade. See Tumours of the Salivary Glands (Section 9).
Acinic cell tumour	See acinic cell carcinoma	
Adenocarcinoma not otherwise specified (NOS)		Carcinoma composed of malignant glands resembling the normal ducts. It is graded, according to the histopathological features into well, moderate, and poorly differentiated types. However this group includes clinically and pathologically heterogeneous unclassifiable adenocarcinomas.
Adenocystic carcinoma	See adenoid cystic carcinoma	
Adenoid cystic carcinoma	Adenocystic carcinoma Cylindroma	The most frequent sinonasal adenocarcinoma. The behaviour of this carcinoma is particularly aggressive at this location.
Adenosquamous carcinoma		A carcinoma composed of both glandular and squamous malignant component.
Alveolar goblet cell carcinoma	See intestinal type adenocarcinoma	
Anaplastic carcinoma	Undifferentiated carcinoma	Used for a heterogeneous group of tumours, composed of pleomorphic cell, spindle cells, and/or small cells.

117

Tumour terminology Recommended terms are in **bold**	Synonyms	Comments
Angiocentric immunoproliferative lesion	See lymphomatoid granulomatosis	
Angiofibroma	Juvenile angiofibroma	Benign rare tumour occurring in the nasopharynx or, less frequently, in the posterior nasal cavity in adolescent males.
Angiosarcoma	Haemangiosarcoma Malignant haemangioendothelioma	Exceptionally rare malignant tumour, which seems to be less aggressive than the same sarcoma at other sites.
Atypical carcinoid	See olfactory neuroblastoma See neuroendocrine carcinoma	
Basal cell adenocarcinoma		Extremely rare. See Tumours of the Salivary Glands (Section 9).
Basal cell adenoma		Extremely rare. See Tumours of the Salivary Glands (Section 9).
Benign mixed tumour	Complex adenoma (obsolete) Mixed tumour Pleomorphic adenoma Pleomorphic sialadenoma (obsolete)	Rare. It is often a "cellular variant" and is not well circumscribed. Recurrences are uncommon.
Blastoma	See teratocarcinoma	
Carcinoid	See neuroendocrine tumour	
Carcinoma arising in pleomorphic adenoma	See malignant mixed tumour	
Carcinoma in situ	Intraepithelial carcinoma Pre-invasive carcinoma	Pre-invasive malignant changes frequently found adjacent to the invasive carcinoma.
Carcinoma with sarcoma-like stroma	See spindle cell carcinoma	
Carcinosarcoma	See metaplastic carcinoma	Rare highly malignant tumour with epithelial and mesenchymal malignant components.
Chordoma		Malignant. Rare in the nasal cavity.

Tumour terminology Recommended terms are in **bold**	Synonyms	Comments
Clear cell carcinoma		Extremely rare histological variant of adenocarcinoma.
Columnar Ringertz carcinoma	See non-keratinising carcinoma	
Complex adenoma	See benign mixed tumour	Obsolete term.
Cylindrical cell carcinoma	See non-keratinising carcinoma	
Cylindrical cell papilloma	See oncocytic Schneiderian sinonasal papilloma	
Cylindroma	See adenoid cystic carcinoma	
Dermal sinus	See dermoid cyst	
Dermoid cyst	Dermal sinus	Rare developmental abnormality containing only ectodermal elements, unlike dermoid at other sites.
Epidermoid carcinoma	See squamous cell carcinoma	
Epithelial-myoepithelial carcinoma		Extremely rare. Low grade malignant.
Esthesioneuroblastoma	See olfactory neuroblastoma	Obsolete term.
Esthesioneurocytoma	See olfactory neuroblastoma	Obsolete term.
Esthesioneuroepithelioma	See olfactory neuroblastoma	Obsolete term.
Esthesioneuroma	See olfactory neuroblastoma	Obsolete term.
Ewing's papilloma	See sinonasal papilloma	Obsolete term.
Ewing's sarcoma		Rare. Malignant small round cell tumour.
Fibroma		Benign. See Tumours of Soft Tissue (Section 42).
Fibromatosis		Rare, locally aggressive myofibroblastic lesion.

Tumour terminology Recommended terms are in **bold**	Synonyms	Comments
Fibrosarcoma		Rare. See Tumours of Soft Tissue (Section 42).
Fungiform papilloma	See sinonasal papilloma	
Glial Heterotopia	Nasal glioma	A congenital central nervous tissue rest without connection with the brain in 80% of cases.
Granuloma gangraenescens	See Wegener's granulomatosis	
Haemangioma		Benign. Common in nasal cavity as lobular capillary haemangioma.
Haemangiopericytoma		Rare. Low rate of recurrence and lack of metastasis at these sites.
Haemangiosarcoma	See angiosarcoma	
Inflammatory pseudotumour		Non-neoplastic mass constituted by a proliferation of myofibroblastic cells and dense inflammatory infiltration with pseudosarcomatous appearance.
Intermediate carcinoma	See non-keratinising carcinoma	
Intestinal-type adenocarcinoma		Histologically similar to adenocarcinoma of the large bowel including the presence of goblet cells. It is associated with long-term exposure to organic dust as well as to leather dust. It has been subclassified into papillary-tubular cylindrical cell (Grades I, II, III), alveolar goblet, and signet ring cell types.
Intraepithelial carcinoma	See carcinoma in situ	
Intranasal neuroblastoma	See olfactory neuroblastoma	
Inverted papilloma	See sinonasal papilloma	
Juvenile angiofibroma	See angiofibroma	
Keratinising carcinoma	See squamous cell carcinoma	
Leiomyoma		Rare, benign. See Tumours of Soft Tissue (Section 42).
Leiomyosarcoma		Rare. See Tumours of Soft Tissue (Section 42).

Tumour terminology Recommended terms are in **bold**	Synonyms	Comments
Lethal midline lethal granulomatosis	See lymphomatoid granulomatosis	Clinical term applied to the destructive process affecting the nose and adjacent structures.
Lipoma		Extremely rare at this location. See Tumours of Soft Tissue (Section 42).
Liposarcoma		Extremely rare at this location. See Tumours of Soft Tissue (Section 42).
Lymphoid hyperplasia		Non-neoplastic mass composed of a massive lymphoid infiltrate which resembles a lymphoma.
Lymphomatoid granulomatosis	Angiocentric immunoproliferative lesion Lethal midline granuloma Midline malignant reticulosis Polymorphic reticulosis	An aggressive morphologically polymorphous lymphoproliferative disease.
Malignant fibrous histiocytoma		Rare. See Tumours of Soft Tissue (Section 42).
Malignant granuloma	See Wegener's granulomatosis	
Malignant haemangioendothelioma	See angiosarcoma	
Malignant lymphoma		See Tumours of the Lymph Nodes and Spleen (Section 24).
Malignant melanoma		Rare; 30% are amelanotic.
Malignant mixed tumour	Carcinoma arising in pleomorphic adenoma	Extremely rare.
Malignant myoepithelioma	Myoepithelial carcinoma	Rare. See Tumours of the Salivary Glands (Section 9).
Malignant neurilemmoma	See malignant schwannoma	
Malignant Schwannoma	Malignant neurilemmoma	Extremely rare. See Tumours of Soft Tissue (Section 42).
Meningioma		Extremely rare. See Tumours of Central Nervous System (Section 2).

Tumour terminology Recommended terms are in **bold**	Synonyms	Comments
Metaplastic carcinoma	Carcinosarcoma	Rare highly malignant tumour with epithelial and mesenchymal malignant components.
Midline malignant reticulosis	See lymphomatoid granulomatosis	
Mixed tumour	See benign mixed tumour	
Mucocystic papillary adenoma	See sinonasal papilloma	
Mucoepidermoid carcinoma	Mucoepidermoid tumour	The second most common sinonasal adenocarcinoma. In this site it is frequently of low grade malignancy. Can be mistaken for benign lesions such as inflammatory polyps and necrotising sialometaplasia.
Mucoepidermoid tumour	See mucoepidermoid carcinoma	
Myoepithelial carcinoma	See malignant myoepithelioma	
Myoepithelioma		Benign. See Tumours of the Salivary Glands (Section 9).
Nasal glioma	See glial heterotopia	
Nasal sympathioma	See olfactory neuroblastoma	Obsolete term.
Neurilemmoma	See schwannoma	
Neuroendocrine carcinoma	See olfactory neuroblastoma	
Neuroendocrine tumour	Carcinoid tumour	Rare. Histologically similar to its bronchial counterpart.
Non-keratinising carcinoma	Columnar Ringertz carcinoma Cylindrical cell carcinoma Intermediate carcinoma Transitional cell carcinoma	Histological variant of squamous carcinoma. It comprises 15–20% of all sinonasal carcinomas. It is characterised by mild to moderate atypia and the absence of keratinisation. Associated with EBV.
Oat cell carcinoma	See small cell carcinoma	

Tumour terminology Recommended terms are in **bold**	Synonyms	Comments
Olfactory neuroblastoma	Atypical carcinoid Esthesioneuroblastoma (obsolete) Esthesioneurocytoma (obsolete) Esthesioneuroepithelioma (obsolete) Esthesioneuroma (obsolete) Intranasal neuroblastoma Nasal sympathioma (obsolete) Neuroendocrine carcinoma Placode tumour (obsolete)	Rare malignant neuroendocrine neoplasm arising from the upper portion of the nasal cavity. Bimodal age peaks of occurrence at 15 and 55 years.
Oncocytic Schneiderian papilloma	See sinonasal papilloma	
Oncocytoma	Oxyphil adenoma	Some authors regard it as low grade adenocarcinoma.
Osteoblastoma		Benign. Rare. Described in the maxilla and in the nasal cavity.
Osteoma		Benign. More frequent in the frontal sinus.
Osteosarcoma		The most common post-radiation malignant tumour.
Oxyphil adenoma	See oncocytoma	
Papillary adenoma	See sinonasal papilloma	Obsolete term.
Papillary sinusitis	See sinonasal papilloma	Obsolete term.
Papillary-tubular cylindrical cell adenocarcinoma	See intestinal-type adenocarcinoma	
Papilloma	See sinonasal papilloma	
Paraganglioma		Extremely rare. Unpredictable behaviour.
Pituitary adenoma		Extremely rare tumour arising from Rathke's pouch remnants.

Tumour terminology Recommended terms are in **bold**	Synonyms	Comments
Placode tumour	See olfactory neuroblastoma	Obsolete term.
Plasmacytoma		The majority of the patients with solitary plasma cell tumours develop disseminated myeloma.
Pleomorphic adenoma	See benign mixed tumour	
Pleomorphic sialadenoma	See benign mixed tumour	Obsolete term.
Polymorphic reticulosis	See lymphomatoid granulomatosis	
Polymorphous low grade adenocarcinoma	Terminal tubule adenocarcinoma	Extremely rare. Low grade malignant.
Pre-invasive carcinoma	See carcinoma in situ	
Pseudosarcomatous carcinoma	See spindle cell carcinoma	
Rhabdomyoma		Benign tumours of striated muscle origin. The foetal type variant has been described in the nasal cavity.
Rhabdomyosarcoma		The nose is one of the most frequent sites of this type of sarcoma in the head and neck region. It has rarely a grossly polypoid, grape-like appearance, referred to as sarcoma botryoides. In this location 85% of rhabdomyosarcomas are embryonal in type.
Ringertz papilloma	See sinonasal papilloma	Obsolete term.
Salivary gland anlage tumour		A polypoid benign hamartomatous lesion that presents at birth.
Schneiderian papilloma	See sinonasal papilloma	
Schwannoma	Neurilemmoma	Extremely rare. See Tumours of the Lymph Nodes and Spleen (Section 24).
Signet ring cell carcinoma	See intestinal type adenocarcinoma	

Tumour terminology Recommended terms are in **bold**	Synonyms	Comments
Sinonasal papilloma	Cylindrical cell papilloma Ewing's papilloma (obsolete) Fungiform papilloma Inverted papilloma Mucocystic papillary adenoma Oncocytic Schneiderian papilloma Papillary adenoma (obsolete) Papillary sinusitis (obsolete) Papilloma Ringertz papilloma (obsolete) Schneiderian papilloma Squamous papilloma Transitional cell papilloma	Unilateral benign tumour either of exophytic or of inverted type.
Small cell carcinoma	Oat cell carcinoma	Rare local aggressive tumour histologically and ultrastructurally similar to pulmonary small cell carcinoma.
Solitary fibrous tumour		Benign. Rare. Histologically analogous to solitary fibrous mesothelioma. See Tumours of the Serous Cavities (Section 21).
Spindle cell carcinoma	Carcinoma with sarcoma-like stromas Pseudosarcomatous carcinoma	High grade histological variant of squamous cell carcinoma.
Squamous cell carcinoma	Epidermoid carcinoma Keratinising carcinoma	The most frequent tumour of the nasal cavity and paranasal sinuses representing about 80–85% of the sinonasal mucosal tumours. It is graded, according to the features, into well, moderate, and poorly differentiated types. Squamous cell carcinoma of the nasal vestibule is a distinct carcinoma arising from the skin of the anterior part of the nasal cavity.

Tumour terminology Recommended terms are in **bold**	Synonyms	Comments
Teratocarcinoma	Blastoma Teratocarcinosarcoma	A rare and very aggressive tumour composed of neuroepithelial, skeletal muscle, cartilaginous, and undifferentiated tissues.
Teratocarcinosarcoma	See teratocarcinoma	
Terminal tubule adenocarcinoma	See polymorphous low grade adenocarcinoma	
Transitional cell carcinoma	See non-keratinising carcinoma	
Transitional cell papilloma	See sinonasal papilloma	
Undifferentiated carcinoma	See anaplastic carcinoma	
Verrucous carcinoma		Rare variant of squamous cell carcinoma with favourable prognosis.
Wegener's granulomatosis	Malignant granuloma Granuloma gangraenescens	This is a necrotising vasculitis, which affects the nose in a destructive manner. The vasculitis may also involve the lungs and kidneys.

Section 19

Tumours of the Larynx and Hypopharynx

J. Sugar

Tumour terminology Recommended terms are in **bold**	Synonyms	Comments
Abrikossoff's tumour	See granular cell tumour	
Acinic cell carcinoma		Rare subtype of adenocarcinoma.
Adenocarcinoma (NOS)		Highly malignant tumour.
Adenocystic carcinoma	See adenoid cystic carcinoma	
Adenoid cystic carcinoma	Adenocystic carcinoma Cribriform adenocarcinoma Cylindroma	Rare. Histologically similar to its salivary gland counterpart.
Adenoid squamous cell carcinoma	Adenosquamous carcinoma	Highly malignant. Some incorporate this tumour with high grade mucoepidermoid carcinoma.
Adenoma		Histologically similar to its bronchial counterpart.
Adenosquamous carcinoma	See adenoid squamous cell carcinoma	
Alveolar soft part sarcoma		See Tumours of Soft Tissue (Section 42).
Amyloid deposits		Tumour-like lesion due to deposition of amyloid.
Angiosarcoma	Haemangiosarcoma	See Tumours of Soft Tissue (Section 42).
Basal cell adenoma	Basaloid adenoma	Rare. Histologically similar to its salivary gland counterpart.
Basaloid adenoma	See basal cell adenoma	

Tumour terminology Recommended terms are in **bold**	Synonyms	Comments
Basaloid squamous cell carcinoma		A highly malignant variant of squamous cell carcinoma.
Carcinoid tumour	See neuroendocrine carcinoma	
Carcinoma in pleomorphic adenoma		Rare. Histologically similar to its salivary gland counterpart.
Carcinoma in situ	In situ carcinoma Intraepithelial carcinoma Non-invasive carcinoma Pre-invasive carcinoma	Neoplastic squamous epithelium, which does not extend beyond the basement membrane.
Chemodectoma	See paraganglioma	
Chondroma		See Tumours of Soft Tissue (Section 42).
Chondrosarcoma		Rare, site of origin is the cricoid.
Chorditis tuberosa	See vocal cord polyp	Obsolete term.
Cribriform adenocarcinoma	See adenoid cystic carcinoma	
Cylindroma	See adenoid cystic carcinoma	
Epithelial–myoepithelial carcinoma		Very rare subtype of adenocarcinoma.
Granular cell myoblastoma	See granular cell tumour	
Granular cell tumour	Abrikossoff's tumour Granular cell myoblastoma	Benign tumour of nerve sheath derivation. See Tumours of Soft Tissue (Section 42).
Haemangioma		Subdivided into adult and infantile form. Adult form is rare. Infantile form is almost always subglottic and may cause airway obstruction.
Haemangiopericytoma		See Tumours of Soft Tissue (Section 42).
Haemangiosarcoma	See angiosarcoma	
Hyperkeratosis	See keratosis without dysplasia	

Tumour terminology Recommended terms are in **bold**	Synonyms	Comments
Hyperplasia	See squamous cell hyperplasia	
In situ carcinoma	See carcinoma in situ	
Intraepithelial carcinoma	See carcinoma in situ	
Intubation granuloma		Tumour-like lesion following prolonged intubation.
Kaposi's sarcoma		See Tumours of Soft Tissue (Section 42).
Keratosis with dysplasia grade 1–3	Leukoplakia Pachydermia	Pre-cancerous (pre-malignant) lesion occurring in smokers.
Keratosis without dysplasia	Hyperkeratosis	Mostly secondary to smoking.
Laryngeal pseudosarcoma	See spindle cell carcinoma	
Leiomyoma		Localisation in the false cords. See Tumours of Soft Tissue (Section 42).
Leiomyosarcoma		See Tumours of Soft Tissue (Section 42).
Leukoplakia	See keratosis with dysplasia	
Lipoglycoproteinosis	See lipoid proteinosis	
Lipoid proteinosis	Lipoglycoproteinosis Lipoidosis cutis et mucosae	Tumour-like lesion.
Lipoidosis cutis et mucosae	See lipoid proteinosis	
Malignant fibrous histiocytoma		See Tumours of Soft Tissue (Section 42).
Malignant lymphoma		Larynx involved secondarily.
Mixed tumour	See pleomorphic adenoma	
Mucoepidermoid carcinoma		Rare. Histologically similar to its salivary gland counterpart.
Myxoma		See Tumours of Soft Tissue (Section 42).
Neurilemmoma	See schwannoma	

Tumour terminology Recommended terms are in **bold**	Synonyms	Comments
Neuroendocrine carcinoma	Carcinoid tumour	Rare. When on larynx, it should be differentiated from a paraganglioma. Large cell and small cell variants.
Neurofibroma		Uncommon, situated mainly in the laryngo-epiglottic fold.
Non-invasive carcinoma	See carcinoma in situ	
Pachydermia	See keratosis with dysplasia	
Papilloma of adult-onset		Benign with low risk of malignancy. May be single or multiple. Papillomas are associated with Human Papilloma Virus (HPV).
Papilloma of juvenile-onset		Benign tumour. May be simple or multiple.
Paraganglioma	Chemodectoma	Rare. See Tumours of the Adrenal Cortex, Adrenal Medulla, and Paraganglia (Section 6).
Pleomorphic adenoma	Mixed tumour	May recur after removal.
Polyps of vocal cord		Tumour-like lesions grow from the anterior two thirds of the cords. Histological variants: fibrous, vascular, hyalinised, myxoid.
Pre-invasive carcinoma	See carcinoma in situ	
Rhabdomyoma		Benign tumour. Histological variants include foetal and adult.
Schwannoma	Neurilemmoma	See Tumours of Soft Tissue (Section 42).
Singer's nodule	See vocal cord polyp	
Spindle cell squamous carcinoma	Laryngeal pseudosarcoma	Highly malignant tumour.
Squamous cell carcinoma		The most frequent malignant tumour of the larynx. Associated with HPV types 16, 18, 30, and 33; referred to as high risk viruses.
Squamous cell dysplasia		Pre-cancerous (pre-malignant) lesion. Histological variants include mild, moderate, and severe.

Tumour terminology Recommended terms are in **bold**	Synonyms	Comments
Squamous cell hyperplasia	Hyperplasia	Tumour-like proliferation of squamous epithelium.
Teacher's nodule	See vocal cord polyp	
Vascular leiomyoma		Rare. Localisation mainly subglottic. See Tumours of Soft Tissue (Section 42).
Verrucous squamous cell carcinoma		Rare, low grade tumour. Recurrences are common.
Vocal cord nodule	See vocal cord polyp	
Vocal cord polyp	Chorditis tuberosa (obsolete) Singer's nodule Teacher's nodule Vocal cord nodule	A non-neoplastic, tumour-like lesion that affects the vocal cords of people who use their voice excessively.
Wegener's granulomatosis		Tumour-like vasculitic lesion of uncertain histogenesis origin.

Section 20

Tumours of the Trachea, Bronchi, and Lungs

M. Sheppard

Tumour terminology Recommended terms are in **bold**	Synonyms	Comments
Acinar adenocarcinoma		This is the most common variant of adenocarcinoma.
Acinic cell carcinoma	Acinic cell tumour	Very rare histological variant of so-called bronchial adenoma. It resembles the salivary gland equivalent. Associated with a good prognosis.
Acinic cell tumour	See acinic cell carcinoma	
Adenocarcinoma		This variant of lung cancer is increasing in incidence and may occur in non-smokers. It is usually peripherally located. Many tumours have a mixed histological pattern. Variants include acinar adenocarcinoma, adenocarcinoma of foetal type, bronchioloalveolar cell, clear cell, hepatoid, mixed, signet ring, papillary, and solid adenocarcinoma with mucin formation.
Adenocarcinoma of foetal type	Adenocarcinoma resembling foetal lung Epithelial blastoma Pulmonary endodermal tumour Well differentiated foetal adenocarcinoma	Rare histological variant of adenocarcinoma characterised by immature epithelial tubules resembling foetal lung.
Adenocarcinoma resembling foetal lung	See adenocarcinoma of foetal type	

Tumour terminology Recommended terms are in **bold**	Synonyms	Comments
Adenocarcinoma with predominant bronchioloalveolar pattern		This variant of adenocarcinoma is characterised by a predominantly bronchioloalveolar cell pattern but shows foci of stromal invasion which by definition involve less than 10% of the whole tumour area.
Adenoid cystic carcinoma		This tumour, which resembles the salivary gland equivalent, arises most frequently in the trachea or major bronchi. Metastases to the regional nodes are common and the ultimate prognosis is poor.
Adenoma	Bronchial adenoma	This obsolete term encompasses a group of tumours resembling the multiple subtypes of salivary gland neoplasms. It includes acinic cell carcinoma, adenoid cystic carcinoma, alveolar adenoma, epithelial myoepithelial carcinoma, mucinous adenoma, mucous gland adenocarcinoma, mucoepidermoid carcinoma, myoepithelioma, oncocytoma, and pleomorphic adenoma.
Adenomatoid proliferation of alveolar epithelium	See alveolar cell hyperplasia	
Adenomyoma		This rare variant of hamartoma consists of smooth muscle enclosing alveolar spaces.
Adenosquamous cell carcinoma		Histological variant of carcinoma composed of both malignant squamous and glandular components. By definition each element must constitute approximately 50% of the whole tumour.
Alveolar adenoma	Papillary adenoma	This is a rare solitary lesion (10–25 mm), which occurs in the periphery of the lung. It is composed of a network of spaces lined by cuboidal pneumocytes with a papillary pattern.
Alveolar atypical hyperplasia	See atypical adenomatous hyperplasia	

Tumour terminology Recommended terms are in **bold**	Synonyms	Comments
Alveolar cell hyperplasia	Adenomatoid proliferation of alveolar epithelium Alveolar hyperplasia Micronodular pneumocyte hyperplasia Nodular alveolar hyperplasia Papillary alveolar hamartoma	Microscopic lesion (<5 mm) consisting of a single row of cuboidal cells along alveolar wall. Can be seen in lymphangiomyomatosis, von Recklinghausen's disease, and atypical alveolar adenomatous hyperplasia.
Alveolar epithelial hyperplasia	See atypical adenomatous hyperplasia	
Alveolar hyperplasia	See alveolar cell hyperplasia	Tumour-like lesion, which may be a feature of lymphangioleiomyomatosis and tuberous sclerosis.
Amyloid tumour		Localised amyloid deposition may present as nodular deposits in the airways and parenchyma. This variant is not associated with systemic amyloidosis.
Anaplastic carcinoma	See large cell carcinoma	
APUD carcinoma	See carcinoid tumour	Obsolete term.
APUD-oma	See carcinoid tumour	Obsolete term.
Atypical adenomatous hyperplasia	Alveolar atypical hyperplasia Alveolar epithelial hyperplasia Atypical alveolar cuboidal cell hyperplasia Atypical alveolar hyperplasia Atypical bronchioloalveolar hyperplasia Bronchioloalveolar adenoma Broncho alveolar cell hyperplasia Pre-invasive lesion	A focal lesion, which may be single or multiple, measuring less than 5 mm in diameter and consisting of alveolar spaces lined by atypical epithelial cells. It is seen in resected lung specimens with carcinoma. The risk of progression to adenocarcinoma, however, is low.

Tumour terminology Recommended terms are in **bold**	Synonyms	Comments
Atypical alveolar cuboidal cell hyperplasia	See atypical adenomatous hyperplasia	
Atypical alveolar hyperplasia	See atypical adenomatous hyperplasia	
Atypical bronchioloalveolar hyperplasia	See atypical adenomatous hyperplasia	
Atypical carcinoid	Well differentiated neuroendocrine carcinoma	This is an extremely rare variant of carcinoid tumour in which pleomorphism, mitotic activity, and necrosis are seen. It is much more likely to metastasise than the typical variant.
Basaloid carcinoma	Small cell squamous cell carcinoma	This aggressive tumour in the elderly is a variant of squamous cell carcinoma characterised by the presence of small cells showing peripheral palisading. If no squamous differentiation is found the tumour is regarded as a variant of large cell carcinoma. Rarely an adenocarcinomatous component may be present. Neuroendocrine features are absent.
Benign clear cell tumour	Clear cell tumour Sugar tumour	This is a rare benign tumour composed of glycogen rich cells thought to be of pericyte derivation. HMB45 expression is common. It presents as a coin lesion on X-ray. Differentiation from clear cell carcinoma and metastatic clear cell carcinoma may be difficult.
Benign sclerosing pneumocytoma	Pneumocytoma Sclerosing haemangioma	This rare usually solitary benign tumour presents as a coin lesion. It is composed of an admixture of papillary, solid, and sclerotic areas. Its histogenesis is uncertain but it probably derives from the pneumocyte. Although vascular, it is not a haemangiomatous lesion.
Biphasic blastoma		This rare tumour of the elderly is composed of epithelial tubules with a primitive malignant stroma. Heterologous differentiation towards skeletal muscle, cartilage, or bone is sometimes seen.

Tumour terminology Recommended terms are in **bold**	Synonyms	Comments
Blastoma	See pulmonary blastoma	
Bronchial adenoma	See adenoma	
Bronchioloalveolar adenoma	See atypical adenomatous hyperplasia	
Bronchioloalveolar carcinoma	Bronchioloalveolar cell carcinoma Goblet cell adenocarcinoma	This tumour is often found in the periphery of the lung. It may arise from pneumocytes, Clara cell, or bronchial goblet cells. Variants include mucinous bronchioloalveolar cell carcinoma, non-mucinous bronchioloalveolar carcinoma, mucinous carcinoma of the lung, and goblet cell carcinoma.
Bronchioloalveolar cell carcinoma	See bronchioloalveolar carcinoma	
Bronchoalveolar cell hyperplasia	See atypical adenomatous hyperplasia	
Carcinoid tumour	APUD-carcinoma (obsolete) APUD-oma (obsolete) Endocrine tumour Neuroendocrine tumour	This is the most common "benign" bronchial tumour. It occurs in young adults and is not associated with smoking. Most often it arises centrally and typically presents as a collar-stud lesion, which protrudes into the lumen of the bronchus. It may be sub-divided on the basis of size, site, and clinical behaviour into tumourlet, typical (central and peripheral) and atypical variants. The last is also known as well differentiated neuroendocrine carcinoma.
Carcinosarcoma	See metaplastic carcinoma	
Chemodectoma	See paraganglioma	
Chondroma		This variant of hamartoma is composed of pure cartilage. It may be a feature of Carney's triad in association with gastric leiomyoblastoma and paraganglioma.
Clear cell adenocarcinoma	See clear cell carcinoma	

Tumour terminology Recommended terms are in **bold**	Synonyms	Comments
Clear cell carcinoma	Clear cell adenocarcinoma	Rare histological variant of carcinoma in which tumour cells are vacuolated due to the presence of glycogen. Commonly clear cell tumours in the lung represent metastases from renal cell carcinoma.
Clear cell squamous cell carcinoma		Histological variant of squamous cell carcinoma in which the tumour cells contains abundant glycogen.
Clear cell tumour	See benign clear cell tumour	
Colloid carcinoma	See mucinous carcinoma	
Combined small cell carcinoma		Histological variant of small cell carcinoma showing foci of glandular and/or squamous differentiation.
Congenital peribronchial myofibroblastic tumour		This rare tumour occurs in children and consists of an atypical myofibroblastic proliferation showing pleomorphism and mitotic activity. The prognosis is good.
Diffuse lymphangiectasis		This rare lesion is characterised by dilatation of benign lymphatic channels associated with congenital heart disease in particular anomalous pulmonary venous drainage. It presents in childhood with chylothorax and is often fatal.
Diffuse neuroendocrine cell hyperplasia		This condition may be seen in association with tumourlets and carcinoid tumours in the peripheral bronchioles. It consists of neuroendocrine cells, confined to bronchiolar epithelium in association with fibrosis or can be idiopathic.
Early squamous cell carcinoma	See microinvasive squamous cell carcinoma	
Embryoma	See pulmonary blastoma	
Endocrine tumour	See carcinoid tumour	
Endometriosis		In the lung this condition may mimic adenocarcinoma and can present as a mass in elderly females taking hormone replacement therapy.

Tumour terminology Recommended terms are in **bold**	Synonyms	Comments
Epidermoid carcinoma	See squamous cell carcinoma	
Epithelial blastoma	See adenocarcinoma of foetal type	
Epithelial myoepithelial carcinoma		This rare tumour is similar to the salivary gland counterpart. It is usually associated with a good prognosis.
Epithelioid haemangioendothelioma	Intravascular bronchioloalveolar tumour IV-BAT	In the lung this tumour commonly presents as multiple nodules infiltrating the bronchovascular bundles. It is characterised by an indolent course but patients may eventually die from respiratory failure.
Fibroxanthoma	See inflammatory pseudotumour	
Germ cell tumour		Primary tumour is extremely rare in the lung and therefore the possibility of metastasis or extension from the mediastinum must always be excluded.
Giant cell carcinoma		This is a rare variant of large cell carcinoma associated with a very poor prognosis.
Glandular papilloma		Very rare, usually solitary papillary lesion.
Glomus tumour		Rare, usually in upper airways. See Tumours of Soft Tissue (Section 42).
Goblet cell adenocarcinoma	See bronchioloalveolar carcinoma	
Granular cell myoblastoma	See granular cell tumour	
Granular cell tumour	Granular cell myoblastoma	See Tumours of Soft Tissue (Section 42).
Hamartoma	See pulmonary hamartoma	
Hepatoid adenocarcinoma		Histological variant of large cell carcinoma in which the tumour cells resemble hepatocytes.
Histiocytoma	See inflammatory pseudotumour	

Tumour terminology Recommended terms are in **bold**	Synonyms	Comments
Hyalinising granuloma		Nodule of hyaline collagen of unknown aetiology but can be associated with retroperitoneal fibrosis.
Inflammatory polyp		Benign reactive lesion in an inflamed airway.
Inflammatory pseudotumour	Fibroxanthoma Histiocytoma Plasma cell granuloma Xanthoma	This is a rare benign tumour-like lesion, which most often presents in the periphery of the lung. It consists of granulation tissue, inflammatory cells, and fibrous tissue. Occasionally plasma cells are very numerous. It sometimes involves the mediastinum.
Intravascular bronchioloalveolar tumour	See epithelioid haemangioendothelioma	
IV-BAT	See epithelioid haemangioendothelioma	
Langerhans cell histiocytosis		In the lung this presents as a diffuse and bilateral nodulo-cystic infiltrate. It may be the only manifestation of disease.
Large cell carcinoma	Anaplastic carcinoma Undifferentiated carcinoma	A pleomorphic tumour showing no evidence of glandular or squamous differentiation. Variants include giant cell carcinoma, large cell carcinoma with rhabdoid features, lymphoepithelioma-like carcinoma, pleomorphic carcinoma, undifferentiated carcinoma.
Large cell carcinoma with neuroendocrine features	Large cell neuroendocrine carcinoma	This is a histological variant of large cell tumour characterised by foci of organoid nesting, peripheral palisading, and trabeculae formation suggesting neuroendocrine differentiation.
Large cell carcinoma with rhabdoid features		This is a very rare aggressive subtype of large cell carcinoma. It is characterised by the presence of intracytoplasmic eosinophilic inclusions.
Large cell neuroendocrine carcinoma	See large cell carcinoma with neuroendocrine features	

Tumour terminology Recommended terms are in **bold**	Synonyms	Comments
Lymphoepithelioma-like carcinoma		This is a variant of large cell carcinoma. It is common in South East Asia and sometimes associated with Epstein-Barr virus. It is probably identical to the nasopharyngeal tumour.
Malignant lymphoma		See Tumours of the Lymph Nodes and Spleen (Section 24).
Melanoma		Primary melanoma in the lung is extremely rare. Metastasis should always be excluded.
Meningioma	See pulmonary meningioma	
Mesenchymal chondroma		This histological variant of hamartoma is composed of an admixture of smooth muscle, connective tissue, and cartilage.
Metaplastic carcinoma	Carcinosarcoma Sarcomatoid carcinoma	This is a rare high grade tumour, which usually presents in the elderly. It is characterised by the presence of both malignant epithelial and mesenchymal components. The former is most commonly squamous in nature but occasionally other subtypes may be represented. The latter may present as a pure spindle cell population but occasionally chondroid, osteoid, leiomyosarcomatous, and rhabomyosarcomatous differentiation may be seen.
Microinvasive squamous cell carcinoma	Early squamous cell carcinoma Superficial squamous cell carcinoma	This tumour is confined to bronchial wall with no infiltration of lung parenchyma. Excellent prognosis with resection.
Micronodular pneumocyte hyperplasia	See alveolar cell hyperplasia	
Mucinous adenoma	Mucinous gland adenoma Mucous gland adenoma	This is a histological variant of adenoma, which presents as a usually solitary lesion in the tracheobronchial tree of children and young adults.

Tumour terminology Recommended terms are in **bold**	Synonyms	Comments
Mucinous bronchioloalveolar carcinoma		Histological variant of bronchioloalveolar carcinoma characterised by massive mucus production and sometimes confused with metastatic adenocarcinoma (particularly from the pancreas).
Mucinous carcinoma of lung	Colloid carcinoma	Histological variant of bronchioloalveolar carcinoma composed of large lakes of mucin containing small groups of non-pleomorphic cells.
Mucinous cystadenocarcinoma		This is a variant of adenocarcinoma characterised by the presence of large cystic spaces lined by atypical mucinous cells showing mitotic activity. Parenchymal invasion is present.
Mucinous cystadenoma	See mucinous cystadenoma of lung	
Mucinous cystadenoma of lung	Mucinous cystadenoma	This benign tumour consists of a large, localised cystic space filled with mucus and lined by uniform columnar mucinous cells. There is no stromal invasion.
Mucinous gland adenoma	See mucinous adenoma	
Mucoepidermoid carcinoma		This is a rare tumour composed of an admixture of squamous and mucus-secreting epithelium similar to salivary gland lesions.
Mucous gland adenoma	See mucinous adenoma	
Multifocal micronodular pneumocyte hyperplasia		This rare condition consists of small foci of pneumocyte proliferation and is seen in tuberous sclerosis.
Multiple meningothelioid nodules		This is a variant of pulmonary meningioma and consists of aggregates of small regular cells in the pulmonary interstitium near to veins. They were previously regarded as chemodectomas but are now recognised as being of meningothelial derivation.

Tumour terminology Recommended terms are in **bold**	Synonyms	Comments
Myoepithelioma		This is an exceedingly rare variant of adenoma composed of a mixture of epithelial and smooth muscle cell proliferation. It presents in the large bronchi.
Neuroendocrine tumour	See carcinoid tumour See small cell carcinoma	
Nodular alveolar hyperplasia	See alveolar cell hyperplasia	
Non–small cell carcinoma		This is a term often used for small biopsies to indicate a tumour that is not a small cell carcinoma and that does not show evidence of glandular or squamous differentiation.
Non-chromaffin paraganglioma	See paraganglioma	
Non-mucinous adenocarcinoma	See non-mucinous bronchioloalveolar carcinoma	
Non-mucinous bronchioloalveolar carcinoma	Non-mucinous adenocarcinoma	Histological variant of bronchioloalveolar carcinoma derived from pneumocytes or Clara cells.
Oat cell carcinoma	See small cell carcinoma	
Oncocytic carcinoid tumour		Histological variant of carcinoid tumour.
Oncocytoma		This variant of adenoma must be distinguished from an oncocytic carcinoid tumour. It is of unpredictable biological behaviour and can behave in a malignant fashion.
Papillary adenocarcinoma		Histological variant of adenocarcinoma characterised by the presence of papillary architecture.
Papillary adenoma	See alveolar adenoma	
Papillary alveolar hamartoma	See alveolar cell hyperplasia	
Papillary squamous cell carcinoma		A variant of squamous cell carcinoma characterised by an endobronchial growth pattern. Stromal invasion is minimal or absent.

Tumour terminology Recommended terms are in **bold**	Synonyms	Comments
Papillomatosis		Multiple squamous papillomas similar to those described in the upper respiratory tract. This usually occurs in children and is related to infection with HPV types 6 or 11.
Paraganglioma	Chemodectoma Non-chromaffin paraganglioma Vagal body tumour	In the lung, these rare tumours arise from chemoreceptors present in the adventitia of the main pulmonary artery branches. See Tumours of the Adrenal Cortex, Adrenal Medulla, and Paraganglia (Section 6).
Plasma cell granuloma	See inflammatory pseudotumour	
Plasmacytoma		This occasionally solitary lesion may very rarely present in the lung. It is often associated with amyloid deposition.
Pleomorphic adenoma		This variant of adenoma may very rarely present in the trachea or lung, similar to salivary gland lesions.
Pleomorphic carcinoma		This tumour is composed of an admixture of malignant epithelial cells and spindle cells. It may be present in association with squamous, glandular, or large cell carcinoma.
Pleuropulmonary blastoma		Childhood variant of pulmonary blastoma. It is composed of cystic or solid sarcoma in which the cysts are lined by metaplastic epithelium. Several variants are recognised, including undifferentiated, rhabdomyosarcomatous, leiomyosarcomatous, chondrosarcomatous, etc.
Pneumocytoma	See benign sclerosing pneumocytoma	
Polypoid carcinoma		A gross descriptive term for a tumour protruding into the lumen. It is sometimes inappropriately used as a synonym for spindle cell squamous carcinoma and carcinosarcoma.
Pre-invasive lesion	See atypical adenomatous hyperplasia	

Tumour terminology Recommended terms are in **bold**	Synonyms	Comments
Pulmonary blastoma	Blastoma Embryoma	This is a malignant tumour composed of immature tubules resembling foetal lung. Adult and childhood variants of this rare tumour are recognised. The former includes adenocarcinoma of foetal type and biphasic blastoma. Childhood variants sometimes involve the pleura in addition to the lung. The latter are known as pleuropulmonary blastomas.
Pulmonary endodermal tumour	See adenocarcinoma of foetal type	
Pulmonary hamartoma	Hamartoma	This is the most common benign tumour of lung. It is composed of an admixture of cartilage, fat, connective tissue, and gland inclusions. It occurs in the elderly. Variants include adenofibroma, chondroma, and mesenchymal chondroma.
Pulmonary lymphangioleiomyo-matosis	See pulmonary lymphangiomyomatosis	
Pulmonary lymphangiomyomatosis	Pulmonary lymphangioleiomyo-matosis	This is a rare hamartomatous condition. It consists of proliferating smooth muscle surrounding dilated lymphatic vessels. Females in the reproductive years are affected suggesting a hormonal pathogenesis.
Pulmonary meningioma	Meningioma	This is an extremely rare tumour, which may present as a solitary coin lesion or as multiple microscopic lesions (multiple meningothelioid nodules). It is histologically identical to the meningeal equivalent and lacks neuroendocrine differentiation.
Sarcomatoid carcinoma	See metaplastic carcinoma	
Sclerosing haemangioma	See benign sclerosing pneumocytoma	
Signet ring carcinoma		This variant of adenocarcinoma is extremely rare in the lung. Always exclude the possibility of metastases.

Tumour terminology Recommended terms are in **bold**	Synonyms	Comments
Small cell carcinoma	Oat cell carcinoma Neuroendocrine tumour	This is a common high grade variant of lung cancer usually associated with smoking. Many tumours are centrally located and exhibit neuroendocrine features.
Small cell squamous cell carcinoma	See basaloid carcinoma	
Solid adenocarcinoma with mucin		Large cell tumour with no obvious gland formation in which there is plentiful mucin.
Spindle cell carcinoma		Histological variant of squamous cell carcinoma. By definition heterologous differentiation is not present.
Squamous cell carcinoma	Epidermoid carcinoma	This is the most common malignant tumour of the trachea and lung. Strongly associated with smoking.
Squamous cell papilloma		This is a very rare lesion, which usually affects the elderly and is associated with smoking and HPV types 6 and 11. It may progress to invasive tumour.
Sugar tumour	See benign clear cell tumour	
Superficial squamous cell carcinoma	See microinvasive squamous cell carcinoma	
Teratoma		Primary involvement of the lung is extremely rare. The possibility of a metastasis or extension from the thymus should always be excluded.
Tumourlet		This not uncommon hyperplastic lesion of neuroendocrine cells by definition measures less than 5 mm in diameter. It may be an incidental finding in normal or scarred lung and is often multiple. Sometimes it presents in association with a typical carcinoid tumour.
Typical carcinoid		This histological variant of carcinoid tumour is the most common. It is characterised by uniform morphology with few mitoses and no necrosis.

Tumour terminology Recommended terms are in **bold**	Synonyms	Comments
Undifferentiated carcinoma	See large cell carcinoma	
Vagal body tumour	See paraganglioma	See also Tumours of the Adrenal Cortex, Adrenal Medulla, and Paraganglia (Section 6).
Verrucous carcinoma		Verrucous carcinoma in the lung is exceptionally rare. It is associated with HPV infection.
Well differentiated foetal carcinoma	See adenocarcinoma of foetal type	
Well differentiated neuroendocrine carcinoma	See atypical carcinoid	
Xanthoma	See inflammatory pseudotumour	

Section 21

Tumours of the Serous Cavities (Pleura, Pericardium, Peritoneum)

M. Sheppard

Tumour terminology Recommended terms are in **bold**	Synonyms	Comments
Adenomatoid tumour		This benign tumour may rarely present in the peritoneum and pleura. See Tumours of the Testis and Epididymis (Section 30).
Anaplastic mesothelioma	Undifferentiated mesothelioma Pleomorphic mesothelioma	A variant of malignant mesothelioma.
Angiosarcoma	Haemangiosarcoma	Exceptionally rare in the pleura and pericardium. In the heart, it arises in the right atrium and then spreads diffusely over the pericardial surface.
Benign epithelial mesothelioma	See well differentiated papillary mesothelioma	
Benign local pleural fibroma	See localised fibrous tumour	
Benign localised mesothelioma	See localised fibrous tumour	
Benign multicystic mesothelioma	Cystic mesothelioma of the peritoneum Multilocular peritoneal inclusion cyst Multicystic mesothelioma	Presents as an intraperitoneal mass that involves both visceral and parietal layers. It is considered benign when with a single layer of mesothelial cells. Recurrence rate is 50%. Very rare in the pleura.

Tumour terminology Recommended terms are in **bold**	Synonyms	Comments
Biphasic malignant mesothelioma	See malignant mesothelioma mixed type	
Blastoma	See pleuropulmonary blastoma	
Calcifying fibrous pseudotumour of the pleura		Tumour-like plaque lesion of visceral pleura. Calcified with psammoma bodies. No relation to asbestos exposure.
Clear cell mesothelioma		A variant of malignant mesothelioma.
Cystic malignant mesothelioma		A variant of malignant mesothelioma.
Cystic mesothelioma of the peritoneum	See benign multicystic mesothelioma	
Deciduoid mesothelioma		Very rare variant of malignant mesothelioma with large decidua-like cells. Occurs in peritoneum of young females. Highly malignant. Not linked to asbestos exposure.
Desmoplastic malignant mesothelioma		A variant of connective tissue (sarcomatous) type malignant mesothelioma with dense collagen.
Desmoplastic round cell tumour	See intra-abdominal desmoplastic small round cell tumour	
Diffuse lymphangiomatosis		Proliferation of benign lymphatic channels usually in pleura but may involve peritoneum.
Diffuse malignant fibrous mesothelioma	See malignant mesothelioma connective tissue type	
Disseminated peritoneal leiomyomatosis	Peritoneal leiomyomatosis Leiomyomatosis peritonalis disseminata	A very rare benign hormone-induced metaplasia of submesothelial connective tissue. It is seen grossly as very large numbers of small nodules diffusely distributed on the peritoneal surface, mimicking metastatic tumour.
Early mesothelioma	See mesothelioma in situ	
Endometrioid carcinoma		Very rare in the peritoneum. Identical to its ovarian counterpart. It is diagnosed only when the ovaries are uninvolved.

Tumour terminology Recommended terms are in **bold**	Synonyms	Comments
Endometrioid stromal sarcoma		Very rare in the peritoneum. Identical to its ovarian counterpart. It is diagnosed only when the ovaries are uninvolved.
Endometriosis		Not a neoplasm. Involves mainly peritoneum but also rarely the pleura. Mimic adenocarcinoma or malignant mesothelioma. Can occur in elderly on hormone replacement therapy.
Endothelioma	See malignant mesothelioma	Obsolete term.
Epithelial mesothelioma	See epithelioid mesothelioma	Obsolete term.
Epithelioid haemangioendothelioma		Rare as primary, which can mimic epithelioid malignant mesothelioma. Keratin negative and endothelial marker positive.
Epithelioid mesothelioma	Epithelial mesothelioma (obsolete)	A rare variant of epithelial-type malignant mesothelioma.
Fibroma	See localised fibrous tumour	
Fibrosarcoma	See localised malignant fibrous tumour	
Giant cell mesothelioma		A variant of malignant mesothelioma.
Glandular mesothelioma	See malignant mesothelioma epithelial type	
Haemangiosarcoma	See angiosarcoma	
Histiocytoma	See inflammatory pseudotumour	
Inflammatory pseudotumour	Plasma cell granuloma Histiocytoma	Can invade pleura and mimic malignant mesothelioma connective tissue type.
Intermediate malignant mesothelioma	See malignant mesothelioma mixed type	
Intra-abdominal desmoplastic small round cell tumour	Desmoplastic round cell tumour Mesothelioblastoma	Rare highly aggressive primitive tumour of mesothelial origin, more common in young males. Extremely rare in pleura.

Tumour terminology Recommended terms are in **bold**	Synonyms	Comments
Kaposi's sarcoma		Can involve the pleura in AIDS. See Tumours of Soft Tissue (Section 42).
Leiomyofibroma	See localised fibrous tumour	
Leiomyoma		Very rare in the pleura. Occasionally found in the peritoneum. See Tumours of Soft Tissue (Section 42).
Leiomyomatosis peritonalis disseminata	See disseminated peritoneal leiomyomatosis	
Leiomyosarcoma		Extremely rare as primary. See Tumours of Soft Tissue (Section 42).
Localised fibrous mesothelioma	See localised fibrous tumour	
Localised fibrous tumour	Benign local pleural fibroma Benign localised mesothelioma Fibroma Leiomyofibroma Localised fibrous mesothelioma Localised solitary monophasic spindle cell tumour Solitary fibrous tumour of the pleura Submesothelial fibroma	Not related to malignant mesothelioma, Slow growing benign unilateral tumour that arises as a solitary mass from the visceral pleura. It is rare in the peritoneum. It is keratin negative and CD34 positive.
Localised malignant fibrous tumour	Fibrosarcoma	Very rare malignant counterpart of localised fibrous tumour.
Localised malignant mesothelioma		Very rare localised tumour, which must histologically, immunohistochemically, and electron microscopically fulfil the criteria of malignant mesothelioma. Can be cured by local resection but is aggressive.
Localised solitary monophasic spindle cell tumour	See benign localised tumour	

Tumour terminology Recommended terms are in **bold**	Synonyms	Comments
Lymphohistiocytic mesothelioma		Variant of malignant mesothelioma.
Malignant fibrous histiocytoma		Very rare. See Tumours of Soft Tissue (Section 42).
Malignant lymphoma		Rare as primary. In the pleura associated with empyema. See Tumours of the Lymph Nodes and Spleen (Section 24).
Malignant mesothelioma	Endothelioma (obsolete) Mesodermoma (obsolete) Mesothelioma	Asbestos associated highly malignant tumour. Histologically is classified into epithelial, mixed, and connective tissue (sarcomatous) type according to the dominating features. The histological, ultrastructural, histochemical, and immunohistochemical features of malignant mesothelioma are the same whether the tumour arises in the pleura, pericardium, peritoneum, or tunica vaginalis. Non-asbestos associated mesotheliomas have been reported. Variants include anaplastic, clear cell, desmoplastic, deciduoid, diffuse malignant fibrous, epithelioid, giant cell, lymphohistiocytic, small cell, transitional.
Malignant mesothelioma connective tissue type	Diffuse malignant fibrous mesothelioma Sarcomatoid mesothelioma Sarcomatous mesothelioma Spindle cell mesothelioma	One of the main types of malignant mesothelioma, with spindle cell predominating. Need immunocytochemistry with cytokeratin positivity.
Malignant mesothelioma epithelial type	Glandular mesothelioma Tubulopapillary mesothelioma	Most common type of malignant mesothelioma. 75% of cases in peritoneum and 50% of cases in pleura.
Malignant mesothelioma mixed type	Biphasic mesothelioma Intermediate mesothelioma	One of the main types of malignant mesothelioma.
Malignant mesothelioma of the tunica vaginalis		Rare tumour divided into high and low grade. Long clinical course with recurrences and spread to peritoneum.

Tumour terminology Recommended terms are in **bold**	Synonyms	Comments
Mesodermoma	See malignant mesothelioma	Obsolete term.
Mesothelioblastoma	See intra-abdominal desmoplastic small round cell tumour	
Mesothelioma	See malignant mesothelioma	
Mesothelioma in situ	Early mesothelioma	Exceptionally rare lesion where atypical cells line the pleural surface with no invasion. Tiny nodules seen. Extensive sampling needed to rule out invasion.
Multicystic mesothelioma	See benign multicystic mesothelioma	
Multilocular peritoneal inclusion cyst	See benign multicystic mesothelioma	
Peritoneal leiomyomatosis	See disseminated peritoneal leiomyomatosis.	
Peritoneal serous psammocarcinoma		Extremely rare variant of peritoneal serous surface carcinoma.
Peritoneal serous surface carcinoma		A high grade tumour with the appearances of an ovarian serous carcinoma. It is diagnosed only when the ovaries are uninvolved.
Peritoneal serous tumour of borderline malignancy	See peritoneal serous tumour of low malignant potential	
Peritoneal serous tumour of low malignant potential	Peritoneal serous tumour of borderline malignancy	Occurs in young women and is identical to its ovarian counterpart. It is diagnosed only when the ovaries are uninvolved.
Plasma cell granuloma	See inflammatory pseudotumour	
Pleomorphic mesothelioma	See anaplastic mesothelioma	
Pleuropulmonary blastoma	Blastoma	Malignant. Occurs in children under 2 years. Often cystic, it can be low or high grade.

Tumour terminology Recommended terms are in **bold**	Synonyms	Comments
Pseudomesotheliomatous adenocarcinoma		Macroscopically mimic malignant mesothelioma with diffuse pleural growth. Glandular tumour with a dense desmoplastic stroma.
Pseudomesotheliomatous angiosarcoma		Extremely rare may mimic diffuse pleural growth of mesothelioma.
Pseudomyxoma of the peritoneum		A condition characterised by masses of gelatinous material within the peritoneal cavity. The source is mucus-secreting serosal cells derived from the rupture of a benign mucocele of the appendix or a mucinous cystic tumour of the ovary. Histologically benign but because of the persistent nature of the lesion there is a fatal outcome in 50% of the cases.
Rhabdomyosarcoma		Extremely rare as primary. Most cases are metastatic. See Tumours of Soft Tissue (Section 42).
Sarcomatoid mesothelioma	See malignant mesothelioma connective tissue type	
Sarcomatous mesothelioma	See malignant mesothelioma connective tissue type	
Serous papillary carcinoma of the peritoneum	See peritoneal serous surface carcinoma	
Serous psammocarcinoma of the peritoneum	See peritoneal serous psammocarcinoma	
Small cell mesothelioma		A variant of malignant mesothelioma. May mimic small cell carcinoma or malignant lymphoma.
Solitary fibrous tumour of the pleura	See localised fibrous tumour	
Solitary fibrous tumour of the pleura	See benign localised mesothelioma	
Spindle cell mesothelioma	See malignant mesothelioma connective tissue type	

Tumour terminology Recommended terms are in **bold**	Synonyms	Comments
Squamous cell carcinoma		Primary squamous cell carcinoma of the pleura is extremely rare associated with pneumothorax for tuberculosis.
Submesothelial fibroma	See localised fibrous tumour	
Synovial sarcoma		Very rare. Mimics malignant mesothelioma both morphologically and immunocytochemically. See Tumours of Soft Tissue (Section 42).
Thymoma		Rare as primary. See Tumours of the Thymus (Section 25).
Transitional mesothelioma		A variant of malignant mesothelioma.
Tubulopapillary adenocarcinoma		Corresponds to the most common metastatic tumour in pleura, either from lung or other systems, such as breast, ovary, gastrointestinal tract.
Tubulopapillary mesothelioma	See malignant mesothelioma epithelial type	
Undifferentiated mesothelioma	See anaplastic mesothelioma	
Well differentiated papillary mesothelioma	Benign epithelial mesothelioma	Relatively common in the peritoneum. Extremely rare in the pleura. Benign. Occurs in females as multiple papillary or nodular lesions. It is not related to asbestos exposure.

Section 22

Tumours of the Heart

M. Sheppard

Tumour terminology Recommended terms are in **bold**	Synonyms	Comments
Angiosarcoma	Haemangiosarcoma	This is the most common malignant tumour of the heart and blood vessels. It is usually associated with a poor prognosis.
Bronchogenic cyst		Primary cardiac involvement is exceedingly rare. The cyst is lined by ciliated epithelium.
Cardiac fibroma		This rare tumour occurs in children as an infiltrating mass in the myocardium. It commonly presents as a solitary lesion but occasionally multiple tumours are found. Regression with age usually occurs.
Cardiac hamartoma		This rare lesion usually presents in the right ventricle and consists of a well defined nodule composed of myocytes and fibrous tissue.
Cardiac paraganglioma	Phaeochromocytoma	Primary cardiac lesions are rare and most often affect the base close to the left atrium and aortic arch.
Cystic tumour of the atrioventricular node	Mesothelioma of the atrioventricular node	This very rare lesion most often arises in the region of the atrioventricular node and presents with heart block and sudden death. It is composed of multiple cysts lined by benign flat, cuboidal, or squamous cells, which express CEA. It is probably of endodermal derivation.
Fibroelastic hamartoma		Histological variant of cardiac fibroma in which elastic fibres are present in addition to collagen.

Tumour terminology Recommended terms are in **bold**	Synonyms	Comments
Fibroelastic papilloma	See papillary fibroelastoma	
Giant Lambl's excrescence	See papillary fibroelastoma	
Granular cell myoblastoma	See granular cell tumour	
Granular cell tumour	Granular cell myoblastoma	Primary cardiac lesions are exceedingly rare. See Tumours of Soft Tissue (Section 42).
Haemangioma		Rare, benign vascular tumour of the heart.
Haemangiosarcoma	See angiosarcoma	
Histiocytoid cardiomyopathy	Oncocytic cardiomyopathy Purkinje cell hamartoma	This rare variant of cardiac hamartoma, which affects infants and children, presents as an arrhythmia. It consists of multiple yellow nodules composed of oncocytic myocytes. The left ventricle is predominantly involved.
Kaposi's sarcoma		The pericardium may be involved in patients with AIDS. See Tumours of Soft Tissue (Section 42).
Leiomyosarcoma		This tumour may exceptionally arise from the vessels in the heart. See Tumours of Soft Tissue (Section 42).
Lipoma		Primary cardiac lipoma is extremely rare. See Tumours of Soft Tissue (Sections 42).
Lipomatous hamartoma of atrial septum	See lipomatous hypertrophy of atrial septum	
Lipomatous hamartoma of cardiac valves		This rare lesion, which is composed of a mixture of mature fat and fibrous tissue predominantly affects the tricuspid and mitral valves. It may present with incompetence.
Lipomatous hypertrophy of atrial septum	Lipomatous hamartoma of the atrial septum Massive fatty deposits of the atrial septum	This lesion represents a non-encapsulated accumulation of mature fat in the interatrial septum. It is not related to obesity or starvation.

Tumour terminology Recommended terms are in **bold**	Synonyms	Comments
Lymphangioma		This very rare tumour is usually located within the pericardial sac. See Tumours of Soft Tissue (Section 42).
Malignant lymphoma		Cardiac lymphoma is extremely rare and is usually of B-cell type. Primary nodal disease should always be excluded.
Malignant mesothelioma of the pericardium		Primary involvement of the pericardium is extremely rare. Patients most often present with dyspnoea and pericardial effusion.
Massive fatty deposits of the atrial septum	See lipomatous hypertrophy of the atrial septum	
Mesothelial cyst	See pericardial cyst	
Mesothelial papilloma		This represents an incidental finding in the pericardium. It is composed of connective tissue covered by plump mesothelial cells.
Mesothelioma of the atrioventricular node	See cystic tumour of the atrioventricular node	
Myxofibrosarcoma	Myxoid malignant fibrous histiocytoma Myxoid MFH Myxosarcoma	This tumour may very rarely arise in the heart. See Tumours of Soft Tissue (Section 42).
Myxoid malignant fibrous histiocytoma	See myxofibrosarcoma	
Myxoid MFH	See myxofibrosarcoma	
Myxoma		This common benign tumour of the heart is of uncertain histogenesis. It frequently presents in the left atrium attached to the fossa ovalis. The valves are not affected.
Myxosarcoma	See myxofibrosarcoma	
Oncocytic cardiomyopathy	See histiocytoid cardiomyopathy	
Papillary fibroelastoma	Fibroelastic papilloma Giant Lambl's excrescence Papilloma of valve	This most commonly affects the aortic valve and is composed of fibroelastic tissue covered by endothelium. Local excision is curative.

Tumour terminology Recommended terms are in **bold**	Synonyms	Comments
Papilloma of valve	See papillary fibroelastoma	
Pericardial cyst	Mesothelial cyst	This rare cystic lesion is lined by benign mesothelial cells.
Pericardial fibroma	See solitary fibrous tumour of the pericardium	
Phaeochromocytoma	See cardiac paraganglioma	
Purkinje cell hamartoma	See histiocytoid cardiomyopathy	
Rhabdomyoma		This is the most common benign cardiac tumour in infants and children. Multiple lesions are most commonly encountered and there is a strong association with tuberous sclerosis.
Rhabdomyosarcoma		This is the second most common sarcoma to affect the heart. It presents in adults. See Tumours of Soft Tissue (Section 42).
Solitary fibrous tumour of the pericardium	Pericardial fibroma	Rarely solitary fibrous tumour may affect the pleura. See Tumours of the Serous Cavities (Section 21).
Struma cordis	See thyroid heterotopia	
Teratoma		This rare tumour, which most often affects females, predominantly arises within the pericardium. Malignant variants are exceptional.
Thymic heterotopia		This very rare lesion is usually an incidental finding.
Thyroid heterotopia	Struma cordis	This very rare lesion is usually an incidental finding. The right ventricular outflow tract is most often affected.

Section 23

Tumours of the Bone Marrow and Leukaemia

C. Matsouka
C.N. Chinyama
M. Kalmanti

Tumour terminology Recommended terms are in **bold**	Synonyms	Comments
Acute lymphoblastic leukaemia		Arises from B or T cells. Affects mostly children. French American British (FAB) classification recognises forms which depend on the size of the lymphoblasts, namely: L1, L2, and L3.
Acute myeloblastic leukaemia	See acute myeloid leukaemia	
Acute myelodysplasia with myelofibrosis	See acute myelofibrosis	
Acute myelofibrosis	Acute myelodysplasia with myelofibrosis Acute myelosclerosis	Distinguished from chronic myelofibrosis by lack of red cell poikilocytosis in the blood smear. Initially associated with proliferation of all three cell lines.
Acute myeloid leukaemia	Acute myeloblastic leukaemia	Affects middle-aged and elderly patients. FAB recognises 8 forms. M0—undifferentiated, M1—without maturation, M2—with granulocytic maturation, M3—acute promyelocytic, M4—granulocytic and monocytic maturation, M5—monoblastic or monocytic, M6—erythroleukaemia, M7—megablastic.

Tumour terminology Recommended terms are in **bold**	Synonyms	Comments
Acute myelosclerosis	See acute myelofibrosis	
Adult T-cell leukaemia/ lymphoma (ATLL)	Caribbean T-cell lymphoma/leukaemia Japanese pleomorphic type T-cell lymphoma	Associated with type C retrovirus (HTLV-1) common in patients of Japanese and Afro-Caribbean origin.
B-chronic lymphocytic leukaemia (B-CLL, CLL)	Chronic lymphatic leukaemia	Most common form of leukaemia in the elderly.
B-prolymphocytic leukaemia (B-PLL)		Variant of CLL, which is characterised by massive splenomegaly and high lymphocytosis.
Caribbean T-cell lymphoma/leukaemia	See adult T-cell leukaemia/lymphoma ATLL	
Chloroma	See granulocytic sarcoma	
Chronic granulocytic leukaemia	See chronic myeloid leukaemia (CML)	
Chronic lymphatic leukaemia	See B-chronic lymphocytic leukaemia (B-CLL, CLL)	
Chronic myelogenous leukaemia	See chronic myeloid leukaemia (CML)	
Chronic myeloid leukaemia (CML)	Chronic granulocytic leukaemia Chronic myelogenous leukaemia	Usually affects middle-aged patients. Associated with Philadelphia chromosome t(22;9).
Chronic myelomonocytic leukaemia	Preleukaemia/ Myelodysplasia	Usually progresses to acute leukaemia.
Chronic neutrophilic leukaemia		Rare form of leukaemia, only diagnosed after all causes of leucocytosis are excluded. Philadelphia chromosome negative.
Eosinophilic leukaemia		Variant of chronic myeloid leukaemia characterised by the predominance of eosinophils in the bone marrow and peripheral blood.

Tumour terminology Recommended terms are in **bold**	Synonyms	Comments
Essential thrombocythaemia		Primary disease, which results from excessive platelets accumulation, which results from excess megakaryocytes in the bone marrow.
Granulocytic sarcoma	Chloroma	A variant of myeloid leukaemia characterised by accumulation of extramedullary myeloblasts. More common in children. The term "chloroma" was applied to the green colouration of the fresh tumour.
Hairy cell leukaemia	Leukaemic reticuloendotheliosis	Rare disease, common in men characterised by proliferation of monoclonal B cell with irregular cytoplasmic outlines "hairy cells" in the spleen and bone marrow.
Japanese pleomorphic type T-cell lymphoma	See adult T-cell leukaemia /lymphoma (ATLL)	
Juvenile chronic myeloid leukaemia		Variant of CML, which occurs in young children. Responds poorly to treatment.
Large granular lymphocyte leukaemia	See T-chronic lymphocytic leukaemia (T-CLL)	
Leukaemic reticuloendotheliosis	See hairy cell leukaemia	
Multiple myeloma	Myelomatosis	Monoclonal proliferation of plasma cells within the bone marrow associated with raised ESR and paraproteinaemia. "Plasmacytoma" is the term used for the localised lesion.
Myelodysplasia	Myelodysplastic syndromes	A group of acquired neoplastic disorders of the bone marrow associated with quantitative and qualitative abnormality of all three cell lines with a tendency to progress to acute leukaemia. Variants include refractory anaemia (RA), RA with ring sideroblasts, RA with excess blasts (RAEB), RAEB in transformation chronic myelomonocytic leukaemia.
Myelodysplastic syndromes	See myelodysplasia	
Myelomatosis	See multiple myeloma	

Tumour terminology Recommended terms are in **bold**	Synonyms	Comments
Polycythaemia rubra vera	See polycythaemia vera	
Polycythaemia vera	Polycythaemia rubra vera	Increase in red cell volume caused by proliferation within the bone marrow. Also associated with proliferation or platelets and granulocytes.
Preleukaemia/ myelodysplasia	See chronic myelomonocytic leukaemia	
RA with excess blasts (RAEB)	See myelodysplasia	
RA with ring sideroblasts		Variant of myelodysplasia.
RAEB in transformation		Variant of myelodysplasia.
Refractory anaemia	See myelodysplasia	
T-chronic lymphocytic leukaemia (T-CLL)	Large granular lymphocyte leukaemia	Rarer than B-CLL.
T-prolymphocyte leukaemia (T-PLL)		Rarer than B-PLL.

Section 24

Tumours of the Lymph Nodes and Spleen

P. Kanavaros
C.N. Chinyama

Due to the complex nature in the classification of lymphomas and use of confusing terms in some classifications, this section does not follow the format of the rest of the book. The REAL classification was used as the main nomenclature and the Kiel and working formulation as the synonym.

R = Revised European-American Lymphoma Classification
K = Kiel
WF = working formulation

B cell lymphomas

Tumour terminology	Synonyms	Comments
Angiotropic large cell lymphoma B-cell (K)		Rare and rapidly fatal disease. The neoplastic cells were thought to be proliferating vascular endothelial cells. High grade lymphoma, which tends to affect elderly patients. Involvement of the CNS results in cerebral symptoms.
B-cell chronic lymphocytic leukaemia (CLL) (R)	B-lymphocytic lymphoma (K) B-lymphocytic leukaemia (K) Small lymphocytic consistent with CLL (WF) Small lymphocytic lymphoma (R)	A disease of the older patient, which comprises 90% chronic lymphocytic lymphoma in the West. Can transform to large cell lymphoma (Ritcher's syndrome).

Tumour terminology	Synonyms	Comments
Burkitt's lymphoma (R)	Burkitt's lymphoma (K) Small non-cleaved cell (WF) Burkitt's lymphoma (WF)	Most common in children. Endemic in Africa. High grade B cell lymphoma associated with Epstein-Barr virus infection and 8:14 chromosome translocation.
Diffuse large cell B-cell lymphoma (R)	Centroblastic (K) B-immunoblastic (K) Large cell anaplastic B cell (K)	A difficult lymphoma to classify, which constitutes 40% of adult non-Hodgkin's lymphoma. An aggressive but potentially curable disease.
Extranodal marginal zone lymphoma (R)	Low grade B-cell lymphoma of Malt type (R)	Most patients have a history of autoimmune disease such as Hashimotos thyroiditis, Sjögren's disease, or Helicobacter gastritis.
Follicle centre lymphoma (R) Grade I, II, III	Centroblastic–centrocytic lymphoma (K) Follicular, predominantly small cleaved cell (WF) Follicular, mixed small, and large cell (WF) Follicular, predominantly large cell (WF) Centroblastic follicular (K)	The lymphoma is composed of centrocytes (cleaved cells) and centroblasts with a follicular pattern, may be diffuse. t (14;18) involving the Bcl-2 gene is present in 70–95% of the lymphomas.
Hairy cell leukaemia (R)	Hairy cell leukaemia (K)	Characterised by hairy projections on smear preparations. Bone marrow always involved. Associated with splenomegaly. Does not respond to ordinary lymphoma chemotherapy but interferon.
High grade B-cell lymphoma, Burkitt's-like (R)	Small non-cleaved cell non-Burkitt's (WF) Diffuse large cell (WF) Large cell immunoblastic (WF)	Lymphoma in which the cell size in intermediate between Burkitt's lymphoma and typical cell lymphoma.
Large cell anaplastic B-cell lymphoma (K)	Ki-1 lymphoma B-cell type (K)	Less common than the T cell type. Cells express CD30 (Ki-1 antibody) and morphologically mimic anaplastic carcinoma.
Lymphoplasmocytoid lymphoma (R)	Lymphoplasmocytoid immunocytoma (K) Small lymphocytic plasmacytoid (WF) Diffuse mixed small and large cell (WF)	Associated with IgM paraproteinaemia and hyperviscosity syndrome (Waldenstrom's syndrome).

Tumour terminology	Synonyms	Comments
Mantle cell lymphoma (R)	Centrocytic (K) Centroblastic, centroid subtype (K) Diffuse, small cleaved cell (WF) Follicular, small cleaved cell (WF) Diffuse, mixed small and large cell (WF) Diffuse, large cleaved cell (WF)	An aggressive form of lymphoma, which affects the lymph nodes, bone marrow, and the gut (lymphomatoid polyposis).
Nodal marginal zone B-cell lymphoma (R)	Monocytoid, including marginal zone (K) Immunocytoma (K) Small lymphocytic (WF) Diffuse, small cleaved cell (WF) Diffuse mixed small and large cell (WF)	Most patients have Sjögren's syndrome or other extranodal Malt-type lymphoma indicating that this may be the same disease process.
Plasmacytoma/myeloma (R)	Plasmacytic (K) Extramedullary plasmacytoma (WF) Multiple myeloma (R)	Neoplasms of the plasma cells, which present as a disseminated bone marrow tumour. May be solitary or extramedullary.
Precursor B-lymphoblastic lymphoma/leukaemia (R)	B-lymphoblastic (K;WF)	Mostly affects children and accounts for 80% acute lymphoblastic leukaemia and 20% of lymphoblastic lymphoma.
Primary mediastinal (thymic) large B-cell lymphoma (R)	Diffuse large cell (WF) Large cell immunoblastic (WF) Immunoblastic (K) Centroblastic (K)	Peaks in the fourth decade. High grade lymphoma of the mediastinum with a propensity for females.
Prolymphocytic leukaemia (R)	Prolymphocytic leukaemia (K)	Variant of B-cell lymphoma characterised by massive splenomegaly and high lymphocytosis.
Splenic marginal zone lymphoma +/- villous lymphocytes (R)	Small lymphocytic (WF) Diffuse small cleaved cell (WF)	Morphologically and clinically distinct from extranodal marginal zone lymphoma. Indolent course and splenectomy is curative.
T-cell rich B-cell lymphoma		Previously mistaken for T-cell lymphoma or Hodgkin's disease. Large B cells are present in the background of reactive T cells. The prognosis is variable.

T-cell lymphomas

Tumour terminology	Synonyms	Comments
Adult T-cell lymphoma/ leukaemia	Pleomorphic small, medium, and large cell— HTLV1+(K) Diffuse small cleaved cell (WF) Diffuse large cell (WF) Large cell immunoblastic (WF)	Affects mostly adults of Japanese or Afro-Caribbean origin who have antibodies of HTLV1. Aggressive disease with median survival of less than a year. Presents with high white cell counts, hypercalcaemia, and hepatosplenomegaly.
Anaplastic large cell lymphoma T and null cell types (R)	T-large cell anaplastic (K) Ki-1 lymphoma (K) Large cell immunoblastic (WF)	A rare lymphoma, which tends to affect patients under the age of 20. The neoplastic cells are large and express CD30 (Ki-1) antigen.
Angiocentric lymphoma (R)	Lethal midline granuloma Lymphomatoid granulomatosis Nasal and nasal type T/ NK cell lymphoma	Characterised by angiocentric and angioinvasive infiltrate. Rare disease in the West, but common in Asia can be indolent or aggressive. Extranodal sites include the nose and palate and are commonly associated with Epstein-Barr virus.
Angioimmunoblastic T-cell lymphoma (R)	Angioimmunoblastic lymphadenopathy (AILD-K) T-cell lymphoma (K) Diffuse small cleaved cell (WF) Diffuse mixed small and large cell (WF) Large cell immunoblastic (WF)	Originally thought to be an abnormal immune reaction. A rare disease in which patients present with lymphadenopathy fever, skin rash, and polyclonal paraproteinaemia.
Hepatosplenic gamma-delta T-cell lymphoma (R)		Recently described variant of T-cell lymphoma, with aggressive behaviour.
Intestinal T-cell lymphoma, with or without enteropathy (R)	Kiel—not listed WF—not listed	The disease was thought to be of histiocytic origin. Affects adults, often with a history of gluten-sensitive enteropathy (coeliac disease).
Large granular lymphocytic leukaemia (R)	Lymphocytic consistent with CLL (WF) T-CLL (K)	Two subtypes of T-cell type (D8+) and natural killer type (NK), characterised by lymphocytosis and indolent course.
Mycosis fungoides/ Sezary syndrome (R)	Small cell cerebriform (K) Mycosis fungoides (WF)	Patients usually present with cutaneous plaques and erythroderma, peripheral blood involvement is late Sezary syndrome.

Tumour terminology	Synonyms	Comments
Peripheral T-cell lymphoma, unspecified (R) (i) Medium sized cell (ii) Mixed medium and large cell (iii) Large cell	T-zone (K) Lymphoepithelioid cell (Lennert's) lymphoma (K) Pleomorphic, small T cell (K) Pleomorphic, medium sized and large T cell (K) T-immunoblastic (K) Diffuse small cleaved cell (K) Diffuse mixed small and large cell (WF) Diffuse large cell (WF) Large cell immunoblastic (WK)	Due to difficult classification, the Real group lumped all these T cell lymphomas under one group. The Kiel group recognized several variants under this category. Constitute 15% of lymphomas in the West. Affects adult patients with involvement of the skin lymph nodes and viscera. More aggressive than B-cell lymphomas.
Subcutaneous panniculitis T-cell lymphoma (R)		T-cell lymphoma, which involves the subcutaneous tissue and is associated with haemophagocytic syndrome.
T-cell chronic lymphocytic leukaemia (R)	T-lymphocytic CLL type (K) Small lymphocytic (WF)	Comprises of 19% CLL. Associated with high white cell count, bone marrow, liver, and lymph node involvement.
T-prolymphocytic leukaemia (R)	T-prolymphocytic leukaemia (K) Prolymphocytic leukacmia (WF)	A variant of T-CLL.

The following terms were used in the past individually or in older classifications not in use anymore. They do not correspond to entities of contemporary classifications and should be considered obsolete.

Angioendotheliomatosis proliferous systematisata

Malignant angioendotheliomatosis

Brill-Symmers disease

Giant follicular lymphadenopathy

Giant lymph follicle hyperplasia

Lymphoblastoma

Lymphocytic reticulosarcoma

Lymphocytoma

Lymphoid follicular reticulosis

Lymphosarcoma

Reticulum cell lymphosarcoma

Reticulum cell sarcoma

Reticulosarcoma

Stem cell lymphoma

Hodgkin's disease

The Reed-Sternberg (RS) cell is the pathognomonic feature in Hodgkin's disease, but the histogenesis of this cell is not clear.

Tumour terminology	Synonyms	Comments
Lymphocyte depletion		Least common variant of HD, which affects older patients. The infiltrate is hypocellular and Reed-Sternberg (RS) are also scanty.
Lymphocyte rich classical HD		This is thought to be a variant of lymphocyte predominance with classical Reed-Sternberg (RS) cells.
Lymphocytic predominance		Affects all ages and involves peripheral lymph nodes with sparing of the mediastinum. The proliferation can be diffuse or nodular. The predominant cell is the lymphocytic and histiocytic. Reed-Sternberg (RS) cells are scanty.
Mixed cellularity		Affects adult patients, males more than females. Follows an aggressive course.
Nodular sclerosis		Mostly affects adolescents and young adults. The lymph nodules exhibit a partially nodular pattern with fibrous bands separating the nodules. Reed-Sternberg (RS) cells are numerous. The dominant cell is the Lacunar type RS.

The following terms were used in the past and should be considered obsolete.

Hodgkin's paragranuloma

Hodgkin's sarcoma

Benign Causes of Lymphadenopathy

Tumour terminology Recommended terms are in **bold**	Synonyms	Comments
Angiofollicular lymph node hyperplasia	See Castleman's disease	
Castleman's disease	Lymph node hamartoma Angiofollicular lymph node hyperplasia	A distinct form of lymph node hyperplasia, which affects mostly the mediastinum. It can be solitary or multicentric. The cause is unknown and may be complicated by lymphoma.

Tumour terminology Recommended terms are in **bold**	Synonyms	Comments
Deciduosis		Decidua can occur in abdominal lymph nodes of pregnant women.
Infections		Viral, bacterial, and fungal infections can cause lymphadenopathy and/or splenomegaly.
Inflammatory pseudotumour		A rare cause of benign lymphadenopathy. The lymph nodes are enlarged due to proliferation of spindle cell fibroblasts and activated macrophages.
Lymph node hamartoma	See Castleman's disease	
Naevus cells in lymph nodes		Naevus cell aggregates are rarely found in lymph nodes.
Rosai-Dorfman disease	See sinus histiocytosis with massive lymphadenopathy	
Sinus histiocytosis with massive lymphadenopathy	Rosai-Dorfman disease	A rare condition of unknown aetiology, which commonly occurs in Africa. Causes massive lymphadenopathy due to proliferation of histiocytes within the sinuses.
Vascular transformation of lymph node sinuses		A reactive condition associated with lymphovascular obstruction. The sinuses are expanded by complex anastomosing vascular channels.

Non-haematolymphoid tumours and tumour-like lesions of the spleen

Tumour terminology Recommended terms are in **bold**	Synonyms	Comments
Angiosarcoma		Primary angiosarcoma of the spleen is a rare and aggressive tumour, which may present with haemoperitoneum.
Bacillary angiomatosis	Epithelioid angiomatosis	A vasoproliferative condition caused by a Rickettsia-like organism, morphologically similar to cat scratch bacillus. Affects exclusively AIDS patients. Affects mostly the skin with spread to lymph nodes and spleen.

Tumour terminology Recommended terms are in **bold**	Synonyms	Comments
Epithelioid angiomatosis	See bacillary angiomatosis	
Haemangioma		Most common primary benign neoplasm of the spleen. Can be single or multiple.
Haemorrhagic spindle cell tumour with amianthoid fibres	Palisaded myofibroblastoma Intranodal myofibroblastoma	A benign spindle cell proliferation, which affects mostly the inguinal lymph nodes. Typically the proliferation forms stellate collagen nodules (amianthoid fibres). Haemorrhage can occur at the periphery.
Intranodal myofibroblastoma	See haemorrhagic spindle cell tumour with amianthoid fibres	
Littoral cell angioma		A rare benign tumour occurring exclusively in the spleen. Associated with splenomegaly and hypersplenism. Tumour consists of anastomosing sinuses lined by bland cells.
Palisaded myofibroblastoma	See haemorrhagic spindle cell tumour with amianthoid fibres	
Splenic cysts		Pseudocysts account for 80% of splenic cysts. They arise due to liquefaction of a hamartoma. Other cysts include epithelial and paracytic cysts.
Splenic hamartoma		Can be solitary or multiple. The tumour is composed of irregularly arranged tortuous vascular channels lined by splenic sinus endothelium and separated by pulp cord-like lesions.

Section 25

Tumours of the Thymus

J. Iakovidou
G.S. Delides

Tumour terminology Recommended terms are in **bold**	Synonyms	Comments
Adenoid cystic carcinoma	See thymic carcinoma	A very rare histological variant of thymic carcinoma.
Adenosquamous carcinoma	See thymic carcinoma	Histological variant of thymic carcinoma.
Anaplastic carcinoma	Undifferentiated carcinoma	A highly malignant carcinoma not readily classified into one of the histological variants of thymic carcinoma.
Basaloid carcinoma		Histological variant of thymic carcinoma.
Benign thymoma	Encapsulated thymoma Medullary thymoma Predominantly epithelial thymoma (obsolete) Predominantly lymphocytic thymoma (obsolete) Spindle cell thymoma Thymoma	*Subclassified to A* a. Predominantly lymphocytic b. Predominantly epithelial c. Mixed and d. spindle cell *Or subclassified B according to* a. Shape of epithelial cells b. Number of lymphocytes c. Ancillary features.
Carcinoid	See neuroendocrine tumour	
Carcinosarcoma	See metaplastic carcinoma	
Clear cell carcinoma		Histological variant of thymic carcinoma.
Combined germ cell tumour	See mixed germ cell tumour	

Tumour terminology Recommended terms are in **bold**	Synonyms	Comments
Cortical thymoma	Mixed thymoma: epithelial-lymphocytic (obsolete)	Histological variant of malignant thymoma.
Encapsulated thymoma	See benign thymoma	
Epithelial thymoma		Histological variant of malignant thymoma.
Germ cell tumour		With the exception of teratoma occur almost exclusively in males, usually in adolescents. Variants include seminoma, embryonal carcinoma, and mixed germ cell tumour. See Tumours of the Testis and Epididymis (Section 30) and Tumours of the Ovary (Section 32).
Germinoma	See seminoma	
Granulomatous thymoma	See Hodgkin's disease	Obsolete term.
Histiocytosis X	See Langerhans cell histiocytosis	
Hodgkin's disease	Granulomatous thymoma (obsolete)	See Tumours of the Lymph Nodes and Spleen (Section 24).
Invasive thymoma	See malignant thymoma	
Langerhans cell histiocytosis	Histiocytosis X	Thymus may be involved as part of systemic disease. See Tumours of the Bone (Section 43).
Large B-cell lymphoma with sclerosis	Sclerosing lymphoma of the mediastinum	More common in young woman. Highly malignant. See Tumours of the Lymph Nodes and Spleen (Section 24).
Leukaemia		See Tumours of the Bone Marrow and Leukaemia (Section 23).
Lymphocytic thymoma (lymphoma)		See Tumours of the Lymph Nodes and Spleen (Section 24).
Lymphoepithelial carcinoma	Lymphoepithelioma-like carcinoma	Histological variant of thymic carcinoma identical to that of nasopharynx.
Lymphoepithelioma-like carcinoma	See lymphoepithelial carcinoma	

Tumour terminology Recommended terms are in **bold**	Synonyms	Comments
Malignant thymoma	Invasive thymoma Malignant thymoma Type I Mixed thymoma: cortical-medullary	Thymoma with capsular/pericapsular invasion. Histological variants: predominantly cortical, cortical, mixed cortical-medullary, well differentiated thymic carcinoma.
Malignant thymoma type I	See malignant thymoma	
Malignant thymoma type II	See thymic carcinoma	
Medullary thymoma	See benign thymoma	
Metaplastic carcinoma	Carcinosarcoma Sarcomatoid carcinoma Spindle cell carcinoma	Histological variant of thymic carcinoma showing mesenchymal differentiation.
Mixed germ cell tumour	Combined germ cell tumour	Histological variant of germ cell tumour.
Mixed myoid-epithelial tumour		Potentially malignant.
Mixed thymoma: cortical-medullary	See malignant thymoma	
Mixed thymoma: epithelial-lymphocytic	See cortical thymoma	Obsolete term.
Mucoepidermoid carcinoma		Histological variant of thymic carcinoma.
Myoid cell tumour		Unpredictable behaviour.
Neuroendocrine carcinoma	See neuroendocrine tumour	
Neuroendocrine tumour	Carcinoid Neuroendocrine carcinoma	Uncommon in thymus heterogeneous group of tumours regarding histology, immunohistochemistry, hormone production, and biological behaviour. Histological variants in thymus: spindle cell, pigmented, sclerotic, diffuse medullary thyroid carcinoma-like, and small cell carcinoma (oat cell carcinoma). Group comprises functioning and non-functioning tumours as well as benign, low grade malignant, and high grade malignant.

Tumour terminology Recommended terms are in **bold**	Synonyms	Comments
Non-Hodgkin's lymphomas		See Tumours of the Lymph Nodes and Spleen (Section 24).
Oat cell carcinoma	See small cell carcinoma	
Predominantly cortical thymoma		Histological variant of malignant thymoma.
Predominantly epithelial thymoma	See benign thymoma	Obsolete term.
Predominantly lymphocytic thymoma	See benign thymoma	Obsolete term.
Rhabdomyosarcoma		See Tumours of Soft Tissue (Section 42).
Sarcomatoid carcinoma	See metaplastic carcinoma	
Sclerosing lymphoma of the mediastinum	See large B-cell lymphoma with sclerosis	
Seminoma	Germinoma	Variant of germ cell tumour.
Small cell carcinoma	Oat cell carcinoma	Highly malignant neuroendocrine tumour. Histologically similar to small cell lung carcinoma.
Spindle cell carcinoma	See metaplastic carcinoma	
Spindle cell thymoma	See benign thymoma	
Squamous cell carcinoma	See thymic carcinoma	The most common histological variant of thymic carcinoma with survival rate over 50%.
Teratoma		Mature teratomas are benign. See Tumours of the Testis and Epididymis (Section 30) and Tumours of the Ovary (Section 32).
Thymic carcinoma	Malignant thymoma type II	With the exception of squamous cell carcinoma all other histological variants highly malignant No association with myasthenia gravis. Histological variants include adenoid cystic carcinoma, adenosquamous carcinoma, basaloid carcinoma, clear cell carcinoma, mucoepidermoid, spindle cell carcinoma, and squamous cell carcinoma.

Tumour terminology Recommended terms are in **bold**	Synonyms	Comments
Thymic cysts		Benign.
Thymolipoma		Rare, benign. Can occasionally be associated with myasthenia gravis.
Thymoliposarcoma		Malignant.
Thymoma	See benign thymoma	
Undifferentiated carcinoma	See anaplastic carcinoma	
Well differentiated thymic carcinoma	Epithelial-predominant carcinoma.	Histological variant of malignant thymoma strongly associated with the occurrence of myasthenia gravis.

Section 26

Tumours of the Mediastinum and Retroperitoneum

W.V. Bogomoletz
G.S. Delides

Tumour terminology Recommended terms are in **bold**	Synonyms	Comments
Adenocarcinoma		Rare as primary in the mediastinum or in the retroperitoneum. May arise in a lymphoepithelial cyst or in a duplicate foregut cyst.
Angiosarcoma		See Tumours of Soft Tissue (Section 42).
Chondrolipoma		See Tumours of Soft Tissue (Section 42).
Dysgerminoma	See seminoma	
Embryonal carcinoma	See malignant teratoma	
Ependymoma		See Tumours of the Central Nervous System (Section 2).
Epithelioid haemangioendothelioma		See Tumours of Soft Tissue (Section 42).
Fibromatosis		See Tumours of Soft Tissue (Section 42).
Germinoma	See seminoma	
Haemangioma		See Tumours of Soft Tissue (Section 42).
Haemangiopericytoma		See Tumours of Soft Tissue (Section 42).
Hodgkin's disease		In mediastinum usually of the nodular sclerosing type. See Tumours of the Lymph Nodes and Spleen(Section 24).
Inflammatory myofibroblastic tumour	Inflammatory pseudotumour	See Tumours of Soft Tissue (Section 42).

Tumour terminology Recommended terms are in **bold**	Synonyms	Comments
Inflammatory pseudotumour	See inflammatory myofibroblastic tumour	
Langerhans cell histiocytosis		See Tumours of the Bone (Section 43).
Leiomyoma		See Tumours of Soft Tissue (Section 42).
Leiomyosarcoma		See Tumours of Soft Tissue (Section 42)
Lipoblastomatosis		See Tumours of Soft Tissue (Section 42).
Lipoma		See Tumours of Soft Tissue (Section 42).
Liposarcoma		See Tumours of Soft Tissue (Section 42).
Lymphangioma		See Tumours of Soft Tissue (Section 42).
Malignant fibrous histiocytoma		See Tumours of Soft Tissue (Section 42).
Malignant lymphoma		See Tumours of the Lymph Nodes and Spleen (Section 24).
Malignant teratoma	Embryonal carcinoma Mixed germ cell tumour	See Tumours of the Testis and Epididymis (Section 30).
Mesothelioma		See Tumours of the Serous Cavities (Section 21).
Mixed germ cell tumour	See malignant teratoma	
Mixed tumour of salivary gland type	See pleomorphic adenoma	
Osteosarcoma		See Tumours of the Bone (Section 43).
Paraganglioma		See Tumours of the Adrenal Cortex, Adrenal Medulla, and Paraganglia (Section 6).
Plasmacytoma		See Tumours of the Lymph Nodes and Spleen(Section 24).
Pleomorphic adenoma	Mixed tumour of salivary gland type	See Tumours of the Salivary Glands (Section 9).
Rhabdoid tumour		See Tumours of Soft Tissue (Section 42).
Rhabdomyoma		See Tumours of Soft Tissue (Section 42).
Rhabdomyosarcoma		See Tumours of Soft Tissue (Section 42).
Seminoma	Dysgerminoma Germinoma	See Tumours of the Testis and Epididymis (Section 30) and Tumours of the Ovary (Section 32).

Tumour terminology Recommended terms are in **bold**	Synonyms	Comments
Solitary fibrous tumour		See Tumours of Soft Tissue (Section 42).
Squamous carcinoma		Rare as primary in the mediastinum or in the retroperitoneum. May arise in a bronchial or in a thymic cyst.
Synovial sarcoma		See Tumours of Soft Tissue (Section 42).
Thymolipoma		See Tumours of the Thymus (Section 25).

Section 27

Tumours of the Kidney

M. Pea
G.M. Mariuzzi

Tumour terminology Recommended terms are in **bold**	Synonyms	Comments
Adenocarcinoma	See renal cell carcinoma clear cell type	
Adenoma	See renal cortical adenoma	
Adenomyosarcoma	See nephroblastoma	Obsolete term.
Adenosarcoma	See nephroblastoma	Obsolete term.
Alveolar adenoma	See renal cortical adenoma	
Anaplastic carcinoma	See renal cell carcinoma sarcomatoid type	
Angioma	See haemangioma	
Angiomyolipoma	Hamartoma Microhamartoma	This rare tumour is composed of an admixture of fat, smooth muscle, and blood vessels. In approximately 50% of cases tumours are multiple and associated with tuberous sclerosis.
Angiosarcoma	Haemangiosarcoma	Primary angiosarcoma of the kidney is exceptionally rare.
Bellini duct carcinoma	See renal cell carcinoma Bellini duct type	
Bone-metastasising renal tumour of childhood	See clear cell sarcoma	
Capsular leiomyoma	See leiomyoma	
Capsuloma	See leiomyoma	

Tumour terminology Recommended terms are in **bold**	Synonyms	Comments
Carcinoid tumour	See neuroendocrine tumour	
Carcinoma of the collecting ducts of Bellini	See renal cell carcinoma Bellini duct type	
Carcinosarcoma	See renal cell carcinoma sarcomatoid type	
Chromophil carcinoma	See renal cell carcinoma papillary cell type	
Chromophil renal cell carcinoma	See renal cell carcinoma papillary cell type	
Chromophobe carcinoma	See renal cell carcinoma chromophobe cell type	
Chromophobe renal cell carcinoma	See renal cell carcinoma chromophobe cell type	
Clear cell carcinoma	See renal cell carcinoma clear cell type	
Clear cell sarcoma	Bone-metastasising renal tumour of childhood	Rare, high grade tumour of childhood associated with a striking propensity for bone metastases. It may be distinguished from nephroblastoma by the absence of blastema and differentiated mesenchymal elements.
Collecting duct carcinoma	See renal cell carcinoma Bellini duct type	
Combined nephroblastomatosis	See nephrogenic rests	
Congenital mesoblastic nephroma	Foetal hamartoma Leiomyomatous hamartoma Mesenchymal hamartoma Mesoblastic nephroma	Rare low grade malignant tumour of early infancy. Very occasional examples have been recorded in adults. Recurrences and metastases are uncommon after surgical resection. It should be distinguished from nephroblastoma.
Cystic nephroma	Multicystic nephroma Multilocular cyst Multilocular cystic nephroma	Uncommon and controversial benign lesion occurring in both adults and children. It must be distinguished from multilocular cystic renal cell carcinoma and cystic partially differentiated nephroblastoma.

Tumour terminology Recommended terms are in **bold**	Synonyms	Comments
Cystic partially differentiated nephroblastoma		This rare lesion is sometimes classified as a variant of cystic nephroma. It can, however, be distinguished by the presence of renal blastema and tubules within the fibrous septa. Incomplete excision may be followed by recurrence.
Dark cell adenocarcinoma	See renal cell carcinoma clear cell type	
Dormant rest	See nephrogenic rests	
Embryoma	See nephroblastoma	Obsolete term.
Fibroma	See renomedullary interstitial cell tumour	
Foetal hamartoma	See congenital mesoblastic nephroma	
Granular cell carcinoma	See renal cell carcinoma clear cell type	Obsolete term.
Grawitz tumour	See renal cell carcinoma clear cell type	Obsolete term.
Haemangioma	Angioma	This tumour only rarely arises in the kidney. Multifocal lesions may form part of Klippel-Trelaunay and Sturge-Weber syndromes. See Tumours of Soft Tissue (Section 42).
Haemangiosarcoma	See angiosarcoma	
Hamartoma	See angiomyolipoma	
Hypernephroma	See renal cell carcinoma clear cell type	Obsolete term.
Hyperplastic diffuse perilobar nephroblastomatosis	See nephrogenic rests	
Hyperplastic rests	See nephrogenic rests	
Incipient rests	See nephrogenic rests	
Intralobar nephroblastomatosis	See nephrogenic rests	
Intrarenal teratoma	See teratoma	
Involuting rests	See nephrogenic rests	

Tumour terminology Recommended terms are in **bold**	Synonyms	Comments
Juxtaglomerular cell tumour	Reninoma	This rare benign tumour is associated with hypertension. Elevated serum renin levels are typically present.
Leiomyoma	Capsular leiomyoma Capsuloma	This tumour rarely presents in the kidney.
Leiomyomatous hamartoma	See congenital mesoblastic nephroma	
Leiomyosarcoma		Although extremely rare, this is the most frequently encountered primary renal sarcoma. There is a predilection for females. See Tumours of Soft Tissue (Section 42).
Lipoma		Primary kidney tumours are very rare and most often affect middle-aged women.
Liposarcoma		Primary tumours of the kidney are extremely rare. Secondary involvement by a retroperitoneal primary is more common. See Tumours of Soft Tissue (Section 42).
Lymphangioma		Most examples of this rare tumour arise in a peripelvic distribution. See Tumours of Soft Tissue (Section 42).
Malakoplakia		A rare inflammatory tumour-like lesion.
Malignant fibrous histiocytoma		Secondary involvement by a retroperitoneal lesion is more commonly encountered than primary tumours. Sarcomatoid-type renal cell carcinoma must always be excluded.
Malignant lymphoma		Primary lesions of the kidney are exceptionally rare. Secondary involvement must always be excluded. See Tumours of the Lymph Nodes and Spleen (Section 24).
Malignant nephroma	See renal cell carcinoma clear cell type	Obsolete term.
Medullary fibroma	See renomedullary interstitial cell tumour	

Tumour terminology Recommended terms are in **bold**	Synonyms	Comments
Medullary fibrous nodule	See renomedullary interstitial cell tumour	
Mesenchymal hamartoma	See congenital mesoblastic nephroma	
Mesoblastic nephroma	See congenital mesoblastic nephroma	
Metanephric adenoma		This is an extremely rare tumour that predominantly affects females, it can be distinguished from adult Wilms' tumour by the absence of renal blastema.
Metanephroma	See renal cell carcinoma clear cell type	Obsolete term.
Microhamartoma	See angiomyolipoma	
Multicystic nephroma	See cystic nephroma	
Multilocular cyst	See cystic nephroma	
Multilocular cystic nephroma	See cystic nephroma	
Multilocular cystic renal cell carcinoma	See renal cell carcinoma clear cell type	
Neoplastic rests	See nephrogenic rests	
Nephroblastoma	Adenomyosarcoma (obsolete) Adenosarcoma (obsolete) Carcinosarcoma Embryoma (obsolete) Teratoid nephroblastoma Wilms' tumour	This malignant tumour predominantly affects young children although occasional cases have been documented in adults. It is characterised by a variable admixture of blastema, stromal mesenchymal elements, and an epithelial component. With current therapy the prognosis is excellent.
Nephroblastomatosis	See nephrogenic rests	
Nephrogenic adenofibroma		This is an extremely rare benign tumour affecting young adults and presenting with hypertension or polycythaemia. It is composed of an admixture of spindle cells and nephrogenic rests.

Tumour terminology Recommended terms are in **bold**	Synonyms	Comments
Nephrogenic rests	Combined nephroblastomatosis Dormant rest Hyperplastic diffuse perilobar nephroblastomatosis Hyperplastic rests Incipient rests Intralobar nephroblastomatosis Involuting rests Neoplastic rests Nephroblastomatosis Obsolescent rests Perilobar nephroblastomatosis Persistent nodular blastema Universal nephroblastomatosis	A pre-malignant lesion consisting of persistent renal blastema, which is capable of developing into nephroblastoma. Multiple histological variants are recognised, any of which, if found in a kidney removed for nephroblastoma, increases the risk of tumour formation in the remaining kidney.
Neuroblastoma		Rare examples arising in the kidney are probably best classified within the spectrum of primitive neuroectodermal tumours.
Neuroendocrine carcinoma	Carcinoid tumour Small cell carcinoma	Primary renal tumours are extremely rare and commonly associated with metastases. Malignant. Extremely rare.
Obsolescent rests	See nephrogenic rests	
Oncocytoma	Renal oncocytoma	This benign tumour comprises about 3% of all renal tumours. It must be differentiated from renal cell carcinoma with oncocytic features.
Ossifying renal tumour	Ossifying renal tumour of infancy	This is an extremely rare benign tumour of uncertain histogenesis, which thus far has been described in male infants and arises adjacent to the renal pelvis.
Ossifying renal tumour of infancy	See ossifying renal tumour	

Tumour terminology Recommended terms are in **bold**	Synonyms	Comments
Osteosarcoma		Primary renal lesion is exceptionally rare. A sarcomatoid renal cell carcinoma must be excluded. See Tumours of the Bone (Section 43).
Papillary adenoma	See renal cortical adenoma	
Papillary carcinoma	See renal cell carcinoma papillary type	
Pelvic fibrolipomatosis	See pelvic lipomatosis	
Pelvic lipomatosis	Pelvic fibrolipomatosis	A tumour-like lesion resulting from excessive proliferation of peripelvic fat.
Perilobar nephroblastomatosis	See nephrogenic rests	
Persistent nodular blastema	See nephrogenic rests	
Plasmacytoma		Primary renal lesions are extremely rare. See Tumours of the Lymph Nodes and Spleen (Section 24).
Renal cell carcinoma	See renal cell carcinoma clear cell type	
Renal cell carcinoma Bellini duct type	Bellini duct carcinoma Carcinoma of the collecting ducts of Bellini Collecting duct carcinoma	This variant comprises 1% of renal cell carcinomas. It is thought to arise from the terminal segment of the renal collecting duct.
Renal cell carcinoma chromophil cell type		Histological variant of renal cell carcinoma. It may be divided into eosinophil and basophil subtypes. This variant often has papillary architecture.
Renal cell carcinoma chromophobe cell type	Chromophobe carcinoma Chromophobe renal cell carcinoma	Histological variant constituting 5% of all renal cell carcinomas. It may be divided into typical and eosinophil (oncocytic features) subtypes. The latter must be distinguished from oncocytoma, which is benign.

Tumour terminology Recommended terms are in **bold**	Synonyms	Comments
Renal cell carcinoma **clear cell type**	Adenocarcinoma Clear cell carcinoma Dark cell adenocarcinoma Granular cell carcinoma (obsolete) Grawitz tumour (obsolete) Hypernephroma (obsolete) Malignant nephroma (obsolete) Metanephroma (obsolete) Multilocular cystic renal cell carcinoma Renal cell carcinoma	The major histological variant of renal cell carcinoma (70%).
Renal cell carcinoma granular cell type		Obsolete term.
Renal cell carcinoma **papillary type**	Papillary carcinoma	Histological variant of renal cell carcinoma (10–15%).
Renal cell carcinoma **sarcomatoid type**	Anaplastic carcinoma Carcinosarcoma Renal cell carcinoma spindle cell type Sarcomatoid carcinoma	High grade variant of renal cell carcinoma. Sarcomatoid change may be found in all of the other subtypes of renal cell carcinoma and when present adversely affects prognosis.
Renal cell carcinoma spindle cell type	See renal cell carcinoma sarcomatoid type	
Renal cell carcinoma **unclassified**		A category that is used to document renal cell carcinomas that do not fit readily in one of the other subtypes. It constitutes 4–5% of cases.
Renal cortical adenoma	Adenoma Alveolar adenoma Papillary adenoma	A controversial small benign lesion, which, by definition, does not exceed 3 cm in diameter and is believed to be a possible precursor of renal cell carcinoma. It may be difficult to distinguish this lesion from a small example of the latter.
Renal oncocytoma	See oncocytoma	

Tumour terminology Recommended terms are in **bold**	Synonyms	Comments
Renal pelvic fibroma	See renomedullary interstitial cell tumour	
Reninoma	See juxtaglomerular cell tumour	
Renomedullary interstitial cell tumour	Fibroma Medullary fibroma Medullary fibrous nodule Renal pelvic fibroma	This is a common lesion of the renal medulla. Symptoms are rare, but it may be related to hypertension. It arises from the renomedullary interstitial cells (which secrete vasoactive substances) but whether it represents a hyperplastic condition or neoplasm is uncertain.
Rhabdoid tumour		This is an extremely high grade rare malignant tumour occurring in children.
Rhabdomyosarcoma		Primary renal tumours are extremely rare and must be distinguished from sarcomatoid renal cell carcinoma and nephroblastoma. See Tumours of Soft Tissue (Section 42).
Sarcomatoid carcinoma	See renal cell carcinoma sarcomatoid type	
Small cell carcinoma	See neuroendocrine carcinoma	
Teratoid nephroblastoma	See nephroblastoma	
Teratoma	Intrarenal teratoma	Primary renal lesions are exceedingly rare and must be distinguished from nephroblastoma.
Universal nephroblastomatosis	See nephrogenic rests	
Wilms' tumour	See nephroblastoma	
Xanthogranulomatous pyelonephritis		Inflammatory tumour-like lesion, which is usually associated with urinary obstruction. It is often mistaken for renal cell carcinoma.

Section 28

Tumours of the Urinary Bladder, Urethra, Ureter, and Renal Pelvis

J. Lekka
G.S. Delides

Tumour terminology Recommended terms are in **bold**	Synonyms	Comments
Abrikossoff's tumour	See granular cell tumour	
Adenocarcinoma	Adenocarcinoma Not Otherwise Specified (NOS)	Rare. A carcinoma in which the glandular component predominates. Poor prognosis.
Adenocarcinoma Not Otherwise Specified (NOS)	See adenocarcinoma	
Adenomatoid metaplasia	See adenomatoid tumour	
Adenomatoid tumour	Adenomatoid metaplasia Nephrogenic adenoma Nephrogenic metaplasia	Tumour-like lesion thought to be a reactive process secondary to inflammation.
Adenosarcoma		Low grade malignant mixed tumour.
Aggressive angiomyxoma	See angiomyxoma	
Angiomyxoma	Aggressive angiomyxoma Superficial angiomyxoma	Presents in the renal peripelvic soft tissue. Locally infiltrative with multiple recurrences.
Angiosarcoma		Rare in the urinary tract malignant tumour. See Tumours of Soft Tissue (Section 42).

Tumour terminology Recommended terms are in **bold**	Synonyms	Comments
Botryoid rhabdomyosarcoma	See embryonal rhabdomyosarcoma	
Brunnian adenoma	See inverted papilloma	Obsolete term.
Carcinoid	See neuroendocrine tumour	
Carcinoma in situ (CIS)	Transitional cell carcinoma in situ Urothelial carcinoma in situ	Non-papillary (flat) and non-invasive transitional cell carcinoma.
Carcinoma in situ pagetoid		Rare histological variant of carcinoma in situ.
Carcinoma with neuroendocrine differentiation	See neuroendocrine tumour	
Carcinoma with trophoblastic differentiation	Choriocarcinoma	High grade, rare histological variant of transitional cell carcinoma.
Carcinosarcoma		High grade malignant mixed tumour with mesenchymal and epithelial component
Caruncle		Tumour-like lesion of the urethra.
Chondrosarcoma		Rare in the urinary tract. See Tumours of the Bone (Section 43).
Choriocarcinoma	See carcinoma with trophoblastic differentiation	
Clear cell adenocarcinoma		Rare histological variant of adenocarcinoma.
Colloid adenocarcinoma	See mucinous adenocarcinoma	
Condyloma acuminatum		Benign human papilloma virus-associated proliferation. Can involve the bladder spreading from external genitalia.
Embryonal rhabdomyosarcoma	Botryoid rhabdomyosarcoma	Histological variant of rhabdomyosarcoma. The most common variant in bladder arising in children less than 5 years old. Botryoid rhabdomyosarcoma represents a macroscopic variant arising in an exophytic grape-like manner.

Tumour terminology Recommended terms are in **bold**	Synonyms	Comments
Enteric adenocarcinoma		Histological variant of adenocarcinoma.
Fibroepithelial polyp		A rare benign mesenchymal tumour of the renal pelvis and ureter.
Fibrosarcoma		Rare in the urinary tract malignant tumour. See Tumours of Soft Tissue (Section 42).
Fibrous histiocytoma		Rare in the urinary tract. See Tumours of Soft Tissue (Section 42).
Giant cell carcinoma	See sarcomatoid carcinoma	
Giant cell transitional cell carcinoma	Transitional cell carcinoma giant cell	Histological variant of transitional cell carcinoma.
Granular cell myoblastoma	See granular cell tumour	
Granular cell tumour	Abrikossoff's tumour Granular cell myoblastoma	Rare in the urinary tract benign tumour. See Tumours of Soft Tissue (Section 42).
Haemangioma		Rare benign polypoid tumour usually seen in children. See Tumours of Soft Tissue (Section 42).
Haemangiopericytoma		Rare in the urinary tract. See Tumours of Soft Tissue (Section 42).
Hamartoma		Tumour-like lesion usually in children.
Inflammatory pseudosarcomatous lesion	See inflammatory pseudotumour	
Inflammatory pseudotumour	Inflammatory pseudosarcomatous lesion Pseudosarcomatous fibromyxoid tumour	·Tumour-like lesion.
Intravascular angiomatosis	Masson's angiomatosis	A benign tumour-like lesion composed of small vessels proliferating within a large vessel. Thought to arise within a thrombus.

Tumour terminology Recommended terms are in **bold**	Synonyms	Comments
Inverted papilloma	Brunnian adenoma (obsolete) Inverted transitional cell papilloma	A benign transitional cell tumour, which occurs in renal pelvis, ureter, and more commonly in the bladder. May be multiple and associated with transitional cell carcinoma at other sites. Divided into trabecular and glandular types.
Inverted transitional cell papilloma	See inverted papilloma	
Leiomyoma		The more common benign tumour of urinary tract. See Tumours of Soft Tissue (Section 42).
Leiomyosarcoma		The more common malignant mesenchymal tumour of urinary tract. See Tumours of Soft Tissue (Section 42).
Leukaemia		See Tumours of the Bone Marrow and Leukaemia (Section 23).
Lipoma		Rare in the urinary tract. See Tumours of Soft Tissue (Section 42).
Liposarcoma		Rare in the urinary tract. See Tumours of Soft Tissue (Section 42).
Lymphoepithelial carcinoma	See Lymphoepithelioma-like carcinoma	
Lymphoepithelioma-like carcinoma	Lymphoepithelial carcinoma	Rare histological variant of transitional cell carcinoma.
Lymphoma-like carcinoma		Histological variant of transitional cell carcinoma.
Malignant lymphoma		Rare primary in the bladder. See Tumours of the Lymph Nodes and Spleen (Section 24).
Malignant melanoma		Primary melanoma of the bladder is exceptionally rare.
Masson's angiomatosis	See intravascular angiomatosis	
Metaplastic carcinoma	See sarcomatoid carcinoma	
Microinvasive transitional cell carcinoma		A transitional cell carcinoma with less than 5 mm invasion.

Tumour terminology Recommended terms are in **bold**	Synonyms	Comments
Mixed carcinoma		A transitional cell carcinoma showing some glandular formation. Obsolete term.
Mucinous adenocarcinoma	Colloid adenocarcinoma	Histological variant of adenocarcinoma.
Nephroblastoma	Wilms' tumour	Malignant tumour in the pelvicalyceal system.
Nephrogenic adenoma	See adenomatoid tumour	
Nephrogenic metaplasia	See adenomatoid tumour	
Nested transitional cell carcinoma		Rare histological variant of transitional cell carcinoma.
Neuroendocrine tumour	Carcinoid Carcinoma with neuroendocrine differentiation	Exceptionally rare in bladder with unpredictable prognosis.
Neurofibroma		Benign, rare in the urinary tract. See Tumours of Soft Tissue (Section 42).
Neurofibrosarcoma		Malignant, rare in the urinary tract. See Tumours of Soft Tissue (Section 42).
Oat cell carcinoma	See small cell carcinoma	
Osteosarcoma		Malignant, rare in the urinary tract See Tumours of the Bone (Section 43).
Papilloma	See transitional cell papilloma	
Paraganglioma	Phaeochromocytoma	Unpredictable behaviour. See Tumours of the Adrenal Cortex (Section 6).
Phaeochromocytoma	See paraganglioma	
Plasmacytoid carcinoma		Rare histological variant of transitional cell carcinoma.
Postoperative spindle cell nodule		Tumour-like lesion.
Pseudosarcomatous fibromyxoid tumour	See inflammatory pseudotumour	
Pseudosarcomatous transitional cell carcinoma	See sarcomatoid carcinoma	

Tumour terminology Recommended terms are in **bold**	Synonyms	Comments
Rhabdoid tumour		Rare malignant tumour. See Tumours of the Kidney (Section 27).
Rhabdomyosarcoma		High grade tumour. In bladder almost always arises in children as embryonal rhabdomyosarcoma.
Sarcomatoid carcinoma	Giant cell carcinoma Metaplastic carcinoma Pseudosarcomatous transitional cell carcinoma	Highly malignant histological variant of transitional cell carcinoma.
Signet ring cell adenocarcinoma		Histological variant of adenocarcinoma. Rare malignant tumour. Poor prognosis.
Small cell carcinoma	Oat cell carcinoma	Highly malignant neuroendocrine tumour. Histologically similar to small cell lung carcinoma.
Squamous cell carcinoma		High grade. Rare in pelvis and ureter. In bladder is common in countries with endemic schistosomiasis.
Superficial angiomyxoma	See angiomyxoma	
Superficial carcinoma	See transitional cell carcinoma	Obsolete term used for tumours that have not invaded into the muscularis propria regardless of their type and grade.
Transitional cell carcinoma	Superficial carcinoma (obsolete) Transitional cell non-papillary carcinoma Transitional cell papillary carcinoma Urothelial carcinoma Urothelial non-papillary carcinoma Urothelial papillary carcinoma	Divided into papillary and non-papillary-invasive. Both types can be present in the same tumour. Papillary carcinomas are graded 1–4. Invasion is usually present in grade 3 tumours and almost always in grade 4.
Transitional cell carcinoma giant cell	See giant cell transitional cell carcinoma	
Transitional cell carcinoma in situ	See carcinoma in situ (CIS)	
Transitional cell carcinoma with gland-like lumina		Rare histological variant of transitional cell carcinoma.

Tumour terminology Recommended terms are in **bold**	Synonyms	Comments
Transitional cell non-papillary carcinoma	See transitional cell carcinoma	
Transitional cell papillary carcinoma	See transitional cell carcinoma	
Transitional cell papilloma	Papilloma Transitional cell tumour grade 0 Urothelial papilloma	A benign tumour which consists of a single papilloma or a cluster of papillomas, covered by urothelium with less than seven cell layers, without cytological atypia, and without or with only few mitotic figures.
Transitional cell tumour grade 0	See transitional cell papilloma	
Urothelial carcinoma	See transitional cell carcinoma	
Urothelial carcinoma in situ	See carcinoma in situ	
Urothelial non-papillary carcinoma	See transitional cell carcinoma	
Urothelial papillary carcinoma	See transitional cell carcinoma	
Urothelial papilloma	See transitional cell papilloma	
Verrucous carcinoma		Rare histological variant of squamous carcinoma with relatively good prognosis. It is common in countries with endemic schistosomiasis.
Villous adenoma		Microscopically similar to its colorectal counterpart. Often associated with cystitis cystica.
Wilms' tumour	See nephroblastoma	

Section 29

Tumours of the Prostate and Seminal Vesicles

R. Montironi
C. Parkinson
G.M. Mariuzzi

Tumour terminology Recommended terms are in **bold**	Synonyms	Comments
Acinar adenocarcinoma		The most common form of prostatic adenocarcinoma.
Adenocarcinoma of the prostate		The most common cancer in males in the USA and second only to lung cancer as a cause of cancer death. It arises in the prostatic ducts, ductules, and acini. Histological variants include acinar adenocarcinoma, adenoid cystic carcinoma, adenosquamous carcinoma, clear cell carcinoma, ductal carcinoma, mucinous adenocarcinoma, signet ring cell adenocarcinoma, and small cell carcinoma.
Adenocarcinoma of the seminal vesicles		Extremely rare.
Adenocarcinoma with endometrioid features	See ductal carcinoma	
Adenofibromyxomatous hyperplasia	See nodular hyperplasia	
Adenoid basal cell tumour	See adenoid cystic carcinoma	
Adenoid cystic carcinoma	Adenoid basal cell tumour Adenoid cystic-like carcinoma Basal cell carcinoma Basaloid carcinoma	Rare low grade variant of prostatic carcinoma, which may represent the malignant end of a morphologic continuum of basal cell proliferations in the prostate that includes basal cell hyperplasia and basal cell adenoma.

Tumour terminology Recommended terms are in **bold**	Synonyms	Comments
Adenoid cystic-like carcinoma	See adenoid cystic carcinoma	
Adenomatoid hyperplasia	See sclerosing adenosis	
Adenomatoid prostatic tumour	See sclerosing adenosis	
Adenosis	See atypical adenomatous hyperplasia	
Adenosquamous carcinoma		Rare histological variant of prostatic carcinoma characterised by a mixture of adenocarcinoma and squamous cell carcinoma. Develops as a complication of radiotherapy or oestrogen therapy.
Atypical adenomatous hyperplasia	Adenosis Atypical adenosis Atypical hyperplasia Small acinar atypical hyperplasia Small gland hyperplasia	Localized proliferation of small acini within the prostate usually in the transition zone and which may be mistaken for adenocarcinoma.
Atypical adenosis	See atypical adenomatous hyperplasia	
Atypical basal cell hyperplasia		Variant of basal cell hyperplasia in which prominent nucleoli are a feature.
Atypical hyperplasia	See atypical adenomatous hyperplasia	
Basal cell adenoma		Relatively small, round, and usually solitary circumscribed nodule made up of acini with basal cell hyperplasia in the setting of nodular hyperplasia.
Basal cell carcinoma	See adenoid cystic carcinoma	
Basal cell hyperplasia		Commonly encountered proliferation of basal cells two or more cells in thickness at the periphery of prostatic acini and often associated with nodular hyperplasia.

Tumour terminology Recommended terms are in **bold**	Synonyms	Comments
Basaloid carcinoma	See adenoid cystic carcinoma	
Benign prostatic hyperplasia	See nodular hyperplasia	
Blue naevus		This rare lesion is characterised by melanin-pigmented dendritic cells in the prostatic stroma. If the glandular epithelium is also pigmented, the term "melanosis" is used.
Carcinoid	See small cell carcinoma	
Carcinoma in situ	See prostatic intraepithelial neoplasia	
Carcinoma of the prostate	See adenocarcinoma of the prostate	
Carcinoma with neuroendocrine differentiation		Histological variant of prostatic adenocarcinoma showing foci of neuroendocrine cells.
Carcinoma with oncocytic features		Morphologic variant of prostatic adenocarcinoma consisting of tumour cells with abundant eosinophilic granular cytoplasm reflecting the presence of numerous mitochondria.
Carcinosarcoma	See metaplastic carcinoma	
Clear cell carcinoma		Adenocarcinoma made up of cells with clear cytoplasm.
Clear cell cribriform hyperplasia	Cribriform hyperplasia Florid benign papillary-cribriform hyperplasia	This is a rare condition characterised by intra-acinar papillary-cribriform hyperplastic epithelium composed of clear, bland cells. Nodular hyperplasia is also invariably present. It should not be mistaken for cribriform carcinoma.
Colloid carcinoma	See mucinous carcinoma	
Comedocarcinoma		Morphological variant of adenocarcinoma characterised by tumour masses, often showing a cribriform pattern and associated with central necrosis.
Cribriform carcinoma		Histologically distinct variant of Gleason 3 adenocarcinoma characterised by epithelial cell masses punctuated by multiple small lumens.

Tumour terminology Recommended terms are in **bold**	Synonyms	Comments
Cribriform hyperplasia	See clear cell cribriform hyperplasia	
Cystadenoleiomyofibroma	See phyllodes tumour	
Cystadenoma of the seminal vesicles		Rare benign tumour composed of cysts lined by a simple columnar epithelium with fibromuscular stroma.
Cystic epithelial-stromal tumour	See phyllodes tumour	
Cystosarcoma phyllodes	See phyllodes tumour	
Ductal carcinoma	Adenocarcinoma with endometrioid features Endometrioid carcinoma Papillary carcinoma	Histological variant of adenocarcinoma that resembles endometrial adenocarcinoma of the female uterus. It arises as a polypoid or papillary mass in periurethral prostatic ducts prolapsing into the urethra. It is frequently associated with typical acinar carcinoma.
Ejaculatory duct adenofibroma		Rare benign tumour, which presents as a polypoid mass of epithelium and stroma that projects into a cystically dilated duct.
Endometrioid carcinoma	See ductal carcinoma	
Endometriosis		This is an extremely rare lesion, which is similar to endometriosis of the female genital tract.
Fibroepithelial nodule	See sclerosing adenosis	
Fibroma		This rare tumour presents as a nodule composed of collagen with few fibroblasts.
Fibromyoglandular hyperplasia	See nodular hyperplasia	
Florid benign papillary-cribriform hyperplasia	See clear cell cribriform hyperplasia	
Germ cell tumour		This malignant tumour is extremely rare in the prostate and exceptional in the seminal vesicles. See Tumours of the Testes and Epididymis (Section 30).
Giant fibroadenoma	See phyllodes tumour	
Giant multilocular prostatic cystadenoma	Multilocular prostatic cystadenoma	This rare tumour is composed of acini and cysts lined by prostatic-type epithelium set in a hypocellular fibrous stroma.

Tumour terminology Recommended terms are in **bold**	Synonyms	Comments
Hyperplasia of mesonephric remnants		Rare. Benign mimic of adenocarcinoma that is usually identified in tissue from transurethral resection of the prostate (TURP) specimens.
Inflammatory myofibroblastic tumour	Inflammatory pseudotumour	Rare benign pathological entity of unknown aetiology similar to that occurring in the bladder, urethra, and other sites without prior surgery.
Inflammatory pseudotumour	See inflammatory myofibroblastic tumour	
Intraductal dysplasia	See prostatic intraepithelial neoplasia	
Leiomyoma		Histologically identical to leiomyoma occurring in other sites. See Tumours of Soft Tissue (Section 42).
Leiomyosarcoma		Histologically identical to leiomyosarcoma occurring in other sites. See Tumours of Soft Tissue (Section 42).
Leukaemia		Infrequent.
Lymphoepithelioma-like carcinoma	Medullary carcinoma	This is an extremely rare variant of carcinoma in which the epithelial element is associated with an intense lymphocytic infiltrate.
Malakoplakia		Rare, chronic inflammatory reaction, which may mimic carcinoma.
Malignant lymphoma		Rare. Histological patterns similar to extranodal lymphomas.
Malignant melanoma		Rare.
Medullary carcinoma	See lymphoepithelioma-like carcinoma	
Melanosis		Benign. Pigmentation of prostatic epithelium (melanin or lipofuscin-like pigment).
Metaplastic carcinoma	Carcinosarcoma Sarcomatoid carcinoma Spindle cell carcinoma	Rare, high grade histological variant of prostatic adenocarcinoma showing both glandular and spindle cell components. Heterologous differentiation may sometimes be present.

Tumour terminology Recommended terms are in **bold**	Synonyms	Comments
Mucinous carcinoma	Colloid carcinoma	Histological variant of adenocarcinoma characterised by at least 25% of the tumour consisting of pools of extracellular mucin. Metastasis or extension of a mucinous carcinoma arising elsewhere must always be excluded.
Mucinous metaplasia		Benign, mucin-producing cells in prostatic epithelium or urothelium.
Multilocular prostatic cystadenoma	See giant multilocular prostatic cystadenoma	
Nephrogenic adenoma	Nephrogenic metaplasia	This rare tumour-like lesion consists of an inflamed papillary mass of cystic or solid tubules replacing or just deep to urethral urothelium. Histologically it may be mistaken for adenocarcinoma.
Nephrogenic metaplasia	See nephrogenic adenoma	
Neuroendocrine carcinoma	See small cell carcinoma	Prostatic adenocarcinoma with neuroendocrine cells. It varies from carcinoid-like pattern to small cell undifferentiated (oat cell) carcinoma.
Nodular hyperplasia	Adenofibromyxomatous hyperplasia Benign prostatic hyperplasia Fibromyoglandular hyperplasia	Benign, frequent, enlargement of the prostate consisting of overgrowth of the epithelium and fibromuscular stroma of the transition zone and periurethral area.
Oat cell carcinoma	See small cell carcinoma	
Papillary carcinoma	See ductal carcinoma	
Phaeochromocytoma / Paraganglioma		See Tumours of the Adrenal Cortex, Adrenal Medulla, and Paraganglia. (Section 6).
Phyllodes tumour	Cystadenoleiomyofibroma Cystic-epithelial-stromal tumour Cystosarcoma phyllodes Giant fibroadenoma Phyllodes type of atypical hyperplasia	An extremely rare tumour similar to that described in the breast. A malignant variant has been described.

Tumour terminology Recommended terms are in **bold**	Synonyms	Comments
Phyllodes-type atypical hyperplasia	See phyllodes tumour	
PIN	See prostatic intraepithelial neoplasia	
Post-atrophic hyperplasia		Benign tumour-like condition consisting of small, distorted glands with flattened epithelium, hyperchromatic nuclei, and stromal fibrosis, closely mimicking adenocarcinoma.
Post-surgical inflammatory myofibroblastic tumour	See postoperative spindle cell nodule	
Postoperative spindle cell nodule	Post-surgical inflammatory myofibroblastic tumour	Rare, benign reparative process, consisting of myofibroblastic proliferation mimicking sarcoma.
Prostatic cyst		Rare cystic tumour-like lesion, which arises from prostatic ducts/acini or from the prostatic utricle (a Müllerian anlage).
Prostatic intraepithelial neoplasia (PIN)	Carcinoma in situ Intraductal dysplasia	The pre-invasive form of carcinoma arising within existing prostatic ducts/acini.
Pseudoadenomatoid hyperplasia	See sclerosing adenosis	
Pseudoadenomatoid tumour	See sclerosing adenosis	
Rhabdoid tumour		Rare. Similar to that originating in the kidney.
Rhabdomyosarcoma		See Tumours of Soft Tissue (Section 42).
Sarcomatoid carcinoma	See metaplastic carcinoma	
Sclerosing adenosis	Adenomatoid hyperplasia Adenomatoid prostatic tumour Fibroepithelial nodule Pseudoadenomatoid hyperplasia Pseudoadenomatoid tumour	Rare, benign circumscribed proliferation of small acini including a distinct myoepithelial component set in a dense spindle cell stroma. Histologically it may be mistaken for adenocarcinoma.

Tumour terminology Recommended terms are in **bold**	Synonyms	Comments
Signet ring cell carcinoma		Extremely rare histological variant of prostatic adenocarcinoma characterised by cytoplasmic vacuoles and displaced nuclei. Mucin and fat vacuoles are not usually present. Metastasis from a signet ring cell carcinoma arising elsewhere should always be excluded.
Small acinar atypical hyperplasia	See atypical adenomatous hyperplasia	
Small cell carcinoma	Carcinoid tumour Neuroendocrine carcinoma Oat cell carcinoma	High grade variant of prostatic adenocarcinoma. Some examples may show neuroendocrine differentiation. It is commonly associated with foci of acinar adenocarcinoma. Metastasis from a small cell carcinoma arising elsewhere should always be excluded.
Small gland hyperplasia	See atypical adenomatous hyperplasia	
Spindle cell carcinoma	See metaplastic carcinoma	
Squamous cell carcinoma		Very rare high grade histological variant of prostatic carcinoma. Direct extension or metastasis from a squamous carcinoma arising elsewhere must always be excluded. Squamous metaplasia associated with infarction or oestrogen therapy also enters the differential diagnosis.
Stromal hyperplasia with atypical giant cells		Rare tumour-like lesion consisting of stromal nodules arising in the transition zone showing increased cellularity and nuclear atypia.
Transitional cell carcinoma	Urothelial carcinoma	May arise in prostatic ducts. Direct spread from the urethra or bladder is more common.
Urothelial carcinoma	See transitional cell carcinoma	
Verumontanum mucosal gland hyperplasia		Uncommon form of small acinar hyperplasia that mimics well differentiated adenocarcinoma.

Section 30

Tumours of the Testis and Epididymis

M. De Nictolis
E. Prete
G.M. Mariuzzi

Tumour terminology Recommended terms are in **bold**	Synonyms	Comments
Adenomatoid tumour		Most frequent in the epididymis. Benign. Mesothelial origin.
Anaplastic seminoma	See seminoma	
Carcinoid tumour		Exceedingly rare. Frequently benign.
Carcinoma of the epididymis		Exceedingly rare.
Choriocarcinoma	See malignant teratoma trophoblastic	
Chorionepithelioma	See malignant teratoma trophoblastic	
Chorionic carcinoma	See malignant teratoma trophoblastic	
Cystadenoma of the epididymis	See papillary cystadenoma of the epididymis	
Dermoid cyst	See teratoma differentiated (TD)	
Dysgerminoma	See seminoma	
Embryonal carcinoma	See malignant teratoma undifferentiated	

Tumour terminology Recommended terms are in **bold**	Synonyms	Comments
Embryonal carcinoma with teratoma	See malignant teratoma intermediate	
Embryonic carcinoma	See malignant teratoma undifferentiated	
Endodermal sinus tumour	See yolk sac tumour	
Germ cell tumours showing more than one histologic pattern	See malignant teratoma intermediate	
Germinoma	See seminoma	
Gonadal stromal tumours	See sex cord-stromal tumours unclassified	
Gonadoblastoma	Gonadocytoma	A mixed germ cell-sex cord tumour, arising in dysgenetic gonads. It may be associated with dysgerminoma or other malignant germ cell tumours.
Gonadocytoma	See gonadoblastoma	
Gonocytoma	See seminoma	
Granulosa cell tumour of the adult type		Exceedingly rare. Generally benign.
Granulosa cell tumour of the juvenile type		Uncommon. Benign. Generally discovered in the first four months of life.
Interstitial cell tumour	See Leydig cell tumour	
Intratubular germ cell neoplasia, unclassified		Cytologically malignant germ cells are present within the testicular tubules. Very frequent in tubules adjacent to invasive germ cell tumours. It may also be observed in apparently normal testes. In this case a clinical follow-up is recommended.
Juvenile embryonal carcinoma	See yolk sac tumour	
Large cell calcifying Sertoli cell tumour		Uncommon. Generally benign. Mean age 16 years. Frequently bilateral and associated with other tumours.
Leiomyoma		Most common benign tumour. See Tumours of Soft Tissue (Section 42).

Tumour terminology Recommended terms are in **bold**	Synonyms	Comments
Leiomyosarcoma		See Tumours of Soft Tissue (Section 42).
Leukaemia		Secondary involvement.
Leydig cell tumour	Interstitial cell tumour	Uncommon. Mainly affects adults 20–50 years. The vast majority are benign, but some tumours may metastasise.
Lipoma		See Tumours of Soft Tissue (Section 42).
Liposarcoma		See Tumours of Soft Tissue (Section 42).
Malignant lymphoma		Advanced age. Generally metastatic.
Malignant mesothelioma		Very rare. Originating from the tunica vaginalis.
Malignant teratoma intermediate (MTI)	Embryonal carcinoma with teratoma Germ cell tumours showing more than one histologic pattern Mixed germ cell tumour Teratocarcinoma Teratoma with malignant transformation	A testicular tumour composed of more than one histological type. It accounts for 50% of all germ cell tumours. Mean age 30 years. Curable.
Malignant teratoma trophoblastic (MTT)	Choriocarcinoma Chorionepithelioma Chorionic carcinoma	Very rare. Elevated levels of HCG. Frequently aggressive.
Malignant teratoma undifferentiated (MTU)	Embryonal carcinoma Embryonic carcinoma	The second most frequent form of pure germ cell tumour. Most common between 25–35 years of age. Frequent spreading via the bloodstream. Curable.
Melanotic hamartoma	See retinal anlage tumour	
Melanotic neuroectodermal tumour	See retinal anlage tumour	
Melanotic progonoma	See retinal anlage tumour	
Mixed germ cell tumour	See malignant teratoma intermediate	
Papillary cystadenoma of the epididymis	Cystadenoma of the epididymis	Rare. Sometimes associated with the von Hippel-Lindau disease.

Tumour terminology Recommended terms are in **bold**	Synonyms	Comments
Polyembryoma		Exceedingly rare.
Primitive neuroectodermal tumour		Exceedingly rare. Malignant.
Retinal anlage tumour	Melanotic hamartoma Melanotic neuroectodermal tumour Melanotic progonoma	Exceedingly rare. Generally benign tumour, which affects infants.
Rhabdomyosarcoma		Paratesticular rhabdomyosarcoma is the most common soft tissue sarcoma. See Tumours of Soft Tissue (Section 42).
Seminoma	Anaplastic seminoma Dysgerminoma Germinoma Gonocytoma	The most frequent germ cell tumour. Peak incidence age: 35–45 years. Curable. Excellent prognosis. Anaplastic seminoma has the same prognosis.
Sertoli cell tumour		Uncommon. Generally well differentiated and benign. Occasional tumours less well differentiated and malignant.
Sex cord-stromal tumours, unclassified	Gonadal stromal tumours	Relatively frequent. All ages. Post-pubertal tumours may pursue a malignant course.
Spermatocytic seminoma		Rare. Benign. Usually over 50 years of age. Exceptionally, associated with a malignant sarcomatous component.
Teratocarcinoma	See malignant teratoma intermediate (MTI)	
Teratoid tumour	See teratoma differentiated (TD)	
Teratoma differentiated (TD)	Dermoid cyst Teratoid tumour Teratoma mature Teratoma pure	Differentiated teratomas are rare and benign in pre-pubertal boys. They can metastasise in post-pubertal males, independently from the mature or immature histologic appearance.
Teratoma mature	See teratoma differentiated (TD)	
Teratoma pure	See teratoma differentiated (TD)	
Teratoma with malignant transformation	See malignant teratoma intermediate (MTI)	

Tumour terminology Recommended terms are in **bold**	Synonyms	Comments
Tumours of ovarian epithelial type		Exceedingly rare. Most are serous tumours of borderline malignancy, which followed a benign clinical course.
Tumours of the rete testis		Rare. Benign or malignant. Carcinomas must be distinguished from metastatic tumours.
Tumours with more than one histological type	See malignant teratoma intermediate	
Yolk sac tumour	Endodermal sinus tumour Juvenile embryonal carcinoma	Pure, in infancy and childhood. Generally benign in the first two years of life. Curable.

Section 31

Tumours of the Penis and Scrotum

M. Pea
G.M. Mariuzzi

Primary cutaneous tumours of the penis and scrotum are dealt with in Skin Melanocytic and Non-melanocytic Tumours Sections 42 and 43.

Tumour terminology Recommended terms are in **bold**	Synonyms	Comments
Aggressive angiomyxoma		This tumour may rarely affect the scrotum and inguinal region. See Tumours of Soft Tissue (Section 42).
Atypical melanotic macule	See mucosal melanosis	
Basaloid carcinoma		This is a rare high grade histological variant of squamous cell carcinoma. Metastases are frequently present.
Bowen's disease	Bowenoid dysplasia Epidermoid carcinoma in situ Erythroplasia of Queyrat Penile intraepithelial neoplasia Squamous cell carcinoma in situ	Lesions arising on the external genitalia are most often associated with HPV 16 and 18. A minority progress to invasive tumour, which is usually high grade.
Bowenoid dysplasia	See Bowen's disease	

Tumour terminology Recommended terms are in **bold**	Synonyms	Comments
Bowenoid papulosis		This benign condition, which is also associated with HPV infection, is sometimes histologically confused with Bowen's disease. Young patients present with rapidly growing and frequently recurrent small papules on both the glans and shaft of the penis. It is characterised by variable dysplasia sometimes amounting to squamous cell carcinoma in situ. In the majority of the cases the lesions regress spontaneously. Invasive squamous cell carcinoma supervenes in only a small percentage of patients.
Buschke-Löwenstein tumour	See verrucous carcinoma	
Condyloma	See condyloma acuminatum	
Condyloma acuminatum	Condyloma Flat condyloma Inverted condyloma Sessile condyloma Squamous papilloma Venereal wart	This represents a genital viral wart, secondary to human papilloma virus infection.
Epidermoid carcinoma	See squamous cell carcinoma	
Epidermoid carcinoma in situ	See Bowen's disease	
Erythroplasia of Queyrat	See Bowen's disease	
Fibrous cavernitis	See Peyronie's disease	
Fibrous sclerosis of the penis	See Peyronie's disease	
Flat condyloma	See condyloma acuminatum	
Genital lentiginosis	See mucosal melanosis	
Giant condyloma	See verrucous carcinoma	
Hirsutoid papillomas	See pearly penile papules	
Idiopathic calcinosis		This is a benign tumour-like lesion, which consists of calcified material and affects the scrotum in childhood and adolescence.

Tumour terminology Recommended terms are in **bold**	Synonyms	Comments
Inverted condyloma	See condyloma acuminatum	
Leiomyoma (scrotum)		This benign smooth muscle tumour is the most common mesenchymal tumour of the scrotum.
Lentiginous melanosis	See mucosal melanosis	
Lentigo	See mucosal melanosis	
Lipogranuloma	See sclerosing lipogranuloma	
Median raphé cyst		This rare tumour-like lesion represents a development abnormality.
Melanoma		Primary genital melanoma is rare. It may affect the glans or prepuce and is usually associated with a poor prognosis.
Mesothelioma of the tunica vaginalis		This rare tumour, which may sometimes be associated with previous asbestos exposure, is associated with a poor prognosis. A hydrocele is often present.
Mucoid cyst		This rare tumour-like lesion develops from ectopic urethral mucosa.
Mucosal melanosis	Atypical melanotic macule Genital lentiginosis Lentiginous melanosis Lentigo	This uncommon lesion is sometimes clinically confused with melanoma. It consists of an irregular pigmented macule and is benign.
Paget's disease		Genital involvement is rare and may represent epidermotropic metastases from an underlying prostatic, bladder, or even rectal primary. See Tumours of Skin (Non-Melanocytic) (Section 41).
Papillomatosis corona penis	See pearly penile papules	Benign. Solitary or multiple fibroepithelial polyps.
Paraffinoma	See sclerosing lipogranuloma	
Pearly penile papules	Hirsutoid papillomas Papillomatosis corona penis	These common benign lesions represent angiofibromas and clinically present as tiny white papules on the corona of the penis.

Tumour terminology Recommended terms are in **bold**	Synonyms	Comments
Penile intraepithelial neoplasia	See Bowen's disease	
Peyronie's disease	Fibrous cavernitis Fibrous sclerosis of the penis Plastic induration of the penis	This rare tumour-like condition presents as a fibrous plaque within the penis. Its aetiology is unknown but it may represent an inflammatory process. There is an association with palmar/plantar fibromatosis.
Plastic induration of the penis	See Peyronie's disease	
Sclerosing lipogranuloma	Lipogranuloma Paraffinoma	Benign tumour-like lesion, which results from the injection of waxy substances to enlarge the penis.
Sessile condyloma	See condyloma acuminatum	
Squamous cell carcinoma (penis)	Epidermoid carcinoma	Penile lesions are related to poor hygiene and occur most often in the uncircumcised. The elderly are most often affected. The prognosis is often poor.
Squamous cell carcinoma (scrotum)		Nowadays this tumour is extremely rare. It is particularly linked to occupational exposure, 3', 4'-benzopyrene has been implicated. See Tumours of Skin (Non-Melanocytic) (Section 41).
Squamous cell carcinoma in situ	See Bowen's disease	
Squamous papilloma	See condyloma acuminatum	
Venereal wart	See condyloma acuminatum	
Verrucous carcinoma	Buschke-Löwenstein tumour Giant condyloma	This rare variant of penile squamous carcinoma is associated with HPV infection. It is often locally aggressive and commonly recurs. Metastasis to regional lymph nodes is extremely rare.

Section 32

Tumours of the Ovary

M. De Nictolis
E. Prete
C.H. Buckley
G.M. Mariuzzi

Tumour terminology Recommended terms are in **bold**	Synonyms	Comments
Adenoacanthofibroma	See endometrioid adenofibroma	Benign endometrioid tumour.
Adenoacanthoma	See endometrioid adenocarcinoma with squamous differentiation	
Adenocarcinoid	See mucinous carcinoid	
Adenocarcinoma		Most common epithelial tumour of the ovary. Variants include endometrioid, clear cell, mucinous carcinoma of intestinal type, mucinous carcinoma NOS, and serous carcinoma, mixed epithelial type.
Adenocarcinoma NOS	Adenocarcinoma	To be used only when the tumour cannot be further classified.
Adenocarcinoma of the rete ovarii	Carcinoma of the rete ovarii	Rare lesion of the rete ovarii.
Adenomatoid tumour		This is more common in the fallopian tube than in the ovary.
Adenofibroma	Benign mixed epithelial tumour Adenofibroma NOS	The classification should specify the epithelial type or mixed epithelial type. If the epithelium cannot be identified, the term "adenofibroma NOS" is appropriate. Variants include clear cell, endometrioid, mucinous adenofibroma of intestinal type, mucinous adenofibroma of Müllerian type, serous adenofibroma.

Tumour terminology Recommended terms are in **bold**	Synonyms	Comments
Adenofibroma NOS	Adenofibroma	To be used only when the epithelial type cannot be classified.
Adenofibroma of mixed epithelial type	See benign mixed epithelial tumour	
Adenoma of the rete ovarii		Rare benign lesion composed of cellular cords and tubules similar to those seen in the normal rete.
Adenomyoma		A mass of endometrium and smooth muscle in the wall of an endometriotic cyst.
Adenosarcoma	Endometrioid adenosarcoma Malignant mixed Müllerian tumour low grade Mixed malignant Müllerian tumour	Benign epithelial elements with homologous or heterologous sarcomatous stroma. Generally unilateral.
Adenosquamous carcinoma		A mixture of squamous and glandular components. Not to be confused with adenoacanthoma. Variants include adenosquamous carcinoma NOS, adenosquamous carcinoma of teratomatous origin, endometrioid adenocarcinoma with squamous differentiation.
Adenosquamous carcinoma NOS		A term to be used only when the histogenesis of the tumour is uncertain.
Adenosquamous carcinoma of teratomatous origin	Adenosquamous carcinoma	A rare unilateral neoplasm occurring generally in the postmenopausal woman in a mature cystic teratoma.
Adrenal cortical-like tumour	See steroid cell tumour NOS	
Adrenal rest tumour	See steroid cell tumour NOS	
Adrenal-like steroid cell tumour	See steroid cell tumour NOS	
Adrenal-like tumour	See steroid cell tumour NOS	
Anaplastic neuroectodermal tumour	Glioblastoma	Histologically resembles high grade glioma (glioblastoma). The contralateral ovary may contain a dermoid cyst.

Tumour terminology Recommended terms are in **bold**	Synonyms	Comments
Androblastoma	See Sertoli-Leydig cell tumour	
Androblastoma with heterologous elements	See Sertoli-Leydig cell tumour	
Androblastoma with lipid storage	See well differentiated Sertoli cell tumour	
Angioma	See haemangioma	
Angiosarcoma	Haemangiosarcoma	A rare, malignant neoplasm reported only in adults. Metastatic disease should be excluded before concluding that this is primary sarcoma.
Apocrine carcinoma	See sweat gland carcinoma	
APUD-oma	See carcinoid tumour	Obsolete term.
Arrhenoblastoma	See Sertoli-Leydig cell tumour	Obsolete term.
Atypical gonadoblastoma	See mixed germ cell sex cord-stromal tumour	
Atypically proliferating clear cell tumour	See clear cell tumour of borderline malignancy	
Atypically proliferating endometrioid tumour	See endometrioid tumour of borderline malignancy	
Atypically proliferating mucinous tumour	See mucinous tumour of borderline malignancy	
Atypically proliferating transitional cell tumour	See Brenner tumour of borderline malignancy	
Atypically proliferating tumour	See borderline tumour	Some people prefer the term "atypically proliferating tumour" to the term "borderline malignancy".
Basal cell carcinoma		Occurs due to malignant transformation in a mature cystic teratoma.
Benign mixed epithelial tumour	Mixed epithelial tumour	Two or more benign epithelia are present: the minor component is 10% or more.
Benign signet ring stromal tumour	Signet ring stromal tumour	Probably a rare variant of sclerosing stromal tumour. Extensive vacuolation of tumour cells leads to the formation of mucin-free signet ring cells. Contrast with Krukenberg-type metastases.

Tumour terminology Recommended terms are in **bold**	Synonyms	Comments
Benign transitional cell tumour	See Brenner tumour	
Borderline Brenner tumour	See Brenner tumour of borderline malignancy	
Borderline mixed epithelial tumour	See mixed epithelial tumour of borderline malignancy	
Borderline tumour	Atypically proliferating tumour Carcinoma of low grade potential Epithelial tumour of borderline malignancy Tumour of borderline malignancy Tumour of low grade potential	The epithelium of these tumours exhibits any two of the following: budding, multilayering, mitotic activity, and nuclear atypia. There is no destructive stromal invasion. Their clinical behaviour varies, some being entirely benign whilst others behave as low grade malignancies or, less commonly, as overtly malignant neoplasms. Primary peritoneal disease may coexist. The epithelial component should always be specified. Variants include Brenner tumour, clear cell tumour, endometrioid tumour, mixed epithelial tumour, mucinous tumour, intestinal type, endocervical type, serous tumour.
Borderline tumour of mixed epithelial type	See mixed epithelial tumour of borderline malignancy	
Brenner tumour	Benign transitional cell tumour	A benign primary tumour made up predominantly by cells resembling urothelial cells, including adenofibromatous and cystadenofibromatous variants. Minor mucinous epithelial elements are common.
Brenner tumour of borderline malignancy	Atypically proliferating transitional cell tumour Borderline Brenner tumour Proliferating Brenner tumour	Including papillary, adenofibromatous, and cystadenofibromatous forms.
Carcinoid tumour	APUD-oma (obsolete) Monodermal teratoma Monophyletic teratoma Neuroendocrine tumour	Primary carcinoid tumours are associated with other teratomatous components in many cases. Variants include trabecular, insular, mucinous, and strumal types.

Tumour terminology Recommended terms are in **bold**	Synonyms	Comments
Carcinoma NOS	See undifferentiated carcinoma	
Carcinoma of low malignant potential	See borderline malignancy	
Carcinoma of mixed epithelial type	Malignant mixed epithelial tumour Mixed epithelial carcinoma	Carcinoma with two or more epithelial types in which the minor component is 10% or more. Mucinous carcinomas associated with benign Brenner tumours are classified as carcinomas of mixed epithelial type and not as malignant Brenner tumours.
Carcinoma of the rete ovarii	See adenocarcinoma of the rete ovarii	
Carcinosarcoma	High grade malignant mixed Müllerian tumour Malignant mixed Müllerian tumour high grade Mesodermal mixed tumour Mixed mesodermal tumour Müllerian mixed malignant tumour	Malignant epithelium and malignant sarcomatous stroma including homologous and heterologous variants. Occurs typically in the post-menopausal women and progresses rapidly.
Cellular fibroma	See fibroma	
Chondroma		Pure chondromas are exceptionally rare. Tumours with conspicuous benign cartilage are more likely to be fibromas with metaplasia or teratomas.
Chondrosarcoma		May be of stromal origin, teratomatous or more frequently a component of a carcinosarcoma.
Choriocarcinoma, gestational	Chorionepithelioma (obsolete)	Arises from an ectopic pregnancy.
Choriocarcinoma, non-gestational	See non-gestational choriocarcinoma	
Chorionepithelioma	See choriocarcinoma—gestational See non-gestational choriocarcinoma	Obsolete term.

Tumour terminology Recommended terms are in **bold**	Synonyms	Comments
Clear cell adenocarcinoma	See clear cell carcinoma	
Clear cell adenofibroma	Adenofibroma	Extremely rare, in which the clear cell epithelium is benign.
Clear cell adenofibroma of borderline malignancy	See clear cell tumour of borderline malignancy	
Clear cell carcinoma	Clear cell adenocarcinoma Clear cell cystadenocarcinoma	Clear cell carcinomas are frequently made up of clear cells and hobnail cells. Sometimes they may develop from the lining of endometriotic ovarian cysts.
Clear cell carcinoma of low malignant potential	See clear cell tumour of borderline malignancy	
Clear cell cystadenocarcinoma	See clear cell carcinoma	
Clear cell cystadenofibroma		Benign, extremely rare.
Clear cell cystadenofibroma of borderline malignancy	See clear cell tumour of borderline malignancy	
Clear cell tumour of borderline malignancy	Atypically proliferating clear cell tumour Clear cell adenofibroma of borderline malignancy Clear cell carcinoma of low malignant potential Clear cell cystadenofibroma of borderline malignancy Proliferating clear cell tumour	Rare unilateral neoplasms composed of abundant fibrous stroma containing glands lined by clear cells with moderately atypical nuclei. Areas of clear cell carcinoma may be present; indeed these tumours must be carefully sampled.
Colloid carcinoma	See mucinous carcinoma	
Cystadenocarcinoma		A term applied to malignant epithelial tumours with cystic differentiation. The epithelial component should be specified. Variants include carcinoma of mixed epithelial type, clear cell cystadenocarcinoma, endometrioid cystadenocarcinoma, mucinous cystadenocarcinoma, serous cystadenocarcinoma.

Tumour terminology Recommended terms are in **bold**	Synonyms	Comments
Cystadenoma of the rete ovarii		Microscopic cysts of the rete ovarii are common and not neoplastic. Cysts larger than 1 cm in diameter must be considered cystadenoma of the rete ovarii.
Dermoid cyst	See mature cystic teratoma	
Dysgenetic gonadoma	See gonadoblastoma	
Dysgerminoma	Germinoma Gonocytoma 1 (obsolete) Gonocytoma 4 (obsolete)	Malignant tumour composed of cells resembling primordial germ cells and homologous with testicular seminoma. Some tumours may contain syncytiotrophoblastic giant cells. If other malignant germ cell elements are present, the tumour should be classified as a malignant mixed germ cell tumour.
Embryonal carcinoma		A rare germ cell tumour characterised by large cells growing in solid, papillary, and glandular pattern. Chemotherapy may be curative.
Endocervical mucinous adenofibroma	See mucinous adenofibroma of Müllerian type	
Endocervical mucinous cystadenofibroma	See mucinous cystadenofibroma of Müllerian type	
Endocervical mucinous cystadenoma	See mucinous cystadenoma of Müllerian type	
Endocervical mucinous cystadenoma of borderline malignancy	See mucinous tumour of borderline malignancy of Müllerian type	
Endocervical mucinous papillary cystadenoma	See mucinous cystadenoma of Müllerian type	
Endocervical mucinous tumour of borderline malignancy	See mucinous tumour of borderline malignancy of Müllerian type	
Endocervical papillary mucinous tumour of borderline malignancy	See mucinous tumour of borderline malignancy of Müllerian type	

Tumour terminology Recommended terms are in **bold**	Synonyms	Comments
Endodermal sinus tumour	See yolk sac tumour	Obsolete term.
Endodermal variant of a mature cystic teratoma	See mature cystic teratoma	
Endolymphatic stromal myosis	See low grade endometrioid stromal sarcoma	
Endometrial stromal nodule of the ovary	See endometrioid stromal nodule	
Endometrial stromal sarcoma (high grade)	See high grade endometrioid stromal sarcoma	
Endometrial stromal sarcoma (low grade)	See low grade endometrioid stromal sarcoma	
Endometrioid adenoacanthoma	See endometrioid adenocarcinoma with squamous metaplasia	
Endometrioid adenocarcinoma	See endometrioid carcinoma	
Endometrioid adenocarcinoma with Sertoliform pattern	See endometrioid carcinoma	
Endometrioid adenocarcinoma with squamous differentiation	Adenoacanthoma Endometrioid adenoacanthoma	Endometrioid adenocarcinoma with areas of squamous metaplasia, which is usually benign.
Endometrioid adenofibroma	Adenoacanthofibroma	Benign endometrioid tumour with cysts lined by epithelium of inactive or proliferative endometrial type set in a fibrovascular stroma in which there may be luteinised cells.
Endometrioid adenofibroma of borderline malignancy	See endometrioid tumour of borderline malignancy	
Endometrioid adenosarcoma	See adenosarcoma	
Endometrioid adenosquamous carcinoma	Adenosquamous carcinoma	Endometrioid adenocarcinoma with malignant squamous epithelial elements. Teratomatous elements indicate a germ cell origin.

Tumour terminology Recommended terms are in **bold**	Synonyms	Comments
Endometrioid carcinoma	Endometrioid adenocarcinoma	Carcinomas, which contain elements resembling those seen in typical carcinomas of the endometrium. Ovarian or pelvic endometriosis is present in 20–30% of cases. Variants include endometrioid carcinoma with Sertoliform pattern, endometrioid secretory adenocarcinoma, malignant endometrioid adenofibroma, malignant endometrioid cystadenofibroma, secretory endometrioid adenocarcinoma.
Endometrioid cystadenofibroma		Benign cystic tumour composed of endometrioid and fibrous components.
Endometrioid cystadenoma		Benign cystic endometrioid tumour.
Endometrioid secretory adenocarcinoma	See endometrioid carcinoma	
Endometrioid stromal nodule	Endometrial stromal nodule of the ovary	Benign tumour composed of stroma of endometrial type. May develop in association with endometriosis.
Endometrioid tumour of borderline malignancy	Atypically proliferating endometrioid tumour Endometrioid adenofibroma of borderline malignancy	Cystic, adenofibromatous, and cystadenofibromatous types are recognised.
Enteroid variant of yolk sac tumour	See yolk sac tumour	
Ependymoma		These are indistinguishable from ependymomas in the CNS and are of teratomatous origin although there are usually no other germ cell elements present. Half have spread beyond the ovary at diagnosis.
Epidermoid cyst of hilar or subcortical origin		This classification should be used when there is no other teratomatous component. Possible sources include coelomic epithelium, endometriotic cysts, and the rete ovarii.
Epidermoid cyst of teratomatous origin	See mature cystic teratoma	Where there is no evidence of teratomatous origin, the tumour should be classified as an epidermoid cyst of hilar or subcortical origin.

Tumour terminology Recommended terms are in **bold**	Synonyms	Comments
Epithelial tumour of borderline malignancy	See borderline tumour	
Epithelioid angiosarcoma		Rare. Probably of teratomatous origin but a case arising in a leiomyoma has been described.
Epithelioma pflugerein	See mixed germ cell sex cord-stromal tumour	Obsolete term.
Extramammary Paget's disease		Rare, and of teratomatous origin. May be associated with invasive carcinoma or may represent adenocarcinoma in situ.
Fetiform teratoma (homonculus)	See mature cystic teratoma	
Fibroma	Cellular fibroma	Includes typical fibroma, fibroma with minor sex cord elements and cellular fibroma. May be associated with ascites and pleural effusion.
Fibrosarcoma		May be of teratomatous or ovarian stromal origin. Cellular fibrous lesions with a mitotic rate of 4 or more per 10 high power fields may behave in a malignant fashion and may be regarded as sarcomas.
Fibrothecoma	Thecafibroma	Almost invariably benign.
Follicular carcinoma of thyroid		A monophyletic or monodermal teratoma or malignant transformation in a mature cystic teratoma.
Ganglioneuroma		Probably hamartomatous rather than neoplastic though a neoplastic form has been described.
Germ cell sex cord-stromal tumour	See mixed germ cell sex cord-stromal tumour	
Germinoma	See dysgerminoma	
Giant cell tumour of the ovary	Osteoclastoma	Morphologically similar to giant cell tumour of bone; benign and malignant variants have been described. A benign cyst of indeterminate type accompanied the benign form.
Glioblastoma	See anaplastic neuroectodermal tumour	
Goblet cell carcinoid	See mucinous carcinoid	

Tumour terminology Recommended terms are in **bold**	Synonyms	Comments
Gonadal anlage tumour	See gonadoblastoma	
Gonadoblastoma	Dysgenetic gonadoma Gonadal anlage tumour Gonocytoma 3 (obsolete) Tumour of dysgenetic gonad	A mixed germ cell-sex cord-stromal tumour usually associated with an underlying gonadal disorder. May undergo malignant transformation, more frequently in a dysgerminoma.
Gonadoblastoma mixed with dysgerminoma or other malignant germ cell elements		These tumours are separately classified as it is the malignant germ cell component that determines the prognosis.
Gonocytoma 1	See dysgerminoma	Obsolete term.
Gonocytoma 2	See mixed germ cell-sex cord-stromal tumour	Obsolete term.
Gonocytoma 3	See gonadoblastoma	Obsolete term.
Gonocytoma 4	See dysgerminoma	Obsolete term.
Granulosa cell tumour (adult type)	Granulosa-theca cell tumour	Accounts for 1% of all ovarian tumours, with a peak incidence age of 50–55 years. Frequently oestrogenic, they have a low malignant potential. Although rare, may be associated with benign mucinous tumour.
Granulosa cell tumour (juvenile type)		Rare and generally benign tumour occurring in the first three decades of life. In pre-pubertal children they frequently cause isosexual pseudoprecocity.
Granulosa-theca cell tumour	See granulosa cell tumour adult type	
Gynandroblastoma		Mixed granulosa cell tumour with Sertoli cell, Leydig cell, or Sertoli-Leydig cell tumour.
Haemangioendothelioma	See angiosarcoma	
Haemangioma	Angioma	Rare, should be distinguished from the normal vascularity of the ovarian medulla. May be associated with stromal luteinisation and hormone effects.
Haemangiopericytoma		Tumour of unknown histogenesis. See Tumours of Soft Tissue (Section 42).
Haemangiosarcoma	See angiosarcoma	

Tumour terminology Recommended terms are in **bold**	Synonyms	Comments
Hepatoid carcinoma	Hepatoid tumour	A surface epithelial carcinoma that must be distinguished from a hepatocellular carcinoma metastatic to the ovary and from the hepatoid yolk sac tumour.
Hepatoid tumour	See hepatoid carcinoma	
Hepatoid variant of yolk sac tumour	See yolk sac tumour	
High grade endometrioid stromal sarcoma	Endolymphatic stromal myosis Endometrial sarcoma of the ovary (high grade) Stromal sarcoma	Tumours closely resembling those developing in the endometrium. Similar synchronous or metachronous uterine tumour may be present.
High grade malignant mixed Müllerian tumour	See carcinosarcoma	
Hilar cell tumour	See Leydig cell tumour	
Hilus cell tumour	See Leydig cell tumour	
Histiocytoid vascular tumour		Malignant transformation in a mature cystic teratoma. A form of epithelioid angiosarcoma.
Hodgkin's disease		See Tumours of the Lymph Nodes and Spleen (Section 24).
Immature teratoma	Malignant teratoma	A rare tumour more frequent in the first two decades of life. Most or all of the immature tissue is composed of neuroectodermal tissue. The amount of the neuroectodermal immature tissue must be histologically graded. May contain a second malignant tumour, e.g., non-gestational choriocarcinoma or yolk sac tumour. If so, it should be classified as a malignant mixed germ cell tumour.
Intestinal mucinous tumour	See mucinous tumour of intestinal type	
Intestinal mucinous tumour of borderline malignancy	See mucinous tumour of borderline malignancy, intestinal type	
Krukenberg tumour	See metastatic tumour	
Leiomyoma		Rare occurrence in the ovary, mainly in pre-menopausal women.

Tumour terminology Recommended terms are in **bold**	Synonyms	Comments
Leiomyosarcoma		Rare, cellular smooth muscle tumours with more than 10 mitoses per 10 high power (hp) fields. They occur usually in older women and may be of ovarian stromal/vascular or teratomatous origin. Criteria for determining prognosis have not been fully established.
Leukaemia		Most commonly a secondary infiltrate of myeloid type.
Leydig cell tumour	Hilar cell tumour Hilus cell tumour Steroid cell tumour Stromal Leydig cell tumour	Usually benign, rare, hormonally active tumours of hilar cell or non-hilar (stromal) type. The majority of hilar cell tumours are masculinising but 10–20% are oestrogenic.
Lipid cell tumour	See Leydig cell tumour See steroid cell tumour NOS See stromal luteoma	
Lipoid cell tumour	See Leydig cell tumour See Steroid cell tumour NOS See stromal luteoma	
Lipoma		May simply be a mature cystic teratoma with conspicuous adipose tissue.
Low grade endometrioid stromal sarcoma	Endometrial stromal sarcoma of the ovary (low grade) Stromal sarcoma	Tumours closely resembling those developing in the endometrium. Between 50 and 85% are associated with endometriosis.
Lymphangioma		Very rare in the ovary. Histologically resembling their counterparts elsewhere in the body.
Lymphangiosarcoma		A single, highly malignant case has been reported.
Malignant adenofibroma		Obsolete term. The epithelial type should be specified. Only when it is impossible to recognise the epithelial type should the term "malignant adenofibroma NOS" be used. Variants include malignant clear cell adenofibroma, malignant endometrioid adenofibroma, malignant mucinous adenofibroma, malignant serous adenofibroma.

Tumour terminology Recommended terms are in **bold**	Synonyms	Comments
Malignant adenofibroma NOS	Malignant adenofibroma	
Malignant Brenner tumour		People may distinguish between a malignant Brenner tumour—a transitional cell carcinoma associated with benign Brenner tumour—and a transitional cell carcinoma in which no benign Brenner element is found.
Malignant clear cell adenofibroma	See clear cell carcinoma	
Malignant cystadenofibroma	See endometrioid carcinoma See clear cell carcinoma See mucinous carcinoma See serous carcinoma	
Malignant diffuse mesothelioma	Malignant mesothelioma	A primary aggressive neoplasm of the peritoneum, which may involve the surface of the ovaries and should be distinguished from the surface epithelial carcinomas of the ovary. Exposure to asbestos may have occurred.
Malignant endometrioid adenofibroma	See endometrioid carcinoma	
Malignant endometrioid cystadenofibroma	See endometrioid carcinoma	
Malignant fibrous histiocytoma		Probably due to malignant transformation in a mature cystic teratoma.
Malignant lymphoma	Non-Hodgkin's lymphoma	Involvement of the ovaries is usually part of disseminated disease but rare instances of primary extranodal lymphoma of the ovary has been described. See Tumours of the Lymph Nodes and Spleen (Section 24).
Malignant melanoma		May be of teratomatous origin, or more frequently metastatic.
Malignant mesothelioma	See malignant diffuse mesothelioma	
Malignant mixed epithelial tumour	See carcinoma of mixed epithelial type	

Tumour terminology Recommended terms are in **bold**	Synonyms	Comments
Malignant mixed germ cell tumour	Mixed germ cell tumour	Malignant tumour with more than one malignant germ cell component, e.g., dysgerminoma, yolk sac tumour, immature teratoma, embryonal carcinoma, and non-gestational choriocarcinoma.
Malignant mixed Müllerian tumour, high grade	See carcinosarcoma	
Malignant mixed Müllerian tumour, low grade	See adenosarcoma	
Malignant mucinous adenofibroma	See mucinous carcinoma	
Malignant mucinous cystadenocarcinoma	See mucinous carcinoma	
Malignant mucinous cystadenofibroma	See mucinous carcinoma	
Malignant neuroectodermal tumour NOS	Anaplastic neuroectodermal tumour Neuroectodermal tumour	A monodermal variant of malignant teratoma.
Malignant serous adenofibroma	See serous carcinoma	
Malignant serous cystadenofibroma	See serous carcinoma	
Malignant teratoma	See immature teratoma See also mature cystic teratoma with malignant transformation	
Malignant thecoma		Exceedingly rare tumour.
Masculinovoblastoma	See steroid cell tumour NOS	
Mature cystic teratoma	Dermoid cyst Endodermal variant of mature cystic teratoma Epidermoid cyst Fetiform teratoma (homonculus)	By definition all tissues in these neoplasms must be mature, and the behaviour is benign. Rarely, malignant transformation occurs. Cysts lined only by stratified squamous epithelium and lacking other teratomatous elements should be classified as epidermoid cysts.

Tumour terminology Recommended terms are in **bold**	Synonyms	Comments
Mature cystic teratoma with malignant transformation		Malignant tumours, which develop in mature cystic teratomas, may be classified according to the nature of the malignant neoplasm or as a mature cystic teratoma with malignant transformation. The nature of the malignant tumour must, however, be specified. Variants of carcinomas include adenocarcinoma, adenosquamous, apocrine, basal cell, carcinoid tumour, clear cell, sebaceous, squamous cell, thyroid, and undifferentiated carcinoma. Other components include: chondrosarcoma, epithelioid angiosarcoma, extramammary Paget's disease, fibrosarcoma, glioblastoma, histiocytoid vascular tumour, leiomyosarcoma, lymphoma, malignant fibrous histiocytoma, malignant melanoma, neuroblastoma, and osteogenic sarcoma.
Mature solid teratoma		Much less common than mature cystic teratoma and with an age distribution similar to that of immature teratoma from which it must be carefully distinguished. Thorough sampling is essential. All tissues must, by definition, be mature. The behaviour is benign.
Melanotic neuroectodermal tumour		Resembling retinal anlage tumour.
Mesodermal mixed tumour	See carcinosarcoma	
Mesothelioma		Well differentiated papillary and diffuse malignant mesothelioma of the peritoneum may involve the ovary. See Tumours of the Serous Cavities (Section 21).
Metastatic tumour	Krukenberg tumour	Metastatic carcinoma from the large bowel, pancreas, and small intestine or carcinoid tumours may mimic primary ovarian neoplasms.
Mixed epithelial carcinoma	See carcinoma of mixed epithelial type	
Mixed epithelial tumour		The term "mixed epithelial tumour" is inadequate to indicate the behaviour of the neoplasm. Tumours can be benign, borderline, or malignant (carcinoma).

Tumour terminology Recommended terms are in **bold**	Synonyms	Comments
Mixed epithelial tumour of borderline malignancy	Borderline mixed epithelial tumour Borderline tumour of mixed epithelial type	Two or more ovarian surface epithelial types are present. The classification is appropriate only when the minor component comprises 10% or more.
Mixed germ cell sex cord-stromal tumour	Atypical gonadoblastoma Epithelioma pflugerein (obsolete) Germ cell sex cord-stromal tumour Gonocytoma 2 (obsolete) Pflügerome (obsolete)	Rare tumours including gonadoblastoma and an unclassified heterogeneous group.
Mixed germ cell tumour	See malignant mixed germ cell tumour	
Mixed malignant Müllerian tumour, high grade	See carcinosarcoma	
Mixed malignant Müllerian tumour, low grade	See adenosarcoma	
Mixed mesodermal tumour	See carcinosarcoma	
Monodermal teratoma	Monophyletic teratoma	These tumours are classified according to the specific tumour type to differentiate them from mature cystic teratoma with mixed elements. Variants include carcinoid tumour, mucinous carcinoid, mucinous tumours of intestinal type, neuroblastoma, primitive neuroectodermal tumour, struma ovarii, strumal carcinoid, and thyroid carcinoma.
Monophyletic teratoma	See monodermal teratoma	
Mucinous adenofibroma of endocervical type	See mucinous adenofibroma of Müllerian type	
Mucinous adenofibroma of intestinal type		Benign mucinous tumour of intestinal type with a fibrous component.
Mucinous adenofibroma of Müllerian type	Endocervical mucinous adenofibroma Mucinous adenofibroma of endocervical type	Benign mucinous tumour of endocervical type with a fibrous component.

Tumour terminology Recommended terms are in **bold**	Synonyms	Comments
Mucinous carcinoid tumour	Adenocarcinoid tumour Goblet cell carcinoid tumour	It is important to exclude the possibility that the lesion is a metastasis from the appendix or elsewhere.
Mucinous carcinoma	Colloid carcinoma	Tumours with destructive stromal invasion made up of intestinal or endocervical-type cells or a combination of the two or of mucinous unclassifiable mucinous cells. They must be distinguished from mucinous carcinomas metastatic to the ovary. Most of the tumours are cystic mucinous cystadenocarcinoma.
Mucinous carcinoma of low malignant potential	See borderline tumour	
Mucinous cyst of intestinal type	See mucinous cystadenoma of intestinal type	
Mucinous cyst of Müllerian type	See mucinous cystadenoma of endocervical type	
Mucinous cystadenocarcinoma	See mucinous carcinoma	
Mucinous cystadenofibroma of endocervical type	See mucinous cystadenofibroma of endocervical type	
Mucinous cystadenofibroma of intestinal type		Benign mucinous tumour of intestinal type. In those rare instances where a malignant germ cell tumour is present, the tumour should be classified according to the malignant germ cell element.
Mucinous cystadenofibroma of Müllerian type	Endocervical mucinous cystadenofibroma Mucinous cystadenofibroma of endocervical type	Benign mucinous tumour of Müllerian type.
Mucinous cystadenoma of endocervical type	See mucinous cystadenoma of Müllerian type	
Mucinous cystadenoma of intestinal type	Mucinous cyst of intestinal type	Benign mucinous tumour of intestinal type.

Tumour terminology Recommended terms are in **bold**	Synonyms	Comments
Mucinous cystadenoma of Müllerian type	Endocervical mucinous cystadenoma Mucinous cystadenoma of endocervical type Mucinous cyst of Müllerian type	Benign mucinous tumour of endocervical type. Variants include endocervical mucinous papillary cystadenoma of Müllerian type, papillary mucinous cystadenoma of Müllerian type.
Mucinous papillary cystadenoma of endocervical type	See Mucinous cystadenoma of Müllerian type	
Mucinous tumour of borderline malignancy of Müllerian type	Atypically proliferating mucinous tumour Atypically proliferating tumour Endocervical mucinous cystadenoma of borderline malignancy Endocervical mucinous tumour of borderline malignancy Mucinous carcinoma of low malignant potential Mucinous tumour of low malignant potential Müllerian mucinous papillary cystadenoma of borderline malignancy Müllerian mucinous tumour of borderline malignancy Proliferating mucinous tumour	Tumours with architecture similar to that of serous borderline tumours but made up of a mucinous epithelium resembling that of endocervix. These tumours may be associated with endometriosis. They behave benignly also in the presence of peritoneal implants or lymph node metastasis. Variants include papillary mucinous cystadenoma of borderline malignancy.
Mucinous tumour of borderline malignancy with early stromal invasion	Mucinous tumour of borderline malignancy with microinvasion	Rare. There are no agreed criteria for defining the limits of this entity and in contrast to similar serous tumours, mucinous tumours in this category may behave like overt carcinomas.
Mucinous tumour of borderline malignancy with microinvasion	See mucinous tumour of borderline malignancy with early stromal invasion	

Tumour terminology Recommended terms are in **bold**	Synonyms	Comments
Mucinous tumour of borderline malignancy, intestinal type	Atypically proliferating tumour Intestinal mucinous tumour of borderline malignancy Mucinous carcinoma of low malignant potential Mucinous tumour of low malignant potential Proliferating mucinous tumour	Generally large, multilocular cystic tumour. The epithelial lining shows a complex villo-glandular pattern with the presence of goblet cells. Destructive stromal invasion is absent. Some of these tumours may have an unusual proliferation and severe cytologic atypia warranting the definition of mucinous borderline tumours with intraepithelial carcinoma. Most cases are diagnosed at stage I and behave as benign neoplasms. A few may be associated with a pseudomyxoma peritoneii. In these cases, the ovarian lesion is a metastasis of an appendiceal or intestinal primary tumour. Mural nodules of various types have been described in the wall of mucinous borderline tumours of intestinal type.
Mucinous tumour of intestinal type	See mucinous tumour of benign, borderline, or malignant categories, intestinal type	
Mucinous tumour of low malignant potential	See mucinous tumour of borderline malignancy, intestinal type	
Mucinous tumour of Müllerian type	See mucinous tumour of benign, borderline, or malignant categories	
Müllerian mixed malignant tumour	See carcinosarcoma	
Müllerian mucinous papillary cystadenoma of borderline malignancy	See mucinous tumour of borderline malignancy of endocervical type	
Müllerian mucinous tumour of borderline malignancy	See mucinous tumour of borderline malignancy of endocervical type	
Myxoma		Rare benign tumour probably of the thecoma-fibroma group.
Nephroblastoma		Has been described as a constituent of a juvenile granulosa cell tumour. Renal Wilm's tumour may also metastasise to the ovary. See Tumours of the Kidney (Section 27).

Tumour terminology Recommended terms are in **bold**	Synonyms	Comments
Neurilemmoma	Schwannoma	Exceedingly rare. See Tumours of Soft Tissue (Section 42).
Neuroblastoma		May develop in a mature or immature teratoma.
Neuroectodermal tumour NOS	See malignant neuroectodermal tumour NOS	
Neuroendocrine tumour	See carcinoid tumour	
Neurofibroma		Exceedingly rare. See Tumours of Soft Tissue (Section 42).
Non-chromaffin paraganglioma		Of teratomatous origin.
Non-gestational choriocarcinoma	Choriocarcinoma, non-gestational type Chorionepithelioma	Pure non-gestational choriocarcinomas are rare and highly malignant. More commonly, choriocarcinoma is a component of a mixed germ cell tumour.
Oncocytic tumour		The tumour may represent oncocytic metaplasia in a common epithelial tumour.
Osteoclastoma	See giant cell tumour	
Osteogenic sarcoma		Exceedingly rare. May arise in a teratoma. See Tumours of Soft Tissue (Section 42).
Osteoma		Probably either a fibroma with osseous metaplasia or heterotopic bone formation in the ovarian stroma.
Ovarian goitre	See struma ovarii	Obsolete term.
Papillary cystadenoma of borderline malignancy	See borderline tumour	
Papillary mucinous cystadenoma of Müllerian type	See mucinous cystadenoma of Müllerian type	
Papillary mucinous tumour of borderline malignancy	See mucinous tumour of borderline malignancy of Müllerian type	
Papillary serous carcinoma of low malignant potential	See serous tumour of borderline malignancy	

Tumour terminology Recommended terms are in **bold**	Synonyms	Comments
Papillary serous cystadenoma of borderline malignancy	See serous tumour of borderline malignancy	
Papillary serous tumour of low malignant potential	See serous tumour of borderline malignancy	
Pflügerome	See mixed germ cell sex cord-stromal tumour	Obsolete term.
Phaeochromocytoma		Very rare in ovary.
Pituitary adenoma		Rare, of teratomatous origin.
Polyembryoma		The term should be applied only to those rare malignant pure germ cell tumours characterised by the presence of embryoid bodies. Occasional embryoid bodies may be found in malignant mixed germ cell tumours.
Polyvesicular vitelline tumour	See yolk sac tumour	
Poorly differentiated Sertoli-Leydig cell tumour (sarcomatoid)	Androblastoma with heterologous elements Arrhenoblastoma Sarcomatoid Sertoli-Leydig cell tumour Sertoli-Leydig cell tumour	May contain heterologous elements usually gastrointestinal epithelium, cartilage, or striated muscle.
Primitive neuroectodermal tumour (PNET)		Of teratomatous origin and resembling PNET elsewhere in the body.
Proliferating Brenner tumour	See Brenner tumour of borderline malignancy	
Proliferating clear cell tumour	See clear cell tumour of borderline malignancy	
Proliferating endometrioid adenofibroma	See endometrioid tumour of borderline malignancy	
Proliferating mucinous tumour	See borderline tumour	
Psammomatous carcinoma	Serous carcinoma	Usually well differentiated serous carcinoma characterised by numerous psammoma bodies.

Tumour terminology Recommended terms are in **bold**	Synonyms	Comments
Retiform androblastoma	See retiform variant of Sertoli-stromal cell tumour	
Retiform variant of Sertoli-stromal cell tumour	Androblastoma Arrhenoblastoma Retiform androblastoma	Moderately and poorly differentiated Sertoli-Leydig cell tumours containing areas resembling the rete testis. They occur in younger women and are less likely to be associated with virilisation.
Rhabdomyoma		Rare in the ovary.
Rhabdomyosarcoma		Very rare, generally metastatic. May be of ovarian stromal origin; develop in carcinosarcoma or Sertoli-Leydig cell tumour as well as in a teratoma.
Sarcoma NOS	See undifferentiated sarcoma	To be used only when it proves impossible to identify the type of sarcoma.
Sarcomatoid Sertoli-Leydig cell tumour	See poorly differentiated Sertoli-Leydig cell tumour	
Schwannoma	See neurilemmoma	
Sclerosing stromal tumour		Benign tumour. Most common in the first three decades of life. Similar to fibroma and thecoma.
Sebaceous carcinoma		Of teratomatous origin.
Secretory endometrioid adenocarcinoma	See endometrioid carcinoma	
Serous adenofibroma		Benign serous tumour.
Serous carcinoma		The most common malignant epithelial tumour of the ovary. Mostly cystic differentiation (serous cystadenocarcinoma). Variants include serous papillary cystadenocarcinoma, psammomatous carcinoma.
Serous cyst	See serous cystadenoma	
Serous cystadenocarcinoma of low malignant potential	See serous tumour of borderline malignancy	

Tumour terminology Recommended terms are in **bold**	Synonyms	Comments
Serous cystadenofibroma		Benign serous tumour with prominent fibrous component. Can be papillary.
Serous cystadenoma	Serous cyst	Benign serous tumour with or without papillary pattern.
Serous papillary adenocarcinoma	See serous carcinoma	
Serous papillary cystadenocarcinoma	See serous carcinoma	
Serous papillary cystadenofibroma	See serous cystadenofibroma	Benign serous tumour.
Serous papillary cystadenoma	See serous cystadenoma	Benign serous tumour.
Serous surface carcinoma	Serous surface adenocarcinoma	Primary serous carcinoma arising from the surface of the ovary most often replacing the underlying ovary. Should be distinguished from primary peritoneal serous carcinoma, which may or may not involve the ovarian surface. Can be papillary.
Serous surface papillary adenocarcinoma	See serous surface carcinoma	
Serous surface papilloma		Benign serous tumour with papillary configuration.
Serous surface tumour of borderline malignancy		Serous tumour of borderline malignancy arising from and usually limited to the surface of the ovary.
Serous tumour of borderline malignancy	Atypically proliferating tumour Borderline tumour Carcinoma of low malignant potential Epithelial tumour of borderline malignancy Serous cystadenocarcinoma of low malignant potential	Tumours with excellent prognosis. Generally unicystic with papillae on the inner and/or outer surface (papillary tumours). Serous borderline tumours are associated with peritoneal implants in about one third of the cases. These implants may occasionally be invasive, and therefore must be considered morphologically and prognostically as a low grade serous carcinoma. In some borderline tumours an uncommon epithelial proliferation may be observed, particularly in the form of a micropapillary pattern. In these cases invasive implants are relatively more frequent.

Tumour terminology Recommended terms are in **bold**	Synonyms	Comments
Serous tumour of borderline malignancy with early stromal invasion	Serous tumour of borderline malignancy with microinvasion	Evidence suggests that this minor degree of stromal invasion does not affect the prognosis.
Serous tumour of borderline malignancy with microinvasion	See serous tumour of borderline malignancy with early stromal invasion	
Sertoli cell carcinoma	See well differentiated Sertoli cell tumour	Obsolete term.
Sertoli cell tumour	See well differentiated Sertoli cell tumour	
Sertoli stromal cell tumour	See Sertoli-Leydig cell tumour	
Sertoli-Leydig cell tumour	Androblastoma Arrhenoblastoma (obsolete)	Sex cord-stromal tumour composed of Sertoli cells and cells of stromal derivation, including Leydig cells, in a variable proportion and degree of differentiation. In about one third of cases they are associated with virilisation. These tumours are subdivided in well, moderately, and poorly differentiated and in retiform forms. Well differentiated tumours are benign; some moderately and retiform tumours and poorly differentiated tumours are malignant. Sarcomatoid and heterologous elements can be present in some tumours.
Sertoli-Leydig cell tumour of intermediate differentiation	Androblastoma with heterologous elements	May contain heterologous elements commonly gastrointestinal epithelium, cartilage, and striated muscle.
Sertoli-stromal cell tumour with retiform pattern	See retiform variant of Sertoli-stromal cell tumour	
Sex cord tumour with annular tubules (SCTAT)		Large unilateral tumours 20% of which are malignant. Small, benign, hamartomatous SCTATs are common in the ovaries of women with Peutz-Jeghers' syndrome.
Sex cord-stromal tumour NOS	See unclassified sex cord-stromal tumour	To be used only when a tumour cannot be more definitely classified.

Tumour terminology Recommended terms are in **bold**	Synonyms	Comments
Signet ring stromal tumour	See benign signet ring stromal tumour	
Small cell carcinoma (pulmonary type)		Rare primary neuroendocrine tumour of the ovary. Metastatic bronchial small cell carcinoma should be excluded.
Small cell tumour desmoplastic type	See desmoplastic small round cell tumour	
Small cell undifferentiated carcinoma (hypercalcaemic type)	Undifferentiated small cell tumour associated with hypercalcaemia	Highly malignant tumour of women under the age of 40 years. Of uncertain origin. Two thirds have raised serum calcium.
Solid teratoma	See immature teratoma See mature solid teratoma	
Squamous cell carcinoma		May be of teratomatous origin or develop in an endometrioid or Brenner tumour.
Steroid cell tumour NOS	Adrenal cortical-like tumour Adrenal-like tumour Adrenal rest tumour Adrenal-like steroid cell tumour Masculinovoblastoma	Rare tumour composed of cells resembling Leydig cells, adrenal cortical cells, or lutein cells. Stromal luteomas and Leydig cell tumours are separately classified.
Stromal Leydig cell tumour	See Leydig cell tumour	
Stromal luteoma	Lipid cell tumour Lipoid cell tumour Steroid cell tumour	It is debatable whether these are true neoplasms or foci of hyperplastic stromal-lutein cells. They are frequently associated with stromal hyperthecosis.
Stromal sarcoma	See endometrial stromal sarcoma	
Stromal tumour with minor sex cord elements	See fibroma	
Struma ovarii	Ovarian goitre (obsolete)	A mature teratoma composed only of thyroid tissue or one in which other teratomatous elements are present but thyroid tissue is grossly visible.

Tumour terminology Recommended terms are in **bold**	Synonyms	Comments
Strumal carcinoid tumour		A mature teratoma in which trabecular or insular carcinoid tumour and thyroid tissue are mixed.
Sweat gland carcinoma	Sweat gland carcinoma	Described only as malignant change in a mature cystic teratoma.
Teratoid androblastoma	Poorly differentiated Sertoli-Leydig cell tumour	Sertoli-Leydig cell tumours with heterologous elements.
Teratoma		This term must be used with the qualification benign or malignant.
Theca cell tumour	See thecoma	
Thecafibroma	See fibrothecoma	
Thecoma	Theca cell tumour	Benign sex cord-stromal tumour composed of cells that resemble theca interna cells and usually developing in women over the age of 40 years. Usually oestrogenic, they may be non-functioning or less commonly androgenic. The category includes luteinised thecomas.
Thyroid carcinoma		Follicular or papillary thyroid carcinoma developing in a struma ovarii.
Transitional cell carcinoma		A transitional cell carcinoma resembling those of the urinary bladder and distinguished, by some people, from a malignant Brenner tumour by the absence of a benign Brenner tumour component.
Tubular adenoma of Pick	See well differentiated Sertoli cell tumour	
Tubular adenoma with Leydig cells	See well differentiated Sertoli-Leydig cell tumour	
Tubular adenoma with lipid storage	See well differentiated Sertoli cell tumour	
Tubular androblastoma	See well differentiated Sertoli cell tumour	Distinguish from endometrioid carcinoma with Sertoliform pattern.

Tumour terminology Recommended terms are in **bold**	Synonyms	Comments
Tubular androblastoma with lipid storage (tubular adenoma of Pick)	See well differentiated Sertoli cell tumour	
Tumour of borderline malignancy	See borderline tumour	Epithelial component should always be specified.
Tumour of dysgenetic gonad	See gonadoblastoma	
Tumour of probable Wolffian origin		Tumour so called because of its resemblance to Wolffian duct remnants and tumours of known Wolffian origin. Some have metastasised and led to the patient's death up to 8 years after initial treatment, indicating the necessity of a long-term follow-up.
Unclassified epithelial tumour		Epithelial tumours in which the type of epithelium cannot be defined. The tumours may be benign or malignant.
Unclassified sex cord-stromal tumour		Tumours believed to be of sex cord-stromal origin, which cannot be further classified.
Undifferentiated carcinoma	Carcinoma NOS	To be used only when the tumour cannot be further classified.
Undifferentiated sarcoma		Sarcoma that cannot be classified morphologically.
Undifferentiated small cell carcinoma associated with hypercalcaemia	See small cell undifferentiated carcinoma (hypercalcaemic type)	
Well differentiated Sertoli cell tumour	Androblastoma with lipid storage Sertoli cell carcinoma (obsolete) Sertoli cell tumour	Usually non-functioning, benign sex cord-stromal tumour histologically similar to its testicular counterpart. They contain only few or no Leydig cells. Variants include Sertoli cell tumour with lipid storage, tubular androblastoma, tubular androblastoma with lipid storage, tubular adenoma of Pick, and Sertoli cell tumour.

Tumour terminology Recommended terms are in **bold**	Synonyms	Comments
Well differentiated Sertoli-Leydig cell tumour	Tubular androblastoma with Leydig cells Tubular adenoma with Leydig cells	Almost invariably benign sex cord-stromal tumour distinguished from the well differentiated Sertoli cell tumour by the presence of Leydig cells. The tumours may be associated with virilisation.
Yolk sac tumour	Endodermal sinus tumour (obsolete)	A malignant germ cell tumour developing most commonly under the age of 40 years. Chemotherapy may be curative. Variants: Enteroid variant of yolk sac tumour, hepatoid variant of yolk sac tumour.

Section 33

Tumours of the Fallopian Tube and Para-Adnexal Structures

D.E. Hughes
M. Wells

Tumour terminology Recommended terms are in **bold**	Synonyms	Comments
Adenocarcinoma		A very rare tumour which predominately affects elderly women. The malignant potential is variable depending upon the grade.
Adenofibroma		This benign tumour may rarely affect the fallopian tube.
Adenoma of the rete ovarii		A rare benign tumour.
Adenomatoid mesothelioma	See adenomatoid tumour	
Adenomatoid tumour	Adenomatoid mesothelioma	This is the most common benign tumour of the fallopian tube. It is of mesothelial origin and consists of an admixture of tubules lined by epithelial-like cells and connective tissue. The latter may include smooth muscle.
Adenomyoma		A rare benign tumour combining glandular tissue and smooth muscle.
Adenosarcoma	See metaplastic carcinoma	
Carcinosarcoma	See metaplastic carcinoma	
Dermoid cyst	See mature cystic teratoma	
Fibroid	See leiomyoma	

Tumour terminology Recommended terms are in **bold**	Synonyms	Comments
Fibroleiomyoma	See leiomyoma	
Fibropapilloma	See papilloma	
Leiomyoma	Fibroid Fibroleiomyoma	Uncommon benign tumour of smooth muscle.
Leiomyosarcoma		This is the most common sarcoma of the fallopian tube.
Low grade cystic mesothelioma		Benign tumour, which histologically may mimic a malignancy.
Malignant mixed mesodermal tumour	See metaplastic carcinoma	
Malignant mixed Müllerian tumour	See metaplastic carcinoma	
Mature cystic teratoma	Dermoid cyst	This benign germ cell tumour may rarely affect the fallopian tube.
Metaplastic carcinoma	Adenosarcoma Carcinosarcoma Malignant mixed mesodermal tumour Malignant mixed Müllerian tumour	A rare high grade tumour combining malignant glandular and mesenchymal elements.
Metaplastic papillary tumour		A rare benign tumour of uncertain derivation.
Papillary cystadenoma of the broad ligament		A benign tumour, which may be associated with von-Hippel-Lindau disease.
Papilloma	Fibropapilloma	Benign tumour composed of connective tissue covered by simple epithelium.
Paratubal tumour of probable mesonephric origin	Paratubal tumour of probable Wolffian origin	Usually benign, but behaviour unpredictable.
Paratubal tumour of probable Wolffian origin	See paratubal tumour of probable mesonephric origin	
Serous carcinoma	Serous papillary carcinoma	Malignant tumour similar to serous adenocarcinoma of the ovary. Behaviour unpredictable.

Tumour terminology Recommended terms are in **bold**	Synonyms	Comments
Serous papillary carcinoma	See serous carcinoma	
Struma salpingii		Histopathological variant of mature cystic teratoma consisting of thyroid tissue.
Well differentiated papillary mesothelioma		Rare benign tumour.

Section 34

Tumours of the Corpus Uteri

D.E. Hughes
M. Wells

Tumour terminology Recommended terms are in **bold**	Synonyms	Comments
Adenocarcinoma	Endometrial carcinoma	This is the most common tumour of the corpus uteri. Malignant potential is variable and depends upon grade. Clear cell, ciliated cell, endometrioid, mucinous, papillary, serous, secretory, and villoglandular variants are recognised.
Adenofibroma	Müllerian adenofibroma Papillary adenofibroma Papillary cystadenofibroma	This is a benign tumour of the elderly and combines epithelial and mesenchymal elements.
Adenomatoid mesothelioma	See adenomatoid tumour	
Adenomatoid tumour	Adenomatoid mesothelioma	This tumour is of mesothelial origin and consists of an admixture of tubules lined by epithelial-like cells and connective tissue. The latter may include smooth muscle.
Adenomyoma		This is a benign tumour, which combines glandular and smooth muscle elements.
Adenosarcoma	See metaplastic carcinoma	
Adenosquamous carcinoma		A histological variant of adenocarcinoma combining malignant glandular and squamous differentiation. This should not be confused with squamous metaplasia.

Tumour terminology Recommended terms are in **bold**	Synonyms	Comments
Atypical endometrial hyperplasia	Intraendometrial neoplasia	Histological variant of endometrial hyperplasia characterised by severe cytological atypia and papillary buds within glandular lumina. At least 30% of patients progress to carcinoma.
Atypical polypoid adenomyoma		This tumour is composed of pleomorphic endometrial glands admixed with smooth muscle. Despite the worrying histology the lesion is biologically benign.
Carcinofibroma		This is a rare tumour comprising malignant epithelial elements admixed with endometrial stroma. The biological behaviour is unpredictable.
Carcinomesenchymoma	See metaplastic carcinoma	
Carcinosarcoma	See metaplastic carcinoma	
Ciliated cell adenocarcinoma	Ciliated cell carcinoma	This is a very rare histological variant of adenocarcinoma.
Ciliated cell carcinoma	See ciliated cell adenocarcinoma	
Clear cell adenocarcinoma	Clear cell carcinoma	Histological variant of adenocarcinoma characterised by the presence of glycogen rich epithelium or hobnail cells. It is associated with a poor prognosis.
Clear cell carcinoma	See clear cell adenocarcinoma	
Endometrial carcinoma	See adenocarcinoma	
Endometrial polyp		This common tumour-like lesion of the endometrium results from the effects of excessive oestrogen stimulation.
Endometrial stromal nodule		This rare benign tumour most often affects pre-menopausal women and is composed of endometrial stromal cells.
Endometrial stromal sarcoma		This is a rare malignant tumour of the endometrial stroma. The biological behaviour is unpredictable. Prognosis depends upon tumour grade. Low and high forms are recognised. A uterine sex cord-like variant is recognised.

Tumour terminology Recommended terms are in **bold**	Synonyms	Comments
Endometrioid adenocarcinoma	Endometrioid carcinoma	This is the most common histological variant of adenocarcinoma.
Endometrioid adenocarcinoma with squamous metaplasia		Histological variant of adenocarcinoma showing squamous metaplasia. It must be distinguished from adenosquamous carcinoma in which the squamous element is histologically malignant.
Endometrioid carcinoma	See endometrioid adenocarcinoma	
Epidermoid carcinoma	See squamous carcinoma	
Fibroid	See leiomyoma	
Fibroleiomyoma	See leiomyoma	
Giant cell carcinoma		This histological variant of endometrioid carcinoma is characterised by the presence of conspicuous multinucleate tumour giant cells. The prognosis is poor.
High grade papillary adenocarcinoma	See papillary serous adenocarcinoma	
High grade papillary carcinoma	See papillary serous adenocarcinoma	
Inflammatory pseudotumour	Postoperative spindle cell nodule Pseudosarcoma botryoides	This tumour-like lesion very rarely affects the uterus. See Tumours of Soft Tissue (Section 42).
Intraendometrial neoplasia	See atypical endometrial hyperplasia	
Leiomyoma	Fibroid Fibroleiomyoma	This benign tumour of smooth muscle is the most common neoplasm of the female internal genitalia.
Leiomyosarcoma		This is the most common sarcoma of the uterus. Smooth muscle tumours with 10 mitoses or more per 10 high power fields are by definition malignant. The prognosis is poor.
Malignant mixed mesodermal tumour	See metaplastic carcinoma	
Malignant mixed Müllerian tumour	See metaplastic carcinoma	

Tumour terminology Recommended terms are in **bold**	Synonyms	Comments
Metaplastic carcinoma	Adenosarcoma Carcinosarcoma Malignant mixed mesodermal tumour Malignant mixed Müllerian tumour Mixed Müllerian tumour Müllerian adenosarcoma	This is a high grade tumour composed of malignant epithelial and mesenchymal elements. The latter may consist of tissue normally present in the uterus (homologous) or comprise foreign components, e.g., skeletal muscle, cartilage, and bone.
Mixed Müllerian tumour	See metaplastic carcinoma	
Mucinous adenocarcinoma	Mucinous carcinoma	Histopathological variant of adenocarcinoma characterised by excessive mucin secretion.
Mucinous carcinoma	See mucinous adenocarcinoma	
Müllerian adenofibroma	See adenofibroma	
Müllerian adenosarcoma	See metaplastic carcinoma	
Neuroendocrine carcinoma	See small cell carcinoma	
Papillary adenofibroma	See adenofibroma	
Papillary cystadenofibroma	See adenofibroma	
Papillary serous adenocarcinoma	High grade papillary adenocarcinoma High grade papillary carcinoma Papillary serous carcinoma Serous papillary carcinoma	This variant of adenocarcinoma, which shows tubal differentiation, is associated with widespread lymphatic and vascular spread. The prognosis is poor.
Papillary serous carcinoma	See papillary serous adenocarcinoma	
Postoperative spindle cell nodule	See inflammatory pseudotumour	

Tumour terminology Recommended terms are in **bold**	Synonyms	Comments
Primitive neuroectodermal tumour		This highly malignant tumour may rarely arise in the uterus, usually in younger individuals. It may be sensitive to chemotherapy or radiotherapy.
Pseudosarcoma botryoides	See inflammatory pseudotumour	
Secretory adenocarcinoma	Secretory carcinoma	Histological variant of adenocarcinoma characterised by the presence of cytoplasmic vacuolation due to the effects of progesterone.
Secretory carcinoma	See secretory adenocarcinoma	
Serous papillary carcinoma	See papillary serous adenocarcinoma	
Small cell carcinoma	Neuroendocrine carcinoma	This highly malignant tumour is sometimes sensitive to chemotherapy or radiotherapy.
Squamous carcinoma	Epidermoid carcinoma	Primary squamous carcinoma is rare in this site: extension of such lesions from the cervix is far more common. The tumour has a malignant potential similar to adenocarcinoma.
Undifferentiated carcinoma		Histological variant of endometrioid carcinoma showing no specific differentiation. Diagnosis often depends on immunocytochemistry.
Uterine sex cord-like tumour		Histological variant of endometrial stromal sarcoma showing epithelial differentiation mimicking granulosa cell/ Sertoli cell tumour.
Villoglandular adenocarcinoma	Villoglandular carcinoma	Histopathological variant of adenocarcinoma.
Villoglandular carcinoma	See villoglandular adenocarcinoma	

Section 35

Tumours of the Cervix Uteri

D.E. Hughes
M. Wells

Tumour terminology Recommended terms are in **bold**	Synonyms	Comments
Acantholytic squamous cell carcinoma		Histological variant of squamous cell carcinoma showing a pseudoglandular pattern.
Adenocarcinoma		A spectrum of tumours of variable malignant potential depending upon the grade. Clear cell, endocervical, endometrioid, enteric, glassy cell, mesonephroid, minimal deviation, mucinous, papillary, and villoglandular papillary variants are recognised.
Adenocarcinoma in situ	See cervical glandular intraepithelial neoplasia	
Adenofibroma	Müllerian adenofibroma	A rare benign tumour composed of glandular and fibrous tissue components.
Adenoid basal carcinoma	Basaloid carcinoma	A histological variant of squamous cell carcinoma resembling basal cell carcinoma.
Adenoid cystic carcinoma	Cervical carcinoma with adenoid cystic pattern	A rare histological variant of cervical adenocarcinoma, which usually presents in elderly females. It is associated with a poor prognosis.
Adenoma malignum	See minimal deviation adenocarcinoma	
Adenosarcoma	See metaplastic carcinoma	
Adenosquamous carcinoma		An uncommon carcinoma of the cervix combining squamous and glandular differentiation. The behaviour of this tumour is similar to that of adenocarcinoma.

Tumour terminology Recommended terms are in **bold**	Synonyms	Comments
Basaloid carcinoma	See adenoid basal carcinoma	
Basaloid squamous carcinoma		Histological variant of squamous cell carcinoma composed of a largely undifferentiated small cell population.
Botryoid rhabdomyosarcoma	See embryonal rhabdomyosarcoma	
Buschke-Löwenstein tumour	See verrucous carcinoma	
Carcinosarcoma	See metaplastic carcinoma	
Cervical adenocarcinoma		
Cervical carcinoma with adenoid cystic pattern	See adenoid cystic carcinoma	
Cervical dysplasia	See cervical intraepithelial neoplasia	
Cervical glandular intraepithelial neoplasia	Adenocarcinoma in situ CGIN Glandular dysplasia	A pre-malignant condition of the cervix, which may be subdivided into three grades. Grade 3 is equivalent to adenocarcinoma in situ.
Cervical intraepithelial neoplasia	Cervical dysplasia CIN Squamous carcinoma in situ Squamous intraepithelial lesion SIL	A pre-malignant lesion, which is divided into grades 1–3 according to increasing severity; CIN 3 is the equivalent of squamous carcinoma in situ. Squamous intraepithelial lesion (SIL) is the equivalent in the American nomenclature of cervical intraepithelial neoplasia and is divided into two grades only—low and high.
CGIN	See cervical glandular intraepithelial neoplasia	
CIN	See cervical intraepithelial neoplasia	
Clear cell adenocarcinoma	Clear cell carcinoma	A histological variant of cervical adenocarcinoma, which may develop in young females in association with vaginal adenosis.
Clear cell carcinoma	See clear cell adenocarcinoma	

Tumour terminology Recommended terms are in **bold**	Synonyms	Comments
Condyloma acuminatum		These genital warts due to human papillomavirus infection may affect the cervix in addition to the vagina and the vulva.
Embryonal rhabdomyosarcoma	Botryoid rhabdomyosarcoma Rhabdomyosarcoma Sarcoma botryoides	A highly malignant sarcoma, which predominantly affects children. Lesions are more often seen in the vagina. It may be sensitive to radiotherapy or chemotherapy.
Endocervical adenocarcinoma	Endocervical carcinoma	A histological variant of cervical adenocarcinoma.
Endocervical carcinoma	See endocervical adenocarcinoma	
Endocervical polyp		A benign tumour-like lesion.
Endocervical stromal sarcoma		A rare tumour of unpredictable malignant potential, prognosis depends upon the grade.
Endometrioid adenocarcinoma	Endometrioid carcinoma	A histological variant of cervical adenocarcinoma.
Endometrioid carcinoma	See endometrioid adenocarcinoma	
Enteric adenocarcinoma	Enteric carcinoma	A histological variant of cervical adenocarcinoma showing intestinal differentiation.
Enteric carcinoma	See enteric adenocarcinoma	
Epidermoid carcinoma	See squamous carcinoma	
Fibroid	See leiomyoma	
Fibroleiomyoma	See leiomyoma	
Giant condyloma of Buschke-Löwenstein	See verrucous carcinoma	
Glandular dysplasia	See cervical glandular intraepithelial neoplasia	
Glassy cell adenocarcinoma	Glassy cell carcinoma	A histological variant of cervical adenosquamous carcinoma.
Glassy cell carcinoma	See glassy cell adenocarcinoma	
Leiomyoma	Fibroid Fibroleiomyoma	This benign tumour is more often found in the myometrium.

Tumour terminology Recommended terms are in **bold**	Synonyms	Comments
Lymphoepithelioma-like carcinoma		An exceedingly rare histological variant of squamous carcinoma characterised by an intense lymphocytic infiltrate.
Malignant mixed mesodermal tumour	See metaplastic carcinoma	
Malignant mixed Müllerian tumour	See metaplastic carcinoma	
Mesonephric papilloma	See Müllerian papilloma	
Mesonephroid adenocarcinoma	Mesonephroid carcinoma	A rare histological variant of cervical adenocarcinoma.
Mesonephroid carcinoma	See mesonephroid adenocarcinoma	
Metaplastic carcinoma	Adenosarcoma Carcinosarcoma Malignant mixed mesodermal tumour Malignant mixed Müllerian tumour Müllerian adenosarcoma	A rare malignant tumour, which may show glandular and/or squamous differentiation in addition to malignant heterologous mesenchymal elements such as skeletal muscle, cartilage, and bone.
Microglandular hyperplasia		A tumour-like lesion.
Minimal deviation adenocarcinoma	Adenoma malignum	A low grade histological variant of adenocarcinoma, associated with Peutz-Jeghers' syndrome.
Mucinous adenocarcinoma	Mucinous carcinoma	This is the cervical equivalent of mucinous adenocarcinoma of the colon.
Mucinous carcinoma	See mucinous adenocarcinoma	
Müllerian adenofibroma	See adenofibroma	
Müllerian adenosarcoma	See metaplastic carcinoma	
Müllerian papilloma	Mesonephric papilloma	A benign papillary tumour presenting in children.
Neuroendocrine carcinoma		A histological variant of cervical carcinoma, which varies from carcinoid-like lesions to undifferentiated variants. The latter are high grade. These tumours may be associated with hormonal production.

Tumour terminology Recommended terms are in **bold**	Synonyms	Comments
Papillary adenocarcinoma	Papillary carcinoma	A histological variant of cervical adenocarcinoma.
Papillary carcinoma	See papillary adenocarcinoma	
Rhabdomyoma		This benign tumour of skeletal muscle may very rarely present in the cervix.
Rhabdomyosarcoma	See embryonal rhabdomyosarcoma	
Sarcoma botryoides	See embryonal rhabdomyosarcoma	
SIL	See cervical intraepithelial neoplasia	
Small cell carcinoma	Undifferentiated carcinoma	A highly malignant variant of squamous carcinoma, which may be sensitive to chemotherapy or radiotherapy.
Squamous carcinoma	Epidermoid carcinoma	Basaloid, lymphoepithelioma-like, and verrucous variants recognised. Variable malignant potential, depending upon grade.
Squamous carcinoma in situ	See CIN	
Squamous intraepithelial lesion	See cervical intraepithelial neoplasia	
Undifferentiated carcinoma	See small cell carcinoma	
Verrucous carcinoma	Giant condyloma of Buschke-Löwenstein Buschke-Löwenstein tumour	This low grade variant of squamous cell carcinoma may rarely present in the cervix.
Villoglandular papillary adenocarcinoma	Villoglandular papillary carcinoma	This low grade histological variant of adenocarcinoma predominately affects young women.
Villoglandular papillary carcinoma	See villoglandular papillary adenocarcinoma	

Section 36

Tumours of the Vagina

D.E. Hughes
M. Wells

Tumour terminology Recommended terms are in **bold**	Synonyms	Comments
Adenocarcinoma	See clear cell adenocarcinoma	
Adenocarcinoma in situ		Pre-malignant lesion.
Adenosis		Tumour-like lesion of Müllerian glandular tissue, which may progress to clear cell adenocarcinoma.
Adenosquamous carcinoma		A rare histological variant with behaviour similar to adenocarcinoma.
Angioma	See haemangioma	
Benign mixed tumour	See mixed tumour	
Botryoid rhabdomyosarcoma	See embryonal rhabdomyosarcoma	
Buschke-Löwenstein tumour	See verrucous carcinoma	
Clear cell adenocarcinoma	Adenocarcinoma Clear cell carcinoma	Rare low grade malignant tumour, which develops in young women and is strongly associated with diethylstilboestrol exposure in utero.
Clear cell carcinoma	See adenocarcinoma	
Condyloma acuminatum		Benign tumour-like lesion associated with human papillomavirus infection.
Dysplasia	See vaginal intraepithelial neoplasia	

Tumour terminology Recommended terms are in **bold**	Synonyms	Comments
Embryonal carcinoma	Undifferentiated malignant germ cell tumour	A highly malignant tumour of young children, which may be sensitive to chemotherapy or radiotherapy.
Embryonal rhabdomyosarcoma	Botryoid rhabdomyosarcoma Rhabdomyosarcoma Sarcoma botryoides	A highly malignant tumour of young children, which may be sensitive to chemotherapy or radiotherapy.
Endodermal sinus tumour	See yolk sac tumour	
Epidermoid carcinoma	See squamous carcinoma	
Fibroepithelial stromal polyp	See vaginal polyp	
Fibroid	See leiomyoma	
Fibroleiomyoma	See leiomyoma	
Glandular dysplasia		Pre-malignant lesion, less advanced disease than adenocarcinoma in situ. Represents the vaginal equivalent of CGIN.
Granular cell myoblastoma	See granular cell tumour	
Granular cell tumour	Granular cell myoblastoma	See Tumours of Soft Tissue (Section 42).
Immature teratoma		A highly malignant tumour, which may be sensitive to chemotherapy or radiotherapy.
Leiomyoma	Fibroid Fibroleiomyoma	This is the most common benign connective tissue tumour of the vagina.
Malignant melanoma	See melanoma	
Malignant teratoma, undifferentiated	See embryonal carcinoma	
Melanoma	Malignant melanoma	Primary melanoma of the vagina is an exceedingly rare high grade tumour. Metastatic involvement is more common and should always be excluded.
Mixed epithelial and mesenchymal neoplasm	See mixed tumour	

Tumour terminology Recommended terms are in **bold**	Synonyms	Comments
Mixed tumour	Benign mixed tumour Mixed epithelial mesenchymal neoplasm Spindle cell epithelioma Vaginal spindle cell epithelioma	A rare benign tumour composed of an admixture of spindle cells and epithelium.
Polypoid myofibroblastoma	See vaginal polyp	
Pseudosarcoma botryoides	See vaginal polyp	
Rhabdomyosarcoma	See embryonal rhabdomyosarcoma	
Sarcoma botryoides	See embryonal rhabdomyosarcoma	
Small cell carcinoma		This is a rare highly malignant neuroendocrine tumour, which may be sensitive to chemotherapy or radiotherapy.
Spindle cell epithelioma	See mixed tumour	
Squamous carcinoma	Epidermoid carcinoma	Differentiated and basaloid variants are recognised. The prognosis relates to the histological grade.
Squamous carcinoma in situ	See vaginal intraepithelial neoplasia	Pre-malignant lesion, equivalent to VAIN 3 or severe dysplasia.
Squamous papilloma		Benign tumour.
Undifferentiated malignant germ cell tumour	See embryonal carcinoma	
Vaginal intraepithelial neoplasia	Dysplasia Squamous carcinoma in situ VAIN	Pre-malignant lesion, divided into grades 1–3 according to increasing severity; VAIN 3 is equivalent to squamous carcinoma in situ.
Vaginal polyp	Fibroepithelial stromal polyp Polypoid myofibroblastoma Pseudosarcoma botryoides	This benign tumour commonly contains atypical multinucleate cells, which may cause confusion with a sarcoma.

Tumour terminology Recommended terms are in **bold**	Synonyms	Comments
Vaginal spindle cell epithelioma	See mixed tumour	
VAIN	See vaginal intraepithelial neoplasia	
Verrucous carcinoma	Buschke-Löwenstein tumour	This is a rare variant of squamous carcinoma associated with HPV infection in which recurrences are very common and metastases exceptional.
Yolk sac tumour	Endodermal sinus tumour	This is a highly malignant tumour, which occurs in children and may be sensitive to chemotherapy or radiotherapy.

Section 37

Tumours of the Vulva

D.E. Hughes
M. Wells

Tumour terminology Recommended terms are in **bold**	Synonyms	Comments
Adenocarcinoma		This is an extremely rare vulval tumour and may be of Bartholin or sweat gland derivation.
Adenoid cystic carcinoma		Locally aggressive malignant tumour arising in Bartholin gland. Associated with a poor long-term prognosis.
Adenosquamous carcinoma		Histological variant of Bartholin gland carcinoma.
Aggressive angiomyxoma		See Tumours of Soft Tissue (Section 42).
Angiokeratoma		The vulva is a site of predilection for this benign variant of haemangioma.
Angiomyofibroblastoma		See Tumours of Soft Tissue (Section 42).
Atypical melanotic macule	See mucosal melanosis	
Bartholin gland adenoma		An extremely rare benign proliferation of Bartholin gland tissue.
Bartholin gland carcinoma		Rare high grade malignant tumour, which may be of glandular or squamous type. The latter is often more aggressive than conventional vulval squamous carcinoma. It also includes adenoid cystic carcinoma, transitional cell carcinoma, and adenosquamous variants.
Basal cell carcinoma		This is extremely rare on the vulva.
Basaloid carcinoma		Variant of squamous cell carcinoma often associated with HPV type 16 infection.

Tumour terminology Recommended terms are in **bold**	Synonyms	Comments
Benign mixed tumour	Pleomorphic adenoma	Rare tumour analogous to the pleomorphic adenoma of the salivary gland. Usually benign but local recurrence is often a problem and a malignant variant is occasionally encountered.
Botryoid rhabdomyosarcoma	See embryonal rhabdomyosarcoma	
Buschke-Löwenstein tumour	See verrucous carcinoma	
Carcinoma in situ	See vulvar intraepithelial neoplasia	
Condyloma acuminatum	Genital wart	A variant of viral wart arising on the external genitalia and in the perianal region.
Condylomatous carcinoma	Warty carcinoma	Variant of squamous cell carcinoma arising in association with condyloma acuminatum. Usually associated with a good prognosis.
Embryonal rhabdomyosarcoma	Botryoid Rhabdomyosarcoma Sarcoma botryoides	A highly malignant variant of rhabdomyosarcoma, which predominantly affects infants. It may be responsive to combination chemotherapy or radiotherapy.
Endometriosis		A tumour-like lesion, which may undergo cyclical hormonal changes.
Extramammary Paget's disease	See Paget's disease	
Fibroadenoma		Benign tumour arising in ectopic breast tissue.
Genital lentiginosis	See mucosal melanosis	
Genital wart	See condyloma acuminatum	
Giant condyloma of Buschke-Löwenstein	See verrucous carcinoma	
Hidradenoma papilliferum	Papillary hidradenoma	A tumour of apocrine sweat gland derivation, which almost invariably arises in Caucasian females. Malignant transformation may very rarely be encountered.

Tumour terminology Recommended terms are in **bold**	Synonyms	Comments
Leiomyoma		This is the most common benign connective tissue tumour of the vulva.
Leiomyosarcoma		This is the most common sarcoma to affect the vulva.
Lentiginous melanosis	See mucosal melanosis	
Lentigo	See mucosal melanosis	
Malignant melanoma		Malignant melanoma arising at this site is a high grade tumour, which has commonly metastasised at presentation.
Mucosal melanosis	Atypical melanotic macule Genital lentiginosis Lentiginous melanosis Lentigo	This uncommon lesion is sometimes clinically confused with melanoma. It consists of an irregular pigmented macule and is benign.
Paget's disease	Extramammary Paget's disease	Vulval Paget's disease is analogous to the mammary variant. It may represent primary intraepithelial adenocarcinoma, spread from an underlying malignant sweat gland tumour or intraepithelial metastatic disease.
Papillary hidradenoma	See hidradenoma papilliferum	
Pleomorphic adenoma	See benign mixed tumour	
Sarcoma botryoides	See embryonal rhabdomyosarcoma	
Spindle cell squamous carcinoma		Histological variant of squamous carcinoma.
Squamous cell carcinoma		This is the most common malignant tumour of the vulva. It may be subdivided into microinvasive (tumour thickness 1 mm or less) and frankly invasive variants. In younger people, it is often preceded by VIN. In the older age group it is associated with lichen sclerosus.
Transitional cell carcinoma		Histological variant of Bartholin gland carcinoma.

Tumour terminology Recommended terms are in **bold**	Synonyms	Comments
Verrucous carcinoma	Buschke-Löwenstein tumour Giant condyloma of Buschke-Löwenstein	Rare variant of squamous cell carcinoma due to infection with human papilloma virus, usually type 6. Recurrences are characteristic but metastatic spread is exceptionally rare.
Vestibular gland adenoma		A rare tumour composed of mucous-secreting epithelium.
Vulvar intraepithelial neoplasia (VIN)		Pre-malignant lesion, divided into grades 1–3 according to increasing severity; VIN 3 is the equivalent to carcinoma in situ.
Warty carcinoma	See condylomatous carcinoma	

Section 38

Tumours of the Placenta

D.E. Hughes
M. Wells

Tumour terminology Recommended terms are in **bold**	Synonyms	Comments
Chorangioma	See haemangioma	
Chorioangioma	See haemangioma	
Choriocarcinoma		Malignant, but highly chemosensitive; usually associated with molar gestation.
Haemangioma	Chorangioma Chorioangioma	Common benign tumour, which can affect the placenta or the umbilical cord. Solitary lesions are often an incidental finding. Multiple lesions are frequently associated with polyhydramnios.
Placental site nodule		This represents a localised benign form of placental site trophoblastic tumour.
Placental site trophoblastic tumour		Usually follows a normal gestation. Although most examples are benign, occasional malignant cases have been recorded.
Teratoma		Primary tumours of the placenta are extremely rare and invariably located between the amnion and chorion. Benign variants affecting the umbilical cord have also been described.

Section 39

Tumours of the Breast

P.M. Arapantoni-Dadioti
C.N. Chinyama

Tumour terminology Recommended terms are in **bold**	Synonyms	Comments
Acute mammary carcinomatosis	See inflammatory carcinoma	Obsolete term.
Adenofibroma	See fibroadenoma	
Adenoid cystic carcinoma	Cylindroma	Rare. Histologically similar to its salivary gland counterpart.
Adenolipoma		A benign tumour composed of fat with normal lobules and ducts interspersed.
Adenoma of the nipple	Erosive adenomatosis of the nipple Florid papillomatosis of the nipple Subareolar papillomatosis	A benign epithelial tumour arising in the nipple ducts.
Adenoma pleomorphic	See pleomorphic adenoma	
Adenomyoepithelioma		A mixed proliferation of myoepithelial and duct epithelial cells. Most cases are benign. A malignant variant has been described.
Adenosis tumour	Nodular adenosis Tumoural adenosis	Descriptive term for a tumour-like lesion composed of multiple nodules of sclerosing adenosis.
Adenosquamous carcinoma		A combined malignant tumour showing mixed glandular and squamous differentiation.

Tumour terminology Recommended terms are in **bold**	Synonyms	Comments
ADH	See atypical ductal hyperplasia	
ALH	See atypical lobular hyperplasia	
Alveolar lobular carcinoma	Alveolar lobular invasive carcinoma	Histological variant of invasive lobular carcinoma.
Amyloid pseudotumour	See amyloid tumour	
Amyloid tumour	Amyloid pseudotumour	Tumour-like condition composed of amyloid.
Angiosarcoma	Haemangiosarcoma Post-mastectomy angiosarcoma Stewart-Treves syndrome	Angiosarcoma may arise de novo but more often occurs as a complication of lymph oedema following mastectomy or radiotherapy. See Tumours of Soft Tissue (Section 42).
Apocrine adenoma		A rare tumour-like lesion composed of ducts and lobules lined by apocrine epithelium.
Apocrine carcinoma	Oncocytic carcinoma Sweat gland carcinoma	Rare histological variant of invasive ductal carcinoma composed of cells with apocrine features.
Apocrine intraductal papilloma	See ductal papilloma	
Atypical ductal epitheliosis	See atypical ductal hyperplasia	
Atypical ductal hyperplasia	ADH Atypical ductal epitheliosis	An epithelial proliferation with architectural and cytological atypia, which falls short of DCIS. It is associated with an increased risk of subsequently developing breast cancer.
Atypical lobular epitheliosis	See atypical lobular hyperplasia	
Atypical lobular hyperplasia	Atypical lobular epitheliosis ALH	Partial involvement of the lobules by neoplastic cells with increased risk of subsequently developing carcinoma.
Atypical medullary carcinoma		Term used for a carcinoma showing some but not all the features of medullary carcinoma.
Benign mixed tumour	See pleomorphic adenoma	

Tumour terminology Recommended terms are in **bold**	Synonyms	Comments
Carcinoid tumour	See neuroendocrine carcinoma	
Carcinoma erysipelatoides	See inflammatory carcinoma	
Carcinoma in situ	In situ carcinoma Intraepithelial carcinoma Non-invasive carcinoma Pre-invasive carcinoma	May be of duct (DCIS) or of lobular (LCIS) type.
Carcinoma mastoides	See inflammatory carcinoma	Obsolete term.
Carcinoma Not Otherwise Specified (NOS)	See invasive ductal carcinoma NOS	
Carcinoma with osteoclast-like giant cells		Rare histological variant characterised by the presence of bizarre giant cells.
Carcinoma with sarcomatous features	See metaplastic carcinoma	
Carcinoma with sarcomatous metaplasia	See metaplastic carcinoma	
Carcinosarcoma	See metaplastic carcinoma	
Cellular fibroadenoma		A fibroadenoma with increased cellularity, which should be distinguished from a phyllode tumour.
Chondrolipoma		See Tumours of Soft Tissue (Section 42).
Clinging carcinoma	Flat micropapillary DCIS	Histological variant of DCIS.
Colloid carcinoma	See mucinous carcinoma	
Combined carcinoma	See mixed carcinoma	
Comedo carcinoma	See carcinoma in situ	
Comedo carcinoma in situ	Comedo carcinoma	Histological variant of DCIS.
Complex sclerosing lesion	See radial scar	
Cribriform carcinoma	See invasive cribriform carcinoma	

Tumour terminology Recommended terms are in **bold**	Synonyms	Comments
Cribriform carcinoma in situ		Histological variant of DCIS with sieve-like pattern morphologically.
Cylindroma	See adenoid cystic carcinoma	
Cystic hypersecretory carcinoma		Recently described entity characterised by numerous cysts containing eosinophilic material resembling thyroid colloid. The malignant epithelial proliferation has a papillary pattern.
Cystic hypersecretory hyperplasia		Benign counterpart of hypersecretory carcinoma.
Cystic papilloma	See duct papilloma	
Cystosarcoma phyllodes	See phyllodes tumour	
DCIS	See ductal carcinoma in situ	
DCIS with neuroendocrine differentiation		Histological variant of DCIS with neuroendocrine features.
Dermal lymphatic carcinomatosis	See inflammatory carcinoma	
Duct papilloma	Cystic papilloma Ductal cystadenoma Intraductal papilloma Intracystic papilloma Papillary cystadenoma	Benign intraductal proliferation of epithelium forming fronds overlying a fibrovascular core. It may arise centrally from a major nipple duct or it can present peripherally as multiple lesions. The latter is associated with a slight increase in malignancy.
Ductal adenoma	See duct papilloma	
Ductal carcinoma in situ (DCIS)	DCIS Intraductal carcinoma Intraductal carcinoma Non-invasive ductal carcinoma Pre-invasive ductal carcinoma	Common form of carcinoma in situ associated with a 10 times risk of progression to invasive tumour. Calcification is usually evident on mammography. It is classified according to nuclear grade into low, intermediate, and high. Architectural variants include comedo, cribriform, micropapillary, solid, signet ring, neuroendocrine, cystic hypersecretory, and clinging.
Ductal cystadenoma	See duct papilloma	
Ductal invasive carcinoma	Invasive carcinoma NOS	

Tumour terminology Recommended terms are in **bold**	Synonyms	Comments
Erosive adenomatosis of the nipple	See adenoma of the nipple	
Fibroadenoma	Adenofibroma Fibroadenomatous tumour Giant fibroadenoma (obsolete)	This is the most common benign breast tumour in young women. It is composed of fibrous and epithelial elements. Intracanalicular, pericanalicular, and tubular variants are recognised.
Fibroadenomatous tumour	See fibroadenoma	
Flat micropapillary DCIS	Clinging carcinoma	
Florid papillomatosis of the nipple	See adenoma of the nipple	
Galactocoele		Benign cyst containing inspissated milk.
Gelatinous carcinoma	See mucinous carcinoma	
Giant fibroadenoma	See fibroadenoma	Obsolete term used to describe both large fibroadenomas and benign phyllodes tumour.
Glycogen rich carcinoma		A rare form of clear cell carcinoma due to accumulation of glycogen in the cytoplasm. Prognosis is similar to or worse than ductal carcinoma of no special type.
Granular cell myoblastoma	See granular cell tumour	
Granular cell tumour	Granular cell myoblastoma	See Tumours of Soft Tissue (Section 42).
Gynaecomastia		Most common cause of benign enlargement of the male breast, associated with hormonal imbalance, drugs, or after systemic disease.
Haemangioma		See Tumours of Soft Tissue (Section 42).
Haemangiosarcoma	See angiosarcoma	
Histiocytoid carcinoma		A rare histological variant of invasive lobular carcinoma.
In situ carcinoma	See carcinoma in situ	
Indurative mastopathy	See radial scar	

Tumour terminology Recommended terms are in **bold**	Synonyms	Comments
Infiltrating carcinoma	See invasive carcinoma	
Infiltrating epitheliosis	See radial scar	
Infiltrating lobular carcinoma	See invasive lobular carcinoma	
Inflammatory cancer	See inflammatory carcinoma	
Inflammatory carcinoma	Acute mammary carcinomatosis (obsolete) Carcinoma erysipelatoides Carcinoma mastoides (obsolete) Dermal lymphatic carcinomatosis Inflammatory cancer Mastitis carcinomatosa (obsolete)	A descriptive clinical term, which describes the cutaneous erythema overlying the cancer, usually of high grade morphology.
Intracanalicular fibroadenoma	See fibroadenoma	
Intracystic papillary carcinoma	Papillary carcinoma in situ	Non-invasive papillary carcinoma within a cystic space.
Intracystic papilloma	See duct papilloma	
Intraductal carcinoma	See ductal carcinoma in situ	
Intraductal carcinoma	See ductal carcinoma in situ	
Intraductal papilloma	See duct papilloma	
Intraepithelial carcinoma	See carcinoma in situ	
Intralobular carcinoma	See lobular carcinoma in situ	
Invasive comedo carcinoma	See invasive ductal carcinoma with comedo pattern	
Invasive cribriform carcinoma	Invasive ductal carcinoma with cribriform pattern	Histological variant of invasive ductal carcinoma with a cribriform (sieve-like) pattern.

Tumour terminology Recommended terms are in **bold**	Synonyms	Comments
Invasive ductal carcinoma of no special type (NST)	Invasive ductal carcinoma	This is the most common variant of invasive breast cancer. By definition there are no specific morphological features to qualify for a particular category.
Invasive ductal carcinoma with comedo pattern	Invasive comedo carcinoma	Histological variant of invasive ductal carcinoma with necrosis resembling comedo DCIS.
Invasive epitheliosis	See radial scar	
Invasive lobular carcinoma	Infiltrating lobular carcinoma Lobular invasive carcinoma	The second most common cancer after ductal carcinoma. It has an increased tendency to bilaterality. Variants include classical, solid, alveolar, pleomorphic, and tubulolobular.
Invasive mixed carcinoma	See mixed carcinoma	
Invasive papillary carcinoma	Papillary carcinoma	A rare carcinoma whose invasive pattern is predominantly papillary. It has favourable prognosis when compared to ductal carcinoma NST.
Invasive tubulolobular carcinoma		Histological variant of lobular carcinoma with a tubular component. It has favourable prognosis.
Juvenile carcinoma	See secretory carcinoma	Obsolete term.
Juvenile fibroadenoma	See fibroadenoma	
Juvenile papillomatosis		A benign condition affecting young women consisting of cysts and duct hyperplasia with apocrine metaplasia. There is a slight increased risk of developing carcinoma in patients with juvenile papillomatosis.
Lactating adenoma		A tubular adenoma with evidence of milk secretion occurring during pregnancy and lactation.
LCIS	See lobular carcinoma in situ	
Lipid rich carcinoma		A rare variant of clear cell carcinoma due to lipid accumulation in the cytoplasm. Very few patients have been studied for accurate prognostication.

Tumour terminology Recommended terms are in **bold**	Synonyms	Comments
Lobular carcinoma	See invasive lobular carcinoma	
Lobular carcinoma in situ	LCIS Lobular neoplasia	In situ carcinoma, which differs from atypical lobular hyperplasia by complete involvement of the lobule.
Lobular invasive carcinoma	See invasive lobular carcinoma	
Lobular neoplasia		A collective term used when atypical lobular hyperplasia cannot be distinguished from lobular carcinoma in situ.
Mastitis carcinomatosa	See inflammatory carcinoma	Obsolete term.
Medullary carcinoma		A high grade variant of invasive ductal carcinoma. Some believe it to have a favourable prognosis.
Metaplastic carcinoma	Carcinoma with sarcomatous features Carcinoma with sarcomatous metaplasia Carcinosarcoma Sarcomatoid carcinoma Spindle cell carcinoma	A very rare high grade variant of invasive ductal carcinoma combining epithelial and malignant mesenchymal elements. Squamous cell elements can also be present.
Microcystic adnexal carcinoma	See syringomatous adenoma of the nipple	
Microglandular adenosis		Benign glandular proliferation, which may be confused with carcinoma.
Microinvasive carcinoma		An invasive carcinoma, which measures 1 mm or less in diameter, associated with ductal carcinoma in situ.
Micropapillary carcinoma in situ		Histological variant of ductal carcinoma in situ.
Mixed ductal and lobular carcinoma	See mixed carcinoma	
Mixed invasive carcinoma	Combined carcinoma Mixed ductal and lobular carcinoma	An invasive carcinoma composed of two morphological types that constitute 10% of the tumour mass.
Mucinous carcinoma	Colloid carcinoma Gelatinous carcinoma Mucoid carcinoma Mucous carcinoma	A histological variant of invasive ductal carcinoma characterised by an abundant mucinous secretion.

Tumour terminology Recommended terms are in **bold**	Synonyms	Comments
Mucocele-like lesion	See mucocele-like tumour	
Mucocele-like tumour	Mucocele-like lesion	A benign tumour-like lesion consisting of ducts filled with mucin similar to the salivary gland mucocele.
Mucoepidermoid carcinoma		A rare histological variant of breast cancer combining mucous-secreting and squamous epithelial elements.
Mucoid carcinoma	See mucinous carcinoma	
Mucous carcinoma	See mucinous carcinoma	
Multiple papillomas		Multiple intraductal papillomas usually arising at the periphery of the breast.
Myoepithelioma		A benign tumour composed of predominantly myoepithelial cells. Malignant transformation is rare.
Neuroendocrine carcinoma	Carcinoid tumour	Primary carcinoma of the breast with morphological and immunohistochemical properties similar to neuroendocrine carcinoma of the gastrointestinal tract. Prognosis similar to invasive ductal carcinoma NST.
Nodular adenosis	See adenosis tumour	
Non-invasive carcinoma	See carcinoma in situ	
Non-invasive ductal carcinoma	See ductal carcinoma in situ	
Non-encapsulated sclerosing lesion	See radial scar	
Obliterative mastopathy	See radial scar	
Oncocytic carcinoma	See apocrine carcinoma	
Paget's disease of the nipple		Intraepidermal spread from an underlying ductal carcinoma in situ presenting as an eczema-like lesion.
Papillary carcinoma	See invasive papillary carcinoma	
Papillary carcinoma in situ	See intracystic papillary carcinoma	
Papillary cystadenoma	See duct papilloma	

Tumour terminology Recommended terms are in **bold**	Synonyms	Comments
Pericanalicular fibroadenoma	See fibroadenoma	
Periductal sarcoma	See phyllodes tumour	Obsolete term.
Phyllodes tumour	Cystosarcoma phyllodes Periductal sarcoma (obsolete)	A fibroepithelial tumour with a leaf-like gross appearance, which differs from fibroadenoma by the cellular stroma. It may be classified as benign, borderline, or malignant depending on the mitotic activity and degree of cellularity.
Pleomorphic adenoma	Adenoma pleomorphic Benign mixed tumour	Benign tumour analogous to that of the salivary gland.
Post-mastectomy angiosarcoma	See angiosarcoma	
Pre-invasive carcinoma	See carcinoma in situ	
Pre-invasive ductal carcinoma	See ductal carcinoma in situ	
Pseudoangiomatous hyperplasia of the mammary stroma		A benign interlobular stromal proliferation mimicking angiosarcoma.
Pure adenoma	See tubular adenoma	
Radial scar	Complex sclerosing lesion Indurative mastopathy Infiltrating epitheliosis Invasive epitheliosis Non-encapsulated sclerosing lesion Obliterative mastopathy Radial sclerosing lesion Rosette-like lesion Scleroelastic lesion Sclerosing papillary proliferation Sclerosing papillomatosis	A benign stellate lesion consisting of central fibroelastosis with surrounding epithelial proliferative elements. Mammographically indistinguishable from a stellate cancer.
Radial sclerosing lesion	See radial scar	
Rosette-like lesion	See radial scar	

Tumour terminology Recommended terms are in **bold**	Synonyms	Comments
Sarcomatoid carcinoma	See metaplastic carcinoma	
Scleroelastic lesion	See radial scar	
Sclerosing papillary proliferation	See radial scar	
Sclerosing papillomatosis	See radial scar	
Secretory carcinoma	Juvenile carcinoma (obsolete)	Rare histological variant of in situ or invasive ductal carcinoma characterised by eosinophilic secretions in microcystic spaces. Children are more often affected but this variant can also present in adults. It has a favourable prognosis.
Signet ring carcinoma		An extremely rare variant of breast cancer. Occasional signet ring cells may be found in both invasive lobular and mucinous carcinomas.
Spindle cell carcinoma	See metaplastic carcinoma	
Squamous cell carcinoma		An extremely rare variant of breast cancer.
Stewart-Treves syndrome	See angiosarcoma	
Subareolar papillomatosis	See adenoma of the nipple	
Sweat gland carcinoma	See apocrine carcinoma	
Syringomatous adenoma of the nipple	Microcystic adnexal carcinoma	A rare locally infiltrating tumour of the nipple.
Tubular adenoma	Pure adenoma	A rare benign tumour composed of uniform tubular structures. It may represent a variant of fibroadenoma.
Tubular carcinoma	Well differentiated carcinoma	A well differentiated carcinoma composed of tubular structures lined by a single layer of epithelium. Associated with a good prognosis.
Tubular fibroadenoma	See fibroadenoma	
Tubulolobular carcinoma		Histological variant of invasive lobular carcinoma composed of tubular and lobular components.

Tumour terminology Recommended terms are in **bold**	Synonyms	Comments
Tumoural adenosis	See adenosis tumour	
Well differentiated carcinoma	See tubular carcinoma	

Section 40

Tumours of Skin (Melanocytic)

J. Sugar
P.H. McKee

Tumour terminology Recommended terms are in **bold**	Synonyms	Comments
Acquired melanocytic naevus	See melanocytic naevus	
Acral lentiginous melanoma	Plantar lentiginous melanoma	Rare in Caucasians. Presents on the palms, soles, and under the nails.
Agminate Spitz naevi	Disseminated Spitz naevi Multiple Spitz naevi	A rare condition characterised by the development of multiple lesions following trauma or previous excision of a solitary Spitz naevus.
Amelanotic malignant melanoma	See amelanotic melanoma	
Amelanotic melanoma	Amelanotic malignant melanoma	Rare variant of melanoma in which pigment is absent.
Atypical mole syndrome	See dysplastic naevus syndrome	
Atypical naevus	See dysplastic naevus	
Atypical Spitz naevus		A histological variant of Spitz naevus with worrying features and uncertain biological potential.
Balloon cell melanoma		Rare histological variant of melanoma with a propensity for skin metastases.
Balloon cell naevus		Rare histological variant of melanocytic naevus.
Bathing trunk naevus	See congenital melanocytic naevus	
Becker's melanosis	See Becker's naevus	

Tumour terminology Recommended terms are in **bold**	Synonyms	Comments
Becker's naevus	Becker's melanosis Becker's pigmentary hamartoma Pigmented hairy epidermal naevus	Organoid hamartoma of childhood and adolescents sometimes complicated by hypertrichosis.
Becker's pigmentary hamartoma	See Becker's naevus	
B-K mole syndrome	See dysplastic naevus syndrome	
Blue naevus	See common blue naevus	
Café-au-lait macules		Variant of lentigo. When multiple may be associated with systemic disease including neurofibromatosis, tuberous sclerosis, and fibrous dysplasia.
CAMS	See dysplastic naevus syndrome	
Cellular blue naevus		Rare variant of blue naevus presenting on the buttocks or around the sacrococcygeal region.
Clark's naevus	See dysplastic naevus	
Clark's naevus syndrome	See dysplastic naevus syndrome	
Classic atypical mole syndrome	See dysplastic naevus syndrome	
Cocarde naevus (Fr)	Cockade naevus (UK)	Rare variant of melanocytic naevus.
Cockade naevus	See cocarde naevus	
Combined naevus		Histological variant of melanocytic naevus combining junctional, compound, or intradermal elements with a blue naevus. Rarely the melanocytic naevus may be combined with a deep penetrating naevus.
Common acquired melanocytic naevus	See melanocytic naevus	
Common blue naevus	Blue naevus Ordinary blue naevus	Variant of intradermal naevus most often presenting on the face or the backs of the hands. Composed of dendritic cells.

Tumour terminology Recommended terms are in **bold**	Synonyms	Comments
Common melanocytic naevus	See melanocytic naevus	
Complex naevus	See compound naevus	Obsolete term.
Compound naevus	Complex naevus (obsolete)	Histological variant of melanocytic naevus, combining junctional and intradermal elements.
Congenital acral melanocytic naevus		Exceedingly rare variant of congenital melanocytic naevus, which may be clinically mistaken for melanoma.
Congenital malignant melanoma	See congenital melanoma	
Congenital melanocytic naevus	Bathing trunk naevus Garment naevus Giant hairy naevus	Relatively common lesion. Giant variants, e.g., bathing trunk naevus, have a high risk of malignant transformation (up to 10%).
Congenital melanoma	Congenital malignant melanoma	This is an exceedingly rare condition. The melanoma may arise in a congenital melanocytic naevus.
Congenital oculodermal melanocytosis	See naevus of Ota	
Deep penetrating naevus	Plexiform spindle cell naevus	Rare histological variant of melanocytic naevus. Clinically may be confused with melanoma.
Desmoplastic melanoma		Rare variant of melanoma characterised by a dense fibrous component. Recurrences are particularly common due to difficulties with primary excision.
Desmoplastic Spitz naevus	Sclerosing Spitz naevus	Rare histological variant of Spitz naevus characterised by a dense fibrous stroma.
Disseminated Spitz naevi	See agminate Spitz naevi	
Dysplastic naevus	Atypical naevus Clark's naevus Naevus with architectural and cytological disorder	Clinically atypical variant of melanocytic naevus with variable dysplasia. The sporadic variant has only a very slightly increased risk of developing melanoma.

Tumour terminology Recommended terms are in **bold**	Synonyms	Comments
Dysplastic naevus syndrome	Atypical mole syndrome B-K mole syndrome CAMS Clark's naevus syndrome Classic atypical mole syndrome Familial atypical mole and melanoma syndrome FAMMM syndrome Large atypical naevus syndrome	Genetic disorder characterised by clinically atypical naevi and a high risk of developing melanoma.
Ephelis	Freckle	Not a tumour. A common condition associated with sun exposure. Large numbers may predict an increased risk of developing melanoma.
Familial atypical mole and melanoma syndrome	See dysplastic naevus syndrome	
FAMMM syndrome	See dysplastic naevus syndrome	
Freckle	See ephelis	
Garment naevus	See congenital melanocytic naevus	
Giant hairy naevus	See congenital melanocytic naevus	
Halo naevus	Leukoderma acquisitum centrifugum (obsolete) Perinaevoid leukoderma Sutton's naevus	Melanocytic naevus surrounded by a white depigmented band (halo) on the skin.
Hutchinson's freckle	See lentigo maligna	
Hutchinson's melanotic freckle	See lentigo maligna	
In situ malignant melanoma	See radial growth phase melanoma	
Intradermal melanoma		Exceedingly rare variant of melanoma. The possibility of metastases must always be excluded.

Tumour terminology Recommended terms are in **bold**	Synonyms	Comments
Intradermal naevus		Histological variant of melanocytic naevus.
Intraepidermal melanoma	See radial growth phase melanoma	
Junctional naevus		Histological variant of melanocytic naevus.
Juvenile melanoma	See Spitz naevus	
Large atypical naevus syndrome	See dysplastic naevus syndrome	
Lentiginous naevus	Naevoid lentigo	Histological variant of junctional naevus.
Lentigo maligna	Hutchinson's freckle Hutchinson's melanotic freckle Precancerous melanosis of Dubreuilh	Precursor lesion of lentigo maligna melanoma.
Lentigo maligna melanoma	Melanoma arising in Hutchinson's melanotic freckle (obsolete) Melanoma arising in pre-cancerous melanosis of Dubreuilh (obsolete)	Variant of melanoma arising on sun damaged skin particularly of the face.
Lentigo senilis	See solar lentigo	
Lentigo simplex		Common non-tumourous lesion. If present in large numbers may be associated with systemic disease including Peutz-Jeghers', Leopard, and Carney's syndromes.
Leptomeningeal melanocytic lesion	See neurocutaneous melanosis	
Leukoderma acquisitum centrifugum	See halo naevus	Obsolete term.
Liver spot	See solar lentigo	
Malignant blue naevus		Extremely rare variant of melanoma.
Malignant melanoma	See melanoma	
Malignant melanoma in situ	See radial growth phase melanoma	
Melanocarcinoma	See melanoma	Obsolete term.

Tumour terminology Recommended terms are in **bold**	Synonyms	Comments
Melanocytic naevus	Acquired melanocytic naevus Common acquired melanocytic naevus Common melanocytic naevus Naevocellular naevus	Common benign proliferative lesions of melanocytes, which present as pigmented macules, papules, and nodules. Occasionally they may have a warty appearance.
Melanoma	Malignant melanoma Melanocarcinoma (obsolete) Melanosarcoma (obsolete)	A malignant tumour of melanocytes. Most tumours arise as a consequence of excessive exposure to sunlight.
Melanoma arising in Hutchinson's melanotic freckle	See lentigo maligna melanoma	Obsolete term.
Melanoma arising in pre-cancerous melanosis of Dubreuilh	See lentigo maligna melanoma	Obsolete term.
Melanoma in situ	See radial growth phase melanoma	
Melanoma of nail apparatus	See subungual melanoma	
Melanosarcoma	See melanoma	Obsolete term.
Microinvasive radial growth phase melanoma		Rare variant of melanoma showing very early invasion of upper dermis. It is thought to be associated with an excellent prognosis.
Minimal deviation melanoma		Rare histological variant of melanoma, which may be confused with a benign melanocytic lesion. Its biological behaviour is unpredictable.
Mongolian spot		Developmental abnormality characterised by a bluish lesion on the lumbosacral region.
Mucocutaneous melanoma	See primary mucosal melanoma	
Mucosal lentiginous melanoma	See primary mucosal melanoma	
Multiple Spitz naevi	See agminate Spitz naevi	

Tumour terminology Recommended terms are in **bold**	Synonyms	Comments
Myxoid melanoma		Rare histological variant of melanoma with myxoid stroma.
Naevocellular naevus	See melanocytic naevus	
Naevoid lentigo	See lentiginous naevus	
Naevus fuscocoeruleus acromiodeltoideus	See naevus of Ito	
Naevus fuscocoeruleus ophthalmomaxillaris	See naevus of Ota	
Naevus fuscocoeruleus zygomaticus	See Sun's naevus	
Naevus of Ito	Naevus fuscocoeruleus acromiodeltoideus	A hamartomatous condition presenting in the distribution of the supraclavicular and lateral branchial cutaneous nerves.
Naevus of Ota	Congenital oculodermal melanocytosis Naevus fuscocoeruleus ophthalmomaxillaris	A hamartomatous condition in the distribution of the trigeminal nerve.
Naevus spilus	Speckled lentiginous naevus	A hamartomatous condition characterised by pigmented macules presenting on a brown background.
Naevus with architectural and cytological disorder	See dysplastic naevus	
Neural naevus	Neurotised naevus	Neurotisation of a dermal naevus.
Neurocutaneous melanosis	Leptomeningeal melanocytic lesion	Rare melanocytic lesion localised to the cranial and/or spinal leptomeninges.
Neurotised naevus	See neural naevus	
Neurotropic melanoma		Histological variant of desmoplastic melanoma, which characteristically spreads along nerves.
Nodular melanoma		This tumour accounts for 10–15% of melanomas.
Non-pigmented spindle and epithelioid cell naevus	See Spitz naevus	
Non-pigmented spindle and/or epithelial cell naevus in children	See Spitz naevus	

Tumour terminology Recommended terms are in **bold**	Synonyms	Comments
Ordinary blue naevus	See common blue naevus	
Pagetoid melanoma	See superficial spreading melanoma	
Perinaevoid leukoderma	See halo naevus	
Pigmented hairy epidermal naevus	See Becker's naevus	
Pigmented spindle cell naevus	Pigmented spindle cell tumour of Reed Reed's naevus	Uncommon pigmented lesion, which predominantly affects young females. Frequently is clinically confused with melanoma.
Pigmented spindle cell tumour of Reed	See pigmented spindle cell naevus	
Plantar lentiginous melanoma	See acral lentiginous melanoma	
Plexiform spindle cell naevus	See deep penetrating naevus	
Precancerous melanosis of Dubreuilh	See lentigo maligna	
Pre-malignant melanoma	See radial growth phase melanoma	
Primary mucosal melanoma	Mucocutaneous melanoma Mucosal lentiginous melanoma	A high grade melanoma associated with a very poor prognosis.
Pseudomelanoma	See recurrent melanocytic naevus	
Radial growth phase melanoma	In situ malignant melanoma Intraepidermal melanoma Malignant melanoma in situ Melanoma in situ Pre-malignant melanoma	Melanoma restricted to the epidermis. Complete excision is curative.

Tumour terminology Recommended terms are in **bold**	Synonyms	Comments
Recurrent melanocytic naevus	Pseudomelanoma	This lesion may follow an incompletely excised benign melanocytic naevus. It is important in that it is sometimes confused with melanoma.
Reed's naevus	See pigmented spindle cell naevus	
Sclerosing Spitz naevus	See desmoplastic Spitz naevus	
Small cell melanoma		A histological variant of melanoma with a poor prognosis.
Solar lentigo	Lentigo senilis Liver spot	A benign pigmented macule, which occurs in older individuals on sun-exposed skin.
Speckled lentiginous naevus	See naevus spilus	
Spindle and epithelioid cell naevus	See Spitz naevus	
Spitz naevus	Juvenile melanoma Non-pigmented spindle and epithelioid cell naevus Non-pigmented spindle and/or epithelioid cell naevus in children Spindle and epithelioid cell naevus Spitz tumour	A benign variant of melanocytic naevus, which may be histologically misdiagnosed as melanoma. It most commonly affects children.
Spitz tumour	See Spitz naevus	
Spitzoid melanoma		A rare variant of minimal deviation melanoma, which histologically resembles Spitz naevus. Its biological potential is uncertain.
Sporadic dysplastic naevus		A dysplastic naevus arising in the absence of a family history of dysplastic naevus syndrome. There is a very low risk of developing melanoma.
Subungual melanoma	Melanoma of nail apparatus	A melanoma arising underneath the nail. The prognosis is usually poor.

Tumour terminology Recommended terms are in **bold**	Synonyms	Comments
Sun's naevus	Naevus fuscocoeruleus zygomaticus	A hamartomatous condition presenting in Chinese persons.
Superficial spreading melanoma	Pagetoid melanoma	The most common variant of melanoma.
Sutton's naevus	See halo naevus	
Verrucous keratotic melanoma	See verrucous pseudonaevoid melanoma	
Verrucous pseudonaevoid melanoma	Verrucous keratotic melanoma	A rare variant of minimal deviation melanoma, which histologically resembles a melanocytic naevus. Its biological potential is uncertain.
Vertical growth phase melanoma		Invasive melanoma characterised by a cohesive aggregate of cells in the dermis.

Section 41

Tumours of Skin (Non-Melanocytic)

S.S. Seopela
P.H. McKee

Tumour terminology Recommended terms are in **bold**	Synonyms	Comments
Acantholytic acanthoma		Tumour-like lesion of no clinical significance.
Acanthoma		A benign proliferation of squamous epithelium, which may present clinically as a tumour-like nodule.
Acanthoma fissuratum	Spectacle frame acanthoma	Tumour-like lesion, which may be clinically mistaken for a basal cell or squamous cell carcinoma.
Achrochordon	See fibroepithelial polyp	
Acquired digital fibrokeratoma	Fibrokeratoma	Tumour-like lesion, which may be confused with a supernumerary digit.
Acquired progressive lymphangioma	Benign lymphangioendothelioma	This rare, acquired benign lymphatic tumour, predominantly affects children and most often presents on the limbs.
Acral arteriovenous tumour	See arteriovenous haemangioma	
Acrosyringeal naevus	See eccrine syringofibroadenoma	
Actinic keratosis	Keratosis senilis Senile keratosis Solar keratosis	Pre-malignant lesion of epidermis due to excessive exposure to sunlight.
Adenoid cystic carcinoma	Adenoid cystic eccrine carcinoma	Rare locally aggressive tumour. Usually occurs on scalp or chest. Recurrences are common. Very rarely metastasises.

Tumour terminology Recommended terms are in **bold**	Synonyms	Comments
Adenoid cystic eccrine carcinoma	See adenoid cystic carcinoma	
Adenosquamous carcinoma	See mucoepidermoid carcinoma	
Aggressive digital papillary adenocarcinoma	Aggressive digital papillary adenoma	Rare eccrine sweat gland tumour. Often presents on extremities. High recurrence rate (50%). Commonly metastasises (40%).
Aggressive digital papillary adenoma	See aggressive digital papillary adenocarcinoma	
Aggressive pilomatrixoma	See pilomatrix carcinoma	
Amputation neuroma	See traumatic neuroma	
Anaplastic syringoma	See eccrine ductal carcinoma	
Ancell-Spiegler syndrome	Turban tumour syndrome	Rare disfiguring condition characterised by multiple cylindromas on the head and neck.
Ancient schwannoma		See Tumours of Soft Tissue (Section 42).
Aneurysmal benign fibrous histiocytoma		Variant of fibrous histiocytoma in which blood-filled lakes may result in confusion with a vascular tumour.
Angioblastoma of Nakagawa	See tufted angioma	
Angioendotheliosis	Reactive angioendotheliosis	Reactive vascular proliferation, which may complicate endocarditis, cryoglobulinaemia, or be idiopathic.
Angiofibroma		Tumour-like lesion associated with tuberous sclerosis.
Angiokeratoma		Superficial vascular ectasia. May be associated with Anderson-Fabry's disease.
Angioleiomyoma		See Tumours of Soft Tissue (Section 42).
Angiolipoma		See Tumours of Soft Tissue (Section 42).
Angiolymphoid hyperplasia with eosinophilia	See epithelioid haemangioma	
Angioma	See haemangioma	

Tumour terminology Recommended terms are in **bold**	Synonyms	Comments
Angioma serpiginosum		A unilateral vascular naevus.
Angiomatosis		See Tumours of Soft Tissue (Section 42).
Angiosarcoma	Haemangioblastoma Haemangiosarcoma Lymphangiosarcoma Malignant haemangioendothelioma	Cutaneous variants are high grade with a very poor prognosis. See Tumours of Soft Tissue (Section 42).
Apocrine carcinoma		Rare slowly progressive malignant sweat gland tumour.
Apocrine cystadenoma	Cystic apocrine adenoma	Benign cystic sweat gland tumour usually found on the head and neck.
Apocrine hidrocystoma		Benign cystic sweat gland tumour usually found on the head and neck.
Apocrine tubular adenoma	Tubular apocrine adenoma	Rare sweat gland tumour, which most often presents on the scalp.
Arsenical keratosis		Pre-malignant lesion of epidermis.
Arteriovenous haemangioma	Acral arteriovenous tumour Arteriovenous malformation Cirsoid aneurysm Racemose haemangioma Vascular malformation	See Tumours of Soft Tissue (Section 42).
Arteriovenous malformation	See arteriovenous haemangioma	
Atrophic dermatofibroma	See atrophic fibrous histiocytoma	
Atrophic fibrous histiocytoma	Atrophic dermatofibroma	Regressing or "burnt-out" fibrous histiocytoma.
Atypical benign fibrous histiocytoma	Dermatofibroma with monster cells Pseudosarcomatous benign fibrous histiocytoma	Variant of fibrous histiocytoma showing marked pleomorphism. Recurrence occurs in up to 18% of cases.
Atypical fibroxanthoma	Paradoxical fibrosarcoma Pseudosarcoma of skin	Pseudosarcomatous tumour, which arises on sun-damaged skin of the elderly. It must be distinguished from spindle cell squamous carcinoma and amelanotic melanoma.

Tumour terminology Recommended terms are in **bold**	Synonyms	Comments
Atypical intravenous vascular proliferation	See epithelioid haemangioma	
Atypical pyogenic granuloma	See epithelioid haemangioma	
Basal cell carcinoma	Basal cell epithelioma Basalioma Rodent ulcer	Most common skin cancer, which often presents on sun-damaged skin of the face. Recurrences are very common. Exceptionally rarely metastasises.
Basal cell carcinoma with sebaceous differentiation	See sebaceous epithelioma	
Basal cell epithelioma	See basal cell carcinoma	
Basal cell hamartoma with follicular differentiation	See follicular infundibulum tumour	
Basalioma	See basal cell carcinoma	
Basaloid squamous cell carcinoma		High grade histological variant of squamous cell carcinoma.
Basosebaceous epithelioma	See sebaceous epithelioma	
Bednár tumour	See pigmented dermatofibrosarcoma protuberans	
Benign cartilaginous exostosis	Osteochondroma Subungual exostosis	See Tumours of the Bone (Section 43).
Benign lymphangioendothelioma	See acquired progressive lymphangioma	
Bilateral acoustic neurofibromatosis	See neurofibromatosis 2 (NF-2)	
Birt-Hogg-Dubé syndrome		The rare association of multiple fibrofolliculomas, trichodiscomas, and fibroepithelial polyps.
Blue rubber bleb naevus syndrome		See Tumours of Soft Tissue (Section 42).
Borst-Jadassohn epithelioma	Intraepidermal epithelioma	Non-specific term implying an intraepidermal clonal proliferation, which may be benign or malignant.

Tumour terminology Recommended terms are in **bold**	Synonyms	Comments
Bowen's disease	Erythroplasia of Queyrat Morbus Bowen Squamous carcinoma in situ	Pre-malignant condition of skin and mucosa.
Bowenoid papulosis	Multicentric pigmented Bowen's disease	Warty pre-malignant condition of anogenital region due to HPV infection. Progression to invasive carcinoma is rare.
Buschke-Löwenstein tumour	See verrucous carcinoma	
Calcifying aponeurotic fibroma		See Tumours of Soft Tissue (Section 42).
Calcifying epithelioma of Malherbe	See pilomatrixoma	
Calcifying fibrous pseudotumour	Childhood fibrous tumour with psammoma bodies	See Tumours of Soft Tissue (Section 42).
Campbell de Morgan spot	See cherry angioma	
Capillary haemangioma	Infantile haemangioendothelioma Juvenile haemangioma Strawberry naevus	Common benign vascular tumour affecting infants.
Carcinoma arising in spiradenoma	See malignant eccrine spiradenoma	
Carcinoma cuniculatum	See verrucous carcinoma	
Carcinoma simplex	See eccrine ductal carcinoma	
Carcinosarcoma	See metaplastic carcinoma	
Cavernous haemangioma		See Tumours of Soft Tissue (Section 42).
Cavernous lymphangioma	Cystic hygroma	See Tumours of Soft Tissue (Section 42).
Cellular benign fibrous histiocytoma		Histological variant of fibrous histiocytoma, which may be confused with a sarcoma. Recurrences are common.

Tumour terminology Recommended terms are in **bold**	Synonyms	Comments
Cellular neurothekeoma		See Tumours of Soft Tissue (Section 42).
Cellular schwannoma		See Tumours of Soft Tissue (Section 42).
Cherry angioma	Campbell de Morgan spot Senile angioma	Small benign cutaneous haemangioma most often affecting the elderly.
Childhood fibrous tumour with psammoma bodies	See calcifying fibrous pseudotumour	
Chondroid lipoma		See Tumours of Soft Tissue (Section 42).
Chondroid syringoma	Mixed tumour of the skin	Slowly growing eccrine sweat gland tumour.
Circumscribed storiform collagenoma	See storiform collagenoma	
Cirsoid aneurysm	See arteriovenous haemangioma	
Classic eccrine carcinoma	See eccrine ductal carcinoma	
Clear cell acanthoma	Degos' acanthoma	Tumour-like lesion most often presenting on the leg.
Clear cell hidradenocarcinoma	See eccrine hidradenocarcinoma	
Clear cell hidradenoma	See eccrine hidradenoma	
Collagenoma	See storiform collagenoma	
Condyloma acuminatum	Genital wart	Viral wart of the anogenital region. Types 16, 18, and 33 are associated with a significant risk of squamous cell carcinoma.
Congenital smooth muscle hamartoma		Rare, usually hair-bearing cutaneous malformation in infants.
Congenital vellus hamartoma	See hair follicle naevus	
Cornu cutaneum	See cutaneous horn	
Cranial fasciitis	Paraosteal fasciitis Periosteal fasciitis	See Tumours of Soft Tissue (Section 42).
Cutaneous adenocystic carcinoma	See mucinous carcinoma	

Tumour terminology Recommended terms are in **bold**	Synonyms	Comments
Cutaneous horn	Cornu cutaneum	A large protuberant mass of keratin, which may complicate a number of skin tumours.
Cutaneous leiomyoma	See pilar leiomyoma	
Cutaneous meningioma		Extremely rare. Represents invasion or metastasis from intracranial meningioma.
Cutaneous myxoid cyst	See digital myxoma	
Cystic apocrine adenoma	See apocrine cystadenoma	
Cystic hygroma	See cavernous lymphangioma	
Dabska's tumour	See malignant endovascular papillary angioendothelioma	
Degos' acanthoma	See clear cell acanthoma	
Dermal cylindroma	Turban tumour	Common benign sweat gland tumour.
Dermal duct tumour	Intradermal eccrine poroma	Benign eccrine sweat gland tumour.
Dermal nerve sheath myxoma	Neurothekeoma	See Tumours of Soft Tissue (Section 42).
Dermatofibroma	See fibrous histiocytoma	
Dermatofibroma with monster cells	See atypical benign fibrous histiocytoma	
Dermatofibrosarcoma protuberans		Low grade tumour of fibroblasts. Recurrences are very common but metastases are extremely rare.
Dermatomyofibroma		Benign tumour of myofibroblasts.
Dermatosis papulosa nigra		Seborrhoeic wart-like lesions, which occur in adult Afro-Caribbeans.
Desmoplastic trichoepithelioma	Sclerosing epithelial hamartoma	A rare benign hair follicle tumour. Most often presents on the face.
Diffuse neurofibroma		See Tumours of Soft Tissue (Section 42).
Digital myxoma	Cutaneous myxoid cyst Myxoma	Myxoid tumour presenting most often on the fingers. Recurrences are common.
Digital pacinian neuroma		Cutaneous variant of traumatic neuroma.

Tumour terminology Recommended terms are in **bold**	Synonyms	Comments
Ductal eccrine carcinoma	See eccrine ductal carcinoma	
Dupuytren's contracture	See palmar fibromatosis	
Dupuytren's disease	See palmar fibromatosis	
Eccrine acrospiroma	See eccrine hidradenoma	
Eccrine ductal carcinoma	Anaplastic syringoma Carcinoma simplex Classic eccrine carcinoma Ductal eccrine carcinoma	Rare high grade sweat gland tumour. Must be distinguished from metastatic carcinoma.
Eccrine epithelioma	Malignant syringoma Syringoid carcinoma Syringomatous carcinoma	Rare low grade malignant sweat gland tumour. Overlaps with microcystic adnexal carcinoma.
Eccrine hidradenocarcinoma	Clear cell hidradenocarcinoma Malignant acrospiroma	Extremely rare sweat gland carcinoma. Behaviour variable.
Eccrine hidradenoma	Clear cell hidradenoma Eccrine acrospiroma Nodular hidradenoma Solid-cystic hidradenoma	Benign sweat gland tumour.
Eccrine hidrocystoma		Tumour-like lesion. Most often presents on the face.
Eccrine porocarcinoma	Malignant eccrine poroma Porocarcinoma	Rare sweat gland tumour. Most often arises on the leg, especially the foot.
Eccrine poroma		Benign sweat gland tumour. Most often presents on the foot.
Eccrine spiradenoma		Frequently tender or painful sweat gland tumour.
Eccrine syringofibroadenoma	Acrosyringeal naevus	Very rare sweat gland tumour. May be associated with hidrotic ectodermal dysplasia.
Eccrine syringoma		Benign sweat gland tumour, commonly multiple. The eyelids and cheeks are often affected.

Tumour terminology Recommended terms are in **bold**	Synonyms	Comments
Ectasia		A general term for dilated blood vessels.
Ectopic meningothelial hamartoma	Meningeal heterotopia Sequestered meningocoele	See Tumours of Soft Tissue (Section 42).
Elastofibroma		See Tumours of Soft Tissue (Section 42).
Endovascular papillary angioendothelioma	See malignant endovascular papillary angioendothelioma	
Epidermoid carcinoma	See squamous cell carcinoma	
Epidermolytic acanthoma		Very rare tumour-like lesion.
Epithelioid angiosarcoma		See Tumours of Soft Tissue (Section 42).
Epithelioid benign fibrous histiocytoma		Rare variant of fibrous histiocytoma. May be confused with a melanocytic tumour.
Epithelioid haemangioendothelioma		See Tumours of Soft Tissue (Section 42).
Epithelioid haemangioma	Angiolymphoid hyperplasia with eosinophilia Atypical intravenous vascular proliferation Atypical pyogenic granuloma Histiocytoid haemangioma Inflammatory angiomatous nodule Intravenous atypical vascular proliferation Papular angiodysplasia Pseudopyogenic granuloma	See Tumours of Soft Tissue (Section 42).
Epithelioid malignant peripheral nerve sheath tumour		See Tumours of Soft Tissue (Section 42).
Epithelioid sarcoma		See Tumours of Soft Tissue (Section 42).

Tumour terminology Recommended terms are in **bold**	Synonyms	Comments
Epithelioma adenoides cysticum [Brooke]		Autosomal dominant condition characterised by multiple trichoepitheliomas.
Erythroplasia of Queyrat	See Bowen's disease	
Extramammary Paget's disease		Intraepidermal carcinoma, which sometimes represents a primary tumour of the sweat duct. It may develop as a consequence of spread from an underlying sweat gland carcinoma or represent an epidermotropic metastasis.
Extraneural perineurioma	See perineurioma	
Extraosseous Ewing's sarcoma	See malignant peripheral primitive neuroectodermal tumour	
Extrarenal rhabdoid tumour		See Tumours of Soft Tissue (Section 42).
Fasciitis	See nodular fasciitis	
Fasciitis ossificans	Fibro-osseous pseudotumour Florid reactive periostitis	See Tumours of Soft Tissue (Section 42).
Faun-tail	See hair follicle naevus	
Ferguson-Smith syndrome		Autosomal dominant condition characterised by multiple keratoacanthomas.
Fibroepithelial polyp	Achrochordon Skin tag Soft fibroma	Extremely common tumour-like lesion.
Fibrofolliculoma		Hair follicle hamartoma. Most often presents on the face.
Fibrokeratoma	See acquired digital fibrokeratoma	
Fibrolipomatous hamartoma of nerve	Perineural fibrolipoma	See Tumours of Soft Tissue (Section 42).
Fibro-osseous pseudotumour	See fasciitis ossificans	
Fibrous hamartoma of infancy		See Tumours of Soft Tissue (Section 42).

Tumour terminology Recommended terms are in **bold**	Synonyms	Comments
Fibrous histiocytoma	Dermatofibroma Histiocytoma cutis Nodular subepidermal fibrosis Sclerosing haemangioma	A large group of tumours the component cells of which often resemble fibroblasts and histiocytes (see specific subtypes).
Florid reactive periostitis	See fasciitis ossificans	
Follicular infundibulum tumour	Basal cell hamartoma with follicular differentiation Infundibuloma	Rare benign tumour of hair follicle. Most often presents on the head and neck.
Generalised eruptive keratoacanthoma of Grzybowski		Multiple (usually hundreds) Keratoacanthomas.
Genital wart	See condyloma acuminatum	
Giant cell fibroblastoma		See Tumours of Soft Tissue (Section 42).
Giant cell tumour of tendon sheath		See Tumours of Soft Tissue (Section 42).
Giant solitary trichoepithelioma	Subcutaneous trichoepithelioma Trichoblastic fibroma	Variant of trichoepithelioma.
Glial heterotopia	Nasal glioma	See Tumours of Soft Tissue (Section 42).
Glomangioma		See Tumours of Soft Tissue (Section 42).
Glomangiomyoma		See Tumours of Soft Tissue (Section 42)
Glomeruloid haemangioma		See Tumours of Soft Tissue (Section 42).
Glomus tumour		See Tumours of Soft Tissue (Section 42).
Granular cell myoblastoma	See granular cell tumour	
Granular cell tumour	Granular cell myoblastoma	See Tumours of Soft Tissue (Section 42).
Granuloma gravidarum	See lobular capillary haemangioma	
Granuloma pyogenicum	See lobular capillary haemangioma	

Tumour terminology Recommended terms are in **bold**	Synonyms	Comments
Haemangioblastoma	See angiosarcoma	
Haemangioma	Angioma	A general term for a benign blood vessel tumour. See Tumours of Soft Tissue (Section 42).
Haemangiosarcoma	See angiosarcoma	
Hair follicle naevus	Congenital vellus hamartoma "Faun-tail"	Hamartomatous condition of hairs. May overly spina bifida.
Hair matrix adenoma	See trichoblastoma	
Hereditary haemorrhagic telangiectasia	See Osler-Weber-Rendu syndrome	
Hibernoma		See Tumours of Soft Tissue (Section 42).
Hidradenoma papilliferum		Benign apocrine sweat gland tumour occurring in females. The vulva is the most common site.
Hidroacanthoma simplex	Intraepidermal eccrine poroma	Benign intraepidermal sweat gland tumour.
Histiocytoid haemangioma	See epithelioid haemangioma	
Histiocytoma cutis	See fibrous histiocytoma	
Hobnail haemangioma	Targetoid haemosiderotic haemangioma	See Tumours of Soft Tissue (Section 42).
Immature trichoepithelioma	See trichoblastoma	
Inclusion body fibromatosis	Infantile digital fibromatosis	See Tumours of Soft Tissue (Section 42).
Infantile digital fibromatosis	See inclusion body fibromatosis	
Infantile haemangioendothelioma	See capillary haemangioma	
Infantile haemangiopericytoma		See Tumours of Soft Tissue (Section 42).
Infantile myofibromatosis		See Tumours of Soft Tissue (Section 42).

Tumour terminology Recommended terms are in **bold**	Synonyms	Comments
Inflammatory angiomatous nodule	See epithelioid haemangioma	
Inflammatory pseudotumour		See Tumours of Soft Tissue (Section 42).
Infundibular adenoma	See sebaceoma	
Infundibuloma	See follicular infundibulum tumour	
Intradermal eccrine poroma	See dermal duct tumour	
Intradermal lipoma	See naevus lipomatosus	
Intraepidermal eccrine poroma	See hidroacanthoma simplex	
Intraepidermal epithelioma	See Borst-Jadassohn epithelioma	
Intraneural perineurioma	See perineurioma	
Intravascular fasciitis		See Tumours of Soft Tissue (Section 42).
Intravascular papillary endothelial hyperplasia	See papillary endothelial hyperplasia	
Intravenous atypical vascular proliferation	See epithelioid haemangioma	
Intravenous pyogenic granuloma		Intravascular variant of lobular capillary haemangioma.
Inverted follicular keratosis	See irritated seborrhoeic wart	
Irritated seborrhoeic wart	Inverted follicular keratosis	A common benign skin tumour of possible follicular derivation.
Juvenile haemangioma	See capillary haemangioma	
Juvenile hyaline fibromatosis		See Tumours of Soft Tissue (Section 42).
Juvenile xanthogranuloma	Naevoxantho-endothelioma Xanthogranuloma	See Tumours of Soft Tissue (Section 42).
Kaposi's sarcoma		See Tumours of Soft Tissue (Section 42).

Tumour terminology Recommended terms are in **bold**	Synonyms	Comments
Kaposiform haemangioendothelioma	Kaposi-like infantile haemangioendothelioma	See Tumours of Soft Tissue (Section 42).
Kaposi-like infantile haemangioendothelioma	See Kaposiform haemangioendothelioma	
Keloid		Exuberant scar tissue usually following trauma.
Keratoacanthoma	Molluscum sebaceum	A self-limiting variant of squamous cell carcinoma.
Keratosis senilis	See actinic keratosis	
Kimura's disease		See Tumours of Soft Tissue (Section 42).
Klippel-Trelaunay syndrome		See Tumours of Soft Tissue (Section 42).
Knuckle pad		Tumour-like fibrous tissue lesion, which may be familial or associated with superficial fibromatosis.
Large cell acanthoma		Tumour-like lesion of epidermis. The face is the most common site.
Ledderhose's disease	See plantar fibromatosis	
Leiomyoma of arrector pili	See pilar leiomyoma	
Lichen planus-like keratosis	See lichenoid keratosis	
Lichenoid keratosis	Lichen planus-like keratosis Solitary lichen planus	Tumour-like lesion, which may be confused with lichen planus.
Lipoblastoma		See Tumours of Soft Tissue (Section 42).
Lipoma		See Tumours of Soft Tissue (Section 42).
Lipomatosis		See Tumours of Soft Tissue (Section 42).
Liposarcoma		See Tumours of Soft Tissue (Section 42).
Lobular capillary haemangioma	Granuloma gravidarum Granuloma pyogenicum Pyogenic granuloma Telangiectatic granuloma	See Tumours of Soft Tissue (Section 42).
Lymphangioma		See Tumours of Soft Tissue (Section 42).

Tumour terminology Recommended terms are in **bold**	Synonyms	Comments
Lymphangioma circumscriptum		A localised superficial cutaneous lymphatic malformation.
Lymphangiomatosis		See Tumours of Soft Tissue (Section 42).
Lymphangiosarcoma	See angiosarcoma	
Malignant acrospiroma	See eccrine hidradenocarcinoma	
Malignant chondroid syringoma	Malignant mixed tumour of the skin	Extremely rare, high grade eccrine sweat gland tumour.
Malignant eccrine poroma	See eccrine porocarcinoma	
Malignant eccrine spiradenoma	Carcinoma arising in spiradenoma	Extremely rare high grade sweat gland tumour.
Malignant endovascular papillary angioendothelioma	Dabska's tumour Endovascular papillary angioendothelioma	See Tumours of Soft Tissue (Section 42).
Malignant haemangioendothelioma	See angiosarcoma	
Malignant hidradenoma papilliferum		Exceptionally rare apocrine sweat gland tumour of the vulva.
Malignant mixed tumour of the skin	See malignant chondroid syringoma	
Malignant peripheral nerve sheath tumour	Malignant schwannoma Neurofibrosarcoma	See Tumours of Soft Tissue (Section 42).
Malignant peripheral primitive neuroectodermal tumour	Extraosseous Ewing's sarcoma MPNET Peripheral primitive neuroepithelioma PPNET Primitive neuroectodermal tumour	See Tumours of Soft Tissue (Section 42).
Malignant pilomatricoma	See pilomatrix carcinoma	
Malignant pilomatrixoma	See pilomatrix carcinoma	

Tumour terminology Recommended terms are in **bold**	Synonyms	Comments
Malignant schwannoma	See malignant peripheral nerve sheath tumour	
Malignant syringoma	See eccrine epithelioma	
Malignant syringoma	See microcystic adnexal carcinoma	
Masson's tumour	See papillary endothelial hyperplasia	
Matrical carcinoma	See pilomatrix carcinoma	
Melanoacanthoma		Pigmented variant of seborrhoeic wart.
Meningeal heterotopia	See ectopic meningothelial hamartoma	
Merkell cell carcinoma	See neuroendocrine tumour	
Metaplastic carcinoma	Carcinosarcoma	An extremely rare tumour combining malignant epithelial and mesenchymal elements.
Metatarsalgia	See Morton's neuroma	
Microcystic adnexal carcinoma	Malignant syringoma. Microcystic eccrine carcinoma Sclerosing carcinoma of sweat ducts Sclerosing sweat duct carcinoma Sweat gland carcinoma with syringomatous features Syringoid carcinoma Syringomatous carcinoma	Slowly growing, locally aggressive eccrine sweat gland tumour. The face is most often affected. Recurrences are very common (60%) but metastases are exceptionally rare.
Microcystic eccrine carcinoma	See microcystic adnexal carcinoma	
Microvenular haemangioma		Rare tumour-like lesion of small veins. Presents on the limbs of young adults as a red-blue papule.

Tumour terminology Recommended terms are in **bold**	Synonyms	Comments
Mixed tumour of the skin	See chondroid syringoma	
Molluscum sebaceum	See keratoacanthoma	
Morbus Bowen	See Bowen's disease	
Morton's metatarsalgia	See Morton's neuroma	
Morton's neuroma	Metatarsalgia Morton's metatarsalgia	See Tumours of Soft Tissue (Section 42).
MPNET	See malignant peripheral primitive neuroectodermal tumour	
Mucinous carcinoma	Cutaneous adenocystic carcinoma	Rare low grade malignant eccrine sweat gland tumour. The face is the most common site.
Mucoepidermoid carcinoma	Adenosquamous carcinoma	Rare aggressive tumour composed of both squamous and mucus-secreting epithelium.
Multicentric pigmented Bowen's disease	See Bowenoid papulosis	
Multicentric reticulohistiocytosis	See reticulohistiocytoma	
Myoepithelioma of the skin		Rare benign tumour of myoepithelial cells.
Myxofibrosarcoma	Myxoid malignant fibrous histiocytoma Myxoid MFH	See Tumours of Soft Tissue (Section 42).
Myxoid malignant fibrous histiocytoma	See myxofibrosarcoma	
Myxoid MFH	See myofibrosarcoma	
Myxolipoma		See Tumours of Soft Tissue (Section 42).
Myxoma	See digital myxoma	
Naevoxantho-endothelioma	See juvenile xanthogranuloma	
Naevus araneus	Spider naevus	See Tumours of Soft Tissue (Section 42).
Naevus flammeus	Salmon patch	See Tumours of Soft Tissue (Section 42).

Tumour terminology Recommended terms are in **bold**	Synonyms	Comments
Naevus lipomatosus	Intradermal lipoma Naevus lipomatosus superficialis	See Tumours of Soft Tissue (Section 42).
Naevus lipomatosus superficialis	See naevus lipomatosus	
Naevus sebaceous	See organoid naevus	
Naevus sebaceous of Jadassohn	See organoid naevus	
Nasal glioma	See glial heterotopia	
Neurilemmoma	See Schwannoma	
Neuroendocrine tumour	Merkell cell carcinoma Trabecular carcinoma	Rare. High grade tumour associated with considerable mortality. The 3 year survival is only about 50%.
Neurofibroma		See Tumours of Soft Tissue (Section 42).
Neurofibromatosis 1 (NF-1)	von Recklinghausen's disease NF-1	See Tumours of Soft Tissue (Section 42).
Neurofibromatosis 2 (NF-2)	Bilateral acoustic neurofibromatosis NF-2	See Tumours of Soft Tissue (Section 42).
Neurofibrosarcoma	See malignant peripheral nerve sheath tumour	
Neurothekeoma	See dermal nerve sheath myxoma	
NF-1	See neurofibromatosis 1	
NF-2	See neurofibromatosis 2	
Nodular fasciitis	Fasciitis	See Tumours of Soft Tissue (Section 42).
Nodular hidradenoma	See eccrine hidradenoma	
Nodular subepidermal fibrosis	See fibrous histiocytoma	
Organoid naevus	Naevus sebaceous Naevus sebaceous of Jadassohn	Tumour-like hamartoma, which may be complicated by the development of basal cell carcinoma and other tumours. The scalp is most often affected.
Osler-Weber-Rendu syndrome	Hereditary haemorrhagic telangiectasia	A rare autosomal dominant condition characterised by the presence of telangiectasias in the skin, mucosae, and internal viscera.

Tumour terminology Recommended terms are in **bold**	Synonyms	Comments
Ossifying fibromyxoid tumour		See Tumours of Soft Tissue (Section 42).
Osteochondroma	See benign cartilaginous exostosis	
Osteoma cutis		Benign dermal tumour composed of mature bone.
Pacinian neurofibroma	See pacinian schwannoma	
Pacinian schwannoma	Pacinian neurofibroma	See Tumours of Soft Tissue (Section 42).
Palisaded encapsulated neuroma	See solitary circumscribed neuroma	
Palmar fibromatosis	Dupuytren's contracture Dupuytren's disease	See Tumours of Soft Tissue (Section 42).
Papillary eccrine adenoma		Rare eccrine sweat gland tumour that typically presents on the extremities. Females are most often affected.
Papillary endothelial hyperplasia	Intravascular papillary endothelial hyperplasia Masson's tumour	See Tumours of Soft Tissue (Section 42).
Papular angiodysplasia	See epithelioid haemangioma	
Paradoxical fibrosarcoma	See atypical fibroxanthoma	
Paraosteal fasciitis	See cranial fasciitis	
Penile fibromatosis	See Peyronie's disease	
Perifollicular fibroma		Extremely rare follicular connective sheath tumour.
Perineural fibrolipoma	See fibrolipomatous hamartoma of nerve	
Perineurioma	Extraneural perineurioma Intraneural perineurioma Storiform perineural fibroma	See Tumours of Soft Tissue (Section 42).
Periosteal fasciitis	See cranial fasciitis	

Tumour terminology Recommended terms are in **bold**	Synonyms	Comments
Peripheral neuroepithelioma	See malignant peripheral primitive neuroectodermal tumour	
Peripheral primitive neuroectodermal tumour	See malignant peripheral primitive neuroectodermal tumour	
Periungual fibroma		Fibrous tissue tumour that develops at the edge or under the nails in patients with tuberous sclerosis.
Peyronie's disease	Penile fibromatosis Plastic induration of penis	See Tumours of Soft Tissue (Section 42).
Pigmented dermatofibrosarcoma protuberans	Bednár tumour Pigmented storiform neurofibroma	See Tumours of Soft Tissue (Section 42).
Pigmented storiform neurofibroma	See pigmented dermatofibrosarcoma protuberans	
Pilar leiomyoma	Cutaneous leiomyoma Leiomyoma of arrector pili	Benign smooth muscle tumour of arrector pili origin; often multiple and painful.
Pilar sheath acanthoma		Benign follicular tumour.
Pilar tumour	See proliferating pilar tumour	
Pilomatricoma	See pilomatrixoma	
Pilomatrix carcinoma	Aggressive pilomatrixoma Malignant pilomatricoma Malignant pilomatrixoma Matrical carcinoma	Extremely rare malignant tumour of hair matrix epithelium.
Pilomatrixoma	Calcifying epithelioma of Malherbe Pilomatricoma	Benign tumour of hair matrix epithelium.
Plantar fibromatosis	Ledderhose's disease	See Tumours of Soft Tissue (Section 42).

Tumour terminology Recommended terms are in **bold**	Synonyms	Comments
Plastic induration of penis	See Peyronie's disease	
Pleomorphic fibroma		See Tumours of Soft Tissue (Section 42).
Pleomorphic lipoma		See Tumours of Soft Tissue (Section 42).
Plexiform fibrohistiocytic tumour		See Tumours of Soft Tissue (Section 42).
Plexiform neurofibroma		See Tumours of Soft Tissue (Section 42).
Plexiform schwannoma		See Tumours of Soft Tissue (Section 42).
Porocarcinoma	See eccrine porocarcinoma	
Poroma-like adnexal neoplasm	See sebaceoma	
Port-wine stain		See Tumours of Soft Tissue (Section 42).
PPNET	See malignant peripheral primitive neuroectodermal tumour	
Primitive neuroectodermal tumour	See malignant peripheral primitive neuroectodermal tumour	
Primitive polypoid granular cell tumour		See Tumours of Soft Tissue (Section 42).
Proliferating pilar tumour	Pilar tumour Proliferating trichilemmal cyst Proliferating trichilemmal tumour	Benign follicular tumour. Recurrences are common. Malignant variants are exceptionally rare.
Proliferating trichilemmal cyst	See proliferating pilar tumour	
Proliferating trichilemmal tumour	See proliferating pilar tumour	
Pseudopyogenic granuloma	See epithelioid haemangioma	
Pseudosarcoma of skin	See atypical fibroxanthoma	

Tumour terminology Recommended terms are in **bold**	Synonyms	Comments
Pseudosarcomatous benign fibrous histiocytoma	See atypical benign fibrous histiocytoma	
Pyogenic granuloma	See lobular capillary haemangioma	
Racemose haemangioma	See arteriovenous haemangioma	
Reactive angioendotheliomatosis	See angioendotheliomatosis	
Reticulohistiocytic granuloma	See reticulohistiocytoma	
Reticulohistiocytoma	Multicentric reticulohistiocytosis Reticulohistiocytic granuloma	See Tumours of Soft Tissue (Section 42)
Retiform haemangioendothelioma		See Tumours of Soft Tissue (Section 42).
Rodent ulcer	See basal cell carcinoma	
Salmon patch	See naevus flammeus	
Schwannoma	Neurilemmoma	See Tumours of Soft Tissue (Section 42).
Sclerosing carcinoma of sweat ducts	See microcystic adnexal carcinoma	
Sclerosing epithelial hamartoma	See desmoplastic trichoepithelioma	
Sclerosing haemangioma	See fibrous histiocytoma	
Sclerosing sweat duct carcinoma	See microcystic adnexal carcinoma	
Sclerotic fibroma	See storiform collagenoma	
Sebaceoma	Infundibular adenoma Poroma-like adnexal neoplasm Sebocrine adenoma	Very rare benign sebaceous gland tumour.
Sebaceous adenoma		Rare sebaceous gland tumour. May be associated with Torre-Muir syndrome.

Tumour terminology Recommended terms are in **bold**	Synonyms	Comments
Sebaceous carcinoma		Rare high grade malignant sebaceous gland tumour. May be associated with Torre-Muir syndrome.
Sebaceous epithelioma	Basal cell carcinoma with sebaceous differentiation Basosebaceous epithelioma Superficial epithelioma with sebaceous differentiation	Histological variant of basal cell carcinoma.
Sebaceous naevus	See organoid naevus	
Sebaceous trichofolliculoma		Histological variant of trichofolliculoma.
Sebocrine adenoma	See sebaceoma	
Seborrhoeic keratosis	Seborrhoeic wart Verruca senilis	Extremely common usually multiple warty skin lesion.
Seborrhoeic wart	See seborrhoeic keratosis	
Senile angioma	See cherry angioma	
Senile keratosis	See actinic keratosis	
Sequestered meningocoele	See ectopic meningothelial hamartoma	
Sinusoidal haemangioma		See Tumours of Soft Tissue (Section 42).
Skin tag	See fibroepithelial polyp	
Soft fibroma	See fibroepithelial polyp	
Solar keratosis	See actinic keratosis	
Solid-cystic hidradenoma	See eccrine hidradenoma	
Solitary circumscribed neuroma	Palisaded encapsulated neuroma	See Tumours of Soft Tissue (Section 42).
Solitary lichen planus	See lichenoid keratosis	
Solitary myofibroma		See Tumours of Soft Tissue (Section 42).
Solitary trichoepithelioma	See trichoepithelioma	

Tumour terminology Recommended terms are in **bold**	Synonyms	Comments
Spectacle frame acanthoma	See acanthoma fissuratum	
Spider naevus	See naevus araneus	
Spindle cell atypical fibroxanthoma		See Tumours of Soft Tissue (Section 42).
Spindle cell haemangioendothelioma	Spindle cell haemangioma	See Tumours of Soft Tissue (Section 42).
Spindle cell haemangioma	See spindle cell haemangioendothelioma	
Spindle cell lipoma		See Tumours of Soft Tissue (Section 42).
Spindle cell squamous carcinoma		A histological variant of squamous cell carcinoma.
Squamous carcinoma in situ	See Bowen's disease	
Squamous cell carcinoma	Epidermoid carcinoma	The second most common skin cancer. The majority arise as a consequence of excessive sun exposure. Scarring conditions, HPV infection, and immunosuppression are additional important predisposing factors.
Stewart Treves syndrome		See Tumours of Soft Tissue (Section 42).
Storiform collagenoma	Circumscribed storiform collagenoma Collagenoma Sclerotic fibroma	See Tumours of Soft Tissue (Section 42).
Storiform perineural fibroma	See perineurioma	
Strawberry naevus	See capillary haemangioma	
Stuccokeratoses		Warty tumour-like lesion most often presenting on the extremities. Usually multiple.
Sturge-Weber syndrome		See Tumours of Soft Tissue (Section 42).
Subcutaneous trichoepithelioma	See giant solitary trichoepithelioma	

Tumour terminology Recommended terms are in **bold**	Synonyms	Comments
Subungual exostosis	See benign cartilaginous exostosis	
Superficial angiomyxoma		See Tumours of Soft Tissue (Section 42).
Superficial epithelioma with sebaceous differentiation	See sebaceous epithelioma	
Sweat gland carcinoma with syringomatous features	See microcystic adnexal carcinoma	
Syringocystadenoma papilliferum		Benign apocrine sweat gland tumour sometimes associated with organoid naevus. Most often present on the scalp.
Syringoid carcinoma	See eccrine epithelioma	
Syringoid carcinoma	See microcystic adnexal carcinoma	
Syringomatous carcinoma	See eccrine epithelioma	
Syringomatous carcinoma	See microcystic adnexal carcinoma	
Targetoid haemosiderotic haemangioma	See hobnail haemangioma	
Telangiectatic granuloma	See lobular capillary haemangioma	
Torre-Muir syndrome		The association of sebaceous tumours and internal malignancy including carcinoma of colon, rectum, and breast.
Trabecular carcinoma	See neuroendocrine tumour	
Traumatic neuroma	Amputation neuroma	See Tumours of Soft Tissue (Section 42).
Trichilemmal carcinoma		Low grade malignant tumour of follicular external root sheath.
Trichilemmoma		Benign tumour of follicular external root sheath. Multiple lesions are typical of Cowden's disease.
Trichoadenoma		Rare benign follicular tumour.

Tumour terminology Recommended terms are in **bold**	Synonyms	Comments
Trichoblastic fibroma	See giant solitary trichoepithelioma	
Trichoblastoma	Hair matrix adenoma Immature trichoepithelioma Trichogenic adnexal tumour Trichogenic trichoblastoma	Extremely rare benign tumour of the hair germ.
Trichodiscoma		Hamartomatous proliferation of the hair disc.
Trichoepithelioma	Solitary trichoepithelioma	Common benign tumour of hair germ, which may be confused with basal cell carcinoma.
Trichofolliculoma		Complex hamartoma of pilosebaceous unit.
Trichogenic adnexal tumour	See trichoblastoma	
Trichogenic trichoblastoma	See trichoblastoma	
Tubular apocrine adenoma	See apocrine tubular adenoma	
Tufted angioblastoma	See tufted angioma	
Tufted angioma	Angioblastoma of Nakagawa Tufted angioblastoma	See Tumours of Soft Tissue (Section 42).
Turban tumour	See dermal cylindroma	
Turban tumour syndrome	See Ancell Spiegler syndrome	
Vascular malformation	See arteriovenous haemangioma	
Venous lake		Vascular ectasia occurring on sun-damaged skin in the elderly.
Verruca senilis	See seborrhoeic keratosis	
Verrucous carcinoma	Buschke-Löwenstein tumour Carcinoma cuniculatum	Rare variant of squamous cell carcinoma. Locally destructive and commonly recurs. Very rarely metastasises. Often HPV associated.

Tumour terminology Recommended terms are in **bold**	Synonyms	Comments
Verrucous haemangioma		See Tumours of Soft Tissue (Section 42).
Von Recklinghausen's disease	See neurofibromatosis 1	
Vulval dysplasia	See vulvar intraepithelial neoplasia (VIN)	
Vulvar intraepithelial neoplasia (VIN)	Vulval dysplasia	In situ, pre-malignant, condition of the vulva. May progress to invasive carcinoma.
Xanthelasma		A lipid-containing plaque, which presents on the eyelids and is often a manifestation of hypercholesteraemia.
Xanthogranuloma	See juvenile xanthogranuloma	
Xanthoma		A benign lipid-containing tumour, which is often a reflection of an underlying hyperlipidaemia.

Section 42

Tumours of Soft Tissue

C.D.M. Fletcher

Tumour terminology Recommended terms are in **bold**	Synonyms	Comments
Abrikossoff's tumour	See granular cell tumour	
Acoustic neuroma	See Schwannoma	
Acral arteriovenous tumour	See arteriovenous haemangioma	
Adiposis dolorosa	See lipomatosis	
Adult rhabdomyoma	Rhabdomyoma	Benign tumour showing skeletal muscle differentiation.
Adult-type myofibroma	See solitary myofibroma	
Aggressive angiomyxoma		Aggressive, locally recurring tumour, which most often affects the vulva.
Alveolar rhabdomyosarcoma		Histological variant of rhabdomyosarcoma with relatively more aggressive behaviour.
Alveolar soft part sarcoma	Non-chromaffin paraganglioma (obsolete)	Sarcoma of uncertain but possible muscular differentiation with a poor long-term prognosis.
Amputation neuroma	See traumatic neuroma	
Amyloid tumour	Amyloidoma	Pseudotumour due to deposition of amyloid.
Amyloidoma	See amyloid tumour	
Ancient schwannoma		Histological variant of Schwannoma showing degenerative changes.
Aneurysmal benign fibrous histiocytoma		See Tumours of Skin (Non-Melanocytic) (Section 41).
Angioblastoma of Nakagawa	See tufted angioma	

Tumour terminology Recommended terms are in **bold**	Synonyms	Comments
Angioendotheliomatosis	Reactive angioendotheliomatosis	The benign variant represents a multifocal reactive intravascular endothelial proliferation.
Angioendotheliomatosis (malignant)	Angiotropic lymphoma	See Tumours of the Lymph Nodes and Spleen (Section 24).
Angiofibroma (cutaneous variant)		See Tumours of Skin (Non-Melanocytic) (Section 41).
Angiofibroma (nasal variant)	See nasopharyngeal angiofibroma	
Angioleiomyoma	Angiomyoma Vascular leiomyoma	Benign smooth muscle tumour of vascular (usually venous) origin.
Angiolipoma		Benign subcutaneous tumour composed of fat and blood vessels.
Angiolymphoid hyperplasia with eosinophilia	See epithelioid haemangioma	
Angiomatoid fibrous histiocytoma	Angiomatoid malignant fibrous histiocytoma	Low grade sarcoma affecting mainly young patients.
Angiomatoid malignant fibrous histiocytoma	See angiomatoid fibrous histiocytoma	
Angiomatosis		Benign but diffuse or extensive proliferation of blood vessels.
Angiomyofibroblastoma		Benign non-recurring tumour, most common in the vulva. Should not be confused with aggressive angiomyxoma.
Angiomyolipoma		Rare tumour affecting kidney, soft tissue, or liver. Sometimes associated with tuberous sclerosis.
Angiomyoma	See angioleiomyoma	
Angiosarcoma	Haemangiosarcoma Lymphangiosarcoma Malignant endothelioma Malignant haemangioendothelioma Stewart-Treves syndrome	Usually aggressive tumour showing vascular endothelial differentiation.

Tumour terminology Recommended terms are in **bold**	Synonyms	Comments
Aponeurotic fibroma	See calcifying aponeurotic fibroma	
Arteriovenous haemangioma	Acral arteriovenous tumour Arteriovenous malformation Cirsoid aneurysm Racemose haemangioma	Benign tumour composed of blood vessels of arterial and venous types; may be superficial or deep seated.
Arteriovenous malformation	See arteriovenous haemangioma	
Askin tumour	See malignant peripheral primitive neuroectodermal tumour	
Atypical benign fibrous histiocytoma	Dermatofibroma with monster cells Pseudosarcomatous fibrous histiocytoma	See Tumours of Skin (Non-Melanocytic) (Section 41).
Atypical decubital fibroplasia	See ischaemic fasciitis	
Atypical fibroxanthoma	Paradoxical fibrosarcoma Pseudosarcoma of skin	See Tumours of Skin (Non-Melanocytic) (Section 41).
Atypical lipoma	Atypical lipomatous tumour Well differentiated liposarcoma	Low grade non-metastasising fatty tumour with frequent local recurrence and potential to dedifferentiate.
Atypical lipomatous tumour	See atypical lipoma	
Bacillary angiomatosis	Epithelioid angiomatosis	Benign reactive vascular proliferation due to Rochalimea quintana infection.
Bannayan syndrome		Syndrome of multiple lipomas and haemangiomas.
Bednár tumour	See pigmented dermatofibrosarcoma protuberans	
Benign fibrous histiocytoma	See fibrous histiocytoma	
Benign synovioma	See giant cell tumour of tendon sheath	

Tumour terminology Recommended terms are in **bold**	Synonyms	Comments
Benign Triton tumour	See neuromuscular hamartoma	
Bilateral acoustic neurofibromatosis	See neurofibromatosis 2	
Biphasic synovial sarcoma		Histological variant of synovial sarcoma showing glandular differentiation.
Bizarre neurofibroma		Histological variant of neurofibroma with nuclear atypia.
Blue rubber bleb naevus syndrome		Multiple cavernous haemangiomas or glomangiomas in skin and gastrointestinal tract.
Botryoid rhabdomyosarcoma		Usually polypoid variant of rhabdomyosarcoma arising beneath a mucosal surface.
Calcifying aponeurotic fibroma	Aponeurotic fibroma Juvenile aponeurotic fibroma	Rare, benign, recurring fibrous tissue tumour.
Calcifying bursitis	See tumoural calcinosis	
Calcifying fibrous pseudotumour		Hyalinised variant of inflammatory myofibroblastic tumour showing calcification.
Campbell de Morgan spot	See cherry angioma	
Capillary haemangioma	Cellular haemangioma of infancy Infantile haemangioendothelioma Juvenile capillary haemangioma Strawberry naevus	See Tumours of Skin (Non-Melanocytic) (Section 41).
Carney's complex	Carney's syndrome LAMB syndrome NAME syndrome	Syndrome of multiple myxomas and other more uncommon tumours.
Carney's syndrome	See Carney's complex	
Carney's triad		Syndrome of epithelioid leiomyosarcoma in stomach, paraganglioma, and pulmonary chondroma.
Cavernous haemangioma		Benign haemangioma with large, dilated blood vessels.

Tumour terminology Recommended terms are in **bold**	Synonyms	Comments
Cavernous lymphangioma	Cystic hygroma Cystic lymphangioma	Benign lymphangioma with dilated vessels.
Cellular angiofibroma		Benign fibrous tumour in the vulvovaginal region.
Cellular benign fibrous histiocytoma	Benign fibrous histiocytoma	See Tumours of Skin (Non-Melanocytic) (Section 41).
Cellular haemangioma of infancy	See capillary haemangioma	
Cellular neurothekeoma		Uncommon benign nerve sheath tumour related to nerve sheath myxoma.
Cellular schwannoma		Variant of benign schwannoma with high cellularity; often mistaken for sarcoma.
Cherry angioma	Campbell de Morgan spot Senile angioma	See Tumours of Skin (Non-Melanocytic) (Section 41).
Chondroid lipoma		Benign lipoma variant with cartilage-like features.
Chondrolipoma		Lipoma with cartilaginous metaplasia.
Chondroma	See soft tissue chondroma	
Chondroma of soft parts	See soft tissue chondroma	
Chordoid sarcoma	See extraskeletal myxoid chondrosarcoma	
Cicatricial fibromatosis		Fibromatosis occurring at the site of previous scarring (trauma/burns etc.).
Circumscribed storiform collagenoma	See storiform collagenoma	
Cirsoid aneurysm	See arteriovenous haemangioma	
Clear cell sarcoma	See malignant melanoma of soft parts	
Collagenous fibroma	See desmoplastic fibroblastoma	
Congenital fibrosarcoma	See infantile fibrosarcoma	
Congenital generalised fibromatosis	See infantile myofibromatosis	

Tumour terminology Recommended terms are in **bold**	Synonyms	Comments
Congenital smooth muscle hamartoma	Smooth muscle hamartoma	See Tumours of Skin (Non-Melanocytic) (Section 41).
Cranial fasciitis	See parosteal fasciitis	Variant of nodular fasciitis with skull erosion, usually presenting in childhood.
Cutaneous leiomyoma	See pilar leiomyoma	
Cutaneous meningioma	Extracranial meningioma	See Tumours of Skin (Non-Melanocytic) (Section 41).
Cystic hygroma	See cavernous lymphangioma	
Cystic lymphangioma	See cavernous lymphangioma	
Dabska's tumour	See endovascular papillary angioendothelioma	
Dedifferentiated liposarcoma		Well differentiated liposarcoma, which has evolved to higher grade non-lipogenic tumour.
Deep benign fibrous histiocytoma		Benign lesion composed of fibroblasts and inflammatory cells.
Deep leiomyoma		Rare variant of leiomyoma occurring in deep soft tissue.
Dercum's disease	See lipomatosis	
Dermal nerve sheath myxoma	Cutaneous neuromyxoma Nerve sheath myxoma Neurothekeoma	Uncommon benign nerve sheath tumour.
Dermatofibroma	See fibrous histiocytoma	
Dermatofibroma with monster cells	See atypical benign fibrous histiocytoma	
Dermatofibrosarcoma protuberans		See Tumours of Skin (Non-Melanocytic) (Section 41).
Dermatomyofibroma		See Tumours of Skin (Non-Melanocytic) (Section 41).
Desmoid fibromatosis	Desmoid tumour Fibromatosis Infantile fibromatosis	Usually deep-seated infiltrative fibrous lesion with high risk of destructive local recurrence but not capable of metastasis.
Desmoid tumour	See desmoid fibromatosis	

Tumour terminology Recommended terms are in **bold**	Synonyms	Comments
Desmoplastic fibroblastoma		Benign fibrous lesion, resembling burnt-out fasciitis.
Desmoplastic small cell tumour	Intra-abdominal desmoplastic small cell tumour	Small round cell sarcoma with divergent differentiation; highly aggressive.
Diffuse neurofibroma		Variant of neurofibroma, usually producing large subcutaneous plaque.
Diffuse-type giant cell tumour	Pigmented villonodular synovitis	Locally recurring tumour, usually affecting large joints. Rarely malignant.
Digital myxoma	Cutaneous myxoid cyst Myxoma	See Tumours of Skin (Non-Melanocytic) (Section 41).
Dupuytren's contracture	See palmar fibromatosis	
Dupuytren's disease	See palmar fibromatosis	
Ectomesenchymal chondromyxoid tumour		Benign neoplasm of tongue with potential to recur.
Ectomesenchymoma		Very rare sarcoma showing neural and rhabdomyoblastic differentiation.
Ectopic meningioma		Usually benign meningothelial neoplasm arising outside the CNS.
Ectopic meningothelial hamartoma	See meningeal hamartoma	
Elastofibroma		Pseudotumour forming elastic tissue, typically beneath the scapula.
Embryonal rhabdomyosarcoma	Sarcoma botryoides	The most common variant of rhabdomyosarcoma, especially occurring in children <10 years.
Endovascular papillary angioendothelioma	Dabska's tumour Malignant endovascular papillary angioendothelioma	Very rare low grade malignant vascular tumour.
Epithelioid angiomatosis	See bacillary angiomatosis	
Epithelioid angiosarcoma		Histological variant of angiosarcoma, which may mimic carcinoma or melanoma.
Epithelioid haemangioendothelioma		Low grade malignant vascular tumour; tendency to multicentricity.

Tumour terminology Recommended terms are in **bold**	Synonyms	Comments
Epithelioid haemangioma	Angiolymphoid hyperplasia with eosinophilia Histiocytoid haemangioma	Benign vascular tumour, most common in head and neck region.
Epithelioid leiomyoma	Leiomyoblastoma (benign variant)	Benign smooth muscle tumour with epithelial-like morphology.
Epithelioid leiomyosarcoma	Leiomyoblastoma (malignant variant)	Malignant smooth muscle tumour with epithelial-like morphology; very rare in non-visceral locations.
Epithelioid malignant peripheral nerve sheath tumour		Uncommon variant of form of malignant peripheral nerve sheath tumour, histologically mimicking carcinoma or melanoma.
Epithelioid sarcoma	Epithelioid sarcoma of Enzinger	Uncommon sarcoma; mainly affects hand/arm; very infiltrative.
Eruptive xanthoma	See xanthoma	
Evans' tumour	See low grade fibromyxoid sarcoma	
Extracranial meningioma	See cutaneous meningioma	
Extracranial meningioma	See meningeal hamartoma	
Extraneural perineurioma	See perineurioma	
Extraosseous Ewing's sarcoma	See malignant peripheral primitive neuroectodermal tumour	
Extraosseous osteosarcoma	See soft tissue osteosarcoma	
Extrarenal rhabdoid tumour	Rhabdoid tumour	Heterogeneous group of aggressive tumours with shared presence of hyaline inclusions and macronucleoli.
Extraskeletal chondroma	See soft tissue chondroma	
Extraskeletal chondrosarcoma	See extraskeletal myxoid chondrosarcoma	

Tumour terminology Recommended terms are in **bold**	Synonyms	Comments
Extraskeletal Ewing's sarcoma	See malignant peripheral primitive neuroectodermal tumour	
Extraskeletal mesenchymal chondrosarcoma	Extraskeletal chondrosarcoma Mesenchymal chondrosarcoma Myxoid chondrosarcoma	Primary chondrosarcoma of soft tissue with small cell morphology and aggressive behaviour.
Extraskeletal myxoid chondrosarcoma	Chordoid sarcoma Extraskeletal chondrosarcoma	Primary chondrosarcoma of soft tissue with copious myxoid matrix.
Extraskeletal osteosarcoma	See soft tissue osteosarcoma	
Extraspinal ependymoma	Extraspinal myxopapillary ependymoma	Ependymoma arising in soft tissue, usually in sacral region.
Extraspinal myxopapillary ependymoma	See extraspinal ependymoma	
Fasciitis		Reactive proliferation of fibroblasts and myofibroblasts, rapidly growing but rarely recurs. Variants include nodular fasciitis, proliferative fasciitis, ischaemic fasciitis, cranial fasciitis, and parosteal fasciitis.
Fasciitis ossificans	Fibro-osseous pseudotumour Florid reactive periostitis	Histological variant of fasciitis with metaplastic ossification.
Fibroblastoma	See desmoplastic fibroblastoma	
Fibroblastoma	See giant cell fibroblastoma	
Fibrodysplasia ossificans progressiva	Myositis ossificans progressiva	Very rare diffuse fibrous proliferation, which undergoes progressive metaplastic ossification.
Fibrolipoma		Histological variant of lipoma.
Fibrolipomatous hamartoma of nerve	Neural fibrolipoma	Very rare intraneural proliferation of fibrofatty tissue; may be associated with digital hypertrophy.

Tumour terminology Recommended terms are in **bold**	Synonyms	Comments
Fibroma		General descriptive term for a benign tumour composed largely of fibrous tissue.
Fibroma of tendon sheath	Tenosynovial fibroma	Benign fibrous tissue tumour usually arising on the hands or feet. Recurrences are common.
Fibromatosis		Locally aggressive, infiltrative, and recurring fibrous neoplasm with no potential for metastasis.
Fibromatosis colli	Sternomastoid tumour Torticollis Wry neck deformity	Tumour-like reactive fibrous tissue in the neck muscle of infants. It usually develops following birth trauma.
Fibromyxoid sarcoma	See low grade fibromyxoid sarcoma	
Fibro-osseous pseudotumour	See fasciitis ossificans	
Fibrosarcoma		Rare sarcoma showing purely fibroblastic differentiation.
Fibrosarcomatous variant of dermatofibrosarcoma		Higher grade form of dermatofibrosarcoma protuberans.
Fibrous hamartoma of infancy		Rare benign fibrous tumour occurring in young infants and children.
Fibrous histiocytoma	Dermatofibroma Histiocytoma (cutis) Nodular subepidermal fibrosis	See Tumours of Skin (Non-Melanocytic) (Section 41).
Fibroxanthosarcoma	See pleomorphic malignant fibrous histiocytoma	
Florid reactive periostitis	See fasciitis ossificans	
Foetal rhabdomyoma		Variant of rhabdomyoma occurring in childhood.
Ganglion	Ganglion cyst Nerve sheath ganglion	Reactive synovial lesion with localised accumulation of mucinous material.
Ganglion cyst	See ganglion	
Ganglioneuroma		Benign neural tumour usually arising from the sympathetic chain.

Tumour terminology Recommended terms are in **bold**	Synonyms	Comments
Gardner's syndrome		The association of adenomatous polyposis coli and desmoid fibromatosis. Other lesions that may sometimes be present include benign osteomas.
Genital leiomyoma		Benign smooth muscle tumour arising in vulva or scrotum.
Genital rhabdomyoma		Benign rhabdomyoblastic tumour arising in vagina or cervix.
Giant cell angiofibroma		Uncommon fibroblastic tumour of adults, usually located in head/neck region.
Giant cell fibroblastoma		Uncommon recurring tumour, which mainly affects children. It is closely related to dermatofibrosarcoma protuberans.
Giant cell malignant fibrous histiocytoma	Malignant giant cell tumour of soft tissues	Aggressive sarcoma with numerous osteoclast-type giant cells; many cases prove to be osteosarcoma.
Giant cell tumour of tendon sheath	Synovioma, benign (obsolete) Localised-type giant cell tumour Nodular tenosynovitis Tenosynovial giant cell tumour	Benign tumour, which occurs most often on the fingers and hand. Recurrences are common.
Gingival fibromatosis	Hereditary gingival fibromatosis Hereditary gingival hyperplasia	Diffuse bilateral gingival fibrosis in children.
Gingival granular cell tumour	Granular cell epulis	Rare benign tumour affecting the gums of neonates.
Glial heterotopia	Nasal glioma	Tumour-like lesion composed of ectopic glial tissue. This hamartomatous condition most often affects children.
Glomangioma		Histological variant of glomus tumour with prominent vessels.
Glomangiomyoma		Histological variant of glomus tumour with prominent blood vessels and smooth muscle.
Glomangiosarcoma	Malignant glomus tumour	Extremely rare malignant variant of glomus tumour.

Tumour terminology Recommended terms are in **bold**	Synonyms	Comments
Glomeruloid haemangioma		Rare benign vascular proliferation associated with Castleman's disease.
Glomus tumour		Benign, often painful tumour composed of specialised perivascular cells.
Granular cell epulis	See gingival granular cell tumour	
Granular cell myoblastoma	See granular cell tumour	
Granular cell tumour	Abrikossoff's tumour Granular cell myoblastoma	Benign tumour composed of cells with copious granular eosinophilic cytoplasm, usually of nerve sheath derivation. Granular cell change may also be seen in leiomyoma and Schwannoma.
Granuloma gravidarum		Variant of lobular capillary haemangioma occurring in pregnancy. Mostly lesions develop in the mouth.
Granuloma pyogenicum	See lobular capillary haemangioma	
Haemangioendothelioma	See angiosarcoma	A term most often used to connote a low grade or borderline malignant vascular tumour; also an outdated term for angiosarcoma and for juvenile capillary haemangioma.
Haemangioma		A benign tumour (hamartomatous, reactive, or neoplastic) composed of blood vessels.
Haemangiopericytoma		A general term for a tumour of unknown histogenesis and variable clinical course characterised by tumour cells arranged around thin-walled branching vessels.
Haemangiosarcoma	See angiosarcoma	
Haemorrhagic spindle cell tumour with amianthoid fibres	See intranodal myofibroblastoma	
Hereditary gingival fibromatosis	See gingival fibromatosis	
Hereditary gingival hyperplasia	See gingival fibromatosis	
Hibernoma		A benign tumour showing brown fat differentiation.

Tumour terminology Recommended terms are in **bold**	Synonyms	Comments
Histiocytoid haemangioma	See epithelioid haemangioma	
Histiocytoma (cutis)	See fibrous histiocytoma	
Hobnail haemangioma	Targetoid haemosiderotic haemangioma	Benign haemangioma with protuberant endothelial cells. ·
Hyalin fibromatosis	See juvenile hyaline fibromatosis	
Hyaline fibromatosis	See juvenile hyaline fibromatosis	
Hyalinosis multiplex congenita	See juvenile hyaline fibromatosis	
Inclusion-body fibromatosis	Infantile digital fibromatosis Infantile digital fibroma	Recurring, sometimes multicentric fibrous tissue lesion, which arises most often on the fingers or toes of children.
Infantile desmoid tumour	See infantile fibromatosis	
Infantile digital fibroma	See inclusion-body fibromatosis	
Infantile digital fibromatosis	See inclusion-body fibromatosis	
Infantile fibromatosis	Infantile desmoid tumour	Variant of desmoid fibromatosis occurring in infants/young children.
Infantile fibrosarcoma	Congenital fibrosarcoma	Fibrosarcoma occurring in infants and young children, usually associated with an excellent prognosis.
Infantile haemangioendothelioma	See capillary haemangioma	
Infantile haemangiopericytoma		Variant of haemangiopericytoma occurring in infants and young children, closely related to infantile myofibromatosis.
Infantile myofibromatosis	Congenital fibromatosis Congenital generalised fibromatosis	Solitary or multicentric benign proliferation of myofibroblasts. Viscera may sometimes be affected. Occasionally the disease presents in adults.
Infiltrating angiolipoma	See intramuscular haemangioma	

Tumour terminology Recommended terms are in **bold**	Synonyms	Comments
Inflammatory fibrosarcoma	See inflammatory myofibroblastic tumour	
Inflammatory leiomyosarcoma		Uncommon histological variant of leiomyosarcoma with a prominent inflammatory cell component.
Inflammatory liposarcoma		Histological variant of well differentiated liposarcoma with a prominent inflammatory cell component.
Inflammatory malignant fibrous histiocytoma		Rare subtype of MFH with prominent neutrophils.
Inflammatory myofibroblastic tumour	Inflammatory fibrosarcoma Inflammatory pseudotumour Omental-mesenteric myxoid hamartoma	Low grade neoplasm occurring most commonly in children. Some cases, however, may be associated with metastatic spread.
Inflammatory pseudotumour	See inflammatory myofibroblastic tumour	
Intermuscular lipoma		Benign lipoma occurring between skeletal muscles.
Intra-abdominal desmoplastic small cell tumour	See desmoplastic small cell tumour	
Intramuscular haemangioma	Infiltrating angiolipoma Vascular malformation	Haemangioma of various types arising in skeletal muscle. Recurrences are common.
Intramuscular lipoma		Benign lipoma arising in skeletal muscle. Recurrences are common.
Intramuscular myxoma		Benign myxomatous lesion arising in skeletal muscle. Recurrences are rare.
Intraneural perineurioma	See perineurioma	
Intranodal haemorrhagic spindle cell tumour with amianthoid fibres	See intranodal myofibroblastoma	
Intranodal myofibroblastoma	Intranodal haemorrhagic spindle cell tumour with amianthoid fibres Palisaded myofibroblastoma	Benign non-recurring myofibroblastic tumour developing in lymph nodes, especially those of the groin.

Tumour terminology Recommended terms are in **bold**	Synonyms	Comments
Intravascular fasciitis		Rare variant of nodular fasciitis occurring in a blood vessel (usually a vein).
Intravascular papillary endothelial hyperplasia	See papillary endothelial hyperplasia	
Intravascular pyogenic granuloma		Rare variant of pyogenic granuloma arising in a vein.
Intravenous leiomyomatosis		Intravenous proliferation of benign smooth muscle, which occurs most often in the uterus.
Ischaemic fasciitis	Atypical decubital fibroplasia	Reactive fibrous proliferation, most common over bony prominences.
Juvenile aponeurotic fibroma	See calcifying aponeurotic fibroma	
Juvenile capillary haemangioma	See capillary haemangioma	
Juvenile hyaline fibromatosis	Hyaline fibromatosis Hyalinosis multiplex congenita	Very rare multicentric fibrous abnormality with systemic features.
Juvenile xanthogranuloma	Naevoxantho-endothelioma Xanthogranuloma	Benign self-limiting histiocytic proliferation. May also occur in adults.
Juxta-articular myxoma		Benign myxoma occurring close to a large joint; prone to recur.
Kaposi's disease	See Kaposi's sarcoma	
Kaposi's sarcoma	Kaposi's disease	Often multicentric vascular tumour. It may be associated with AIDS.
Kaposiform haemangioendothelioma	Kaposi-like infantile haemangioendothelioma	Rare, locally aggressive vascular tumour, most common in infants.
Kaposi-like infantile haemangioendothelioma	See Kaposiform haemangioendothelioma	
Kikuyu bursa	See tumoural calcinosis	
Kimura's disease		Rare inflammatory disorder, most common in oriental patients.
Klippel-Trelaunay syndrome	Vascular malformation	Diffuse vascular malformation of a limb, often with hypertrophy.
LAMB syndrome	See Carney's complex	
Ledderhose's disease	See plantar fibromatosis	

Tumour terminology Recommended terms are in **bold**	Synonyms	Comments
Leiomyoblastoma (benign variant)	See epithelioid leiomyoma	
Leiomyoblastoma (malignant variant)	See epithelioid leiomyosarcoma	
Leiomyoma		Benign tumour showing smooth muscle differentiation.
Leiomyoma of arrector pili	See pilar leiomyoma	
Leiomyomatosis peritonealis disseminata		Multicentric intraperitoneal proliferation of benign smooth muscle.
Leiomyosarcoma		Malignant tumour showing smooth muscle differentiation.
Lipoblastoma		Localised benign proliferation of immature fat in children.
Lipoblastomatosis		Diffuse form of lipoblastoma.
Lipoid dermatoarthritis	See multicentric reticulohistiocytosis	
Lipoma		Benign tumour composed of mature fat cells.
Lipoma arborescens	Synovial lipoma	Benign possibly reactive proliferation of fat in synovium.
Lipoma-like liposarcoma		Histological variant of low grade liposarcoma resembling mature adipose tissue.
Lipomatosis	Adiposis dolorosa Dercum's disease Madelung's disease Pelvic lipomatosis	Diffuse benign proliferation of mature adipose tissue.
Liposarcoma		Malignant tumour showing lipoblastic/ adipocytic differentiation.
Lobular capillary haemangioma	Capillary haemangioma Granuloma gravidarum Granuloma pyogenicum Pyogenic granuloma Telangiectatic granuloma	Histological variant of capillary haemangioma often associated with rapid exophytic growth.
Localised fibrous tumour	See solitary fibrous tumour	

Tumour terminology Recommended terms are in **bold**	Synonyms	Comments
Localised-type giant cell tumour	See giant cell tumour of tendon sheath	
Low grade fibromyxoid sarcoma	Evans' tumour Fibromyxoid sarcoma	Low grade fibroblastic sarcoma with high long-term risk of metastasis.
Lymphangioma		Benign tumour (often hamartomatous) composed of lymphatic vessels.
Lymphangioma circumscriptum		Histological variant of lymphangioma with numerous cutaneous vesicles.
Lymphangiomatosis		Diffuse lymphatic proliferation, often with visceral involvement.
Lymphangiomyomatosis		Rare systemic proliferation of lymphatics and associated myoid cells.
Lymphangiosarcoma	See angiosarcoma	
Madelung's disease	See lipomatosis	
Maffucci's syndrome		Haemangiomas (especially spindle cell haemangiomas) associated with enchondromatosis of bone.
Malignant endovascular papillary angioendothelioma	See endovascular papillary angioendothelioma	
Malignant fibrous histiocytoma	Fibroxanthosarcoma "MFH"	Heterogeneous group of sarcomas occurring mainly in adults (see variants).
Malignant giant cell tumour of soft tissues	See giant cell malignant fibrous histiocytoma	
Malignant glomus tumour	See glomangiosarcoma	
Malignant haemangioendothelioma	See angiosarcoma	
Malignant melanoma of soft parts	Clear cell sarcoma Melanoma of soft parts	Special type of malignant melanoma arising in deep soft tissue of limbs.
Malignant mesenchymoma		Sarcoma showing two or more lines of specific differentiation.
Malignant peripheral nerve sheath tumour	Malignant schwannoma MPNST Neurofibrosarcoma	Malignant tumour showing differentiation into nerve sheath cells and often arising from a nerve.

Tumour terminology Recommended terms are in **bold**	Synonyms	Comments
Malignant peripheral primitive neuroectodermal tumour	Askin tumour Extraosseous Ewing's sarcoma MPNET Extraskeletal Ewing's sarcoma Peripheral neuroepithelioma PPNET Primitive neuroectodermal tumour Thoraco pulmonary small cell tumour	Malignant soft tissue tumour showing variable degree of neuroectodermal differentiation; defined in most cases by t(11;22)(q24;q12) translocation.
Malignant schwannoma	See malignant peripheral nerve sheath tumour	
Malignant synovioma	See synovial sarcoma	Obsolete term.
Malignant Triton tumour		Histological variant of MPNST showing skeletal muscle differentiation; generally aggressive.
Masson's tumour	See papillary endothelial hyperplasia	
Melanocytic schwannoma	See melanotic schwannoma	
Melanoma of soft parts	See malignant melanoma of soft parts	
Melanotic neuroectodermal tumour of infancy	Melanotic progonoma Pigmented neuroectodermal tumour of infancy Retinal anlage tumour	Rare infantile neuroectodermal tumour arising mainly in the maxilla; usually (but not always) benign.
Melanotic progonoma	See melanotic neuroectodermal tumour of infancy	
Melanotic schwannoma	Melanocytic schwannoma	Rare histological variant of schwannoma associated with melanin pigmentation. It may be benign or malignant.
Meningeal hamartoma	Ectopic meningothelial hamartoma Sequestrated meningocoele	Benign extracranial or extraspinal proliferation of meningothelial cells, most likely a malformation.

Tumour terminology Recommended terms are in **bold**	Synonyms	Comments
Mesenchymal chondrosarcoma	See extraskeletal mesenchymal chondrosarcoma	
Metatarsalgia	See Morton's neuroma	
MFH	See malignant fibrous histiocytoma	
Mixed tumour	Myoepithelioma Pleomorphic adenoma	Rare soft tissue tumour comparable to salivary gland counterpart.
Monophasic epithelial synovial sarcoma		Exceedingly rare purely epithelial variant of synovial sarcoma.
Monophasic synovial sarcoma		Variant of synovial sarcoma with purely spindle cell morphology.
Morton's metatarsalgia	See Morton's neuroma	
Morton's neuroma	Metatarsalgia Morton's metatarsalgia	Reactive fibrosis of nerve(s) beneath heads of metatarsal bones in foot.
MPNET	See malignant peripheral primitive neuroectodermal tumour	
MPNST	See malignant peripheral nerve sheath tumour	
Mucosal neuroma		Rare hamartomatous proliferation of nerves associated with multiple endocrine neoplasia, type IIb.
Multicentric reticulohistiocytosis	Lipoid dermatoarthritis	Multifocal reticulohistiocytoma affecting mainly skin and joints, leading to arthropathy.
Myelolipoma		Benign tumour composed of adipose and haemopoietic tissue; rarely occurs outside the adrenal.
Myoblastoma	See granular cell tumour	
Myoepithelioma	See mixed tumour	
Myofibroblastoma		Benign myofibroblastic tumour occurring in lymph node, breast, or soft tissue.
Myofibroma	See solitary myofibroma	
Myolipoma		Rare benign tumour composed of adipose tissue and smooth muscle.

Tumour terminology Recommended terms are in **bold**	Synonyms	Comments
Myositis ossificans		Intramuscular reactive (myo)fibroblastic lesion with bone formation.
Myositis ossificans progressiva	See fibrodysplasia ossificans progressiva	
Myxofibrosarcoma	Myxoid malignant fibrous histiocytoma Myxoid MFH	Common sarcoma of usually older patients showing fibroblastic differentiation and mucin production.
Myxoid chondrosarcoma	See extraskeletal myxoid chondrosarcoma	
Myxoid liposarcoma		Histological variant of liposarcoma with mucinous matrix and of variable grade.
Myxoid malignant fibrous histiocytoma	See myxofibrosarcoma	
Myxoid MFH	See myxofibrosarcoma	
Myxolipoma		Benign lipoma with myxoid degeneration.
Myxoma		Benign fibroblastic tumour associated with copious mucin production.
Myxopapillary ependymoma	See extraspinal ependymoma	
Naevoxantho-endothelioma	See juvenile xanthogranuloma	
Naevus araneus	See spider naevus	
Naevus flammeus	Salmon patch	Birthmark composed of dilated blood vessels; usually regresses.
Naevus lipomatosus	Naevus lipomatosus cutaneous superficialis	Diffuse multinodular lipoma(s) of skin, usually congenital.
Naevus lipomatosus cutaneous superficialis	See naevus lipomatosus	
NAME syndrome	See Carney's complex	
Nasal glioma	See glial heterotopia	
Nasopharyngeal angiofibroma		Locally aggressive fibrovascular tumour, most common in adolescent males.
Nerve sheath ganglion	See ganglion	
Nerve sheath myxoma	See dermal nerve sheath myxoma	

Tumour terminology Recommended terms are in **bold**	Synonyms	Comments
Neural fibrolipoma	See fibrolipomatous hamartoma of nerve	
Neurilemmoma	See schwannoma	
Neurinoma	See schwannoma	
Neuroepithelioma (peripheral)	See malignant peripheral primitive neuroectodermal tumour	
Neurofibroma		Benign nerve sheath tumour, possibly hamartomatous; often multiple and associated with NF-1.
Neurofibromatosis 1 (NF-1)	von Recklinghausen's disease NF-1	An inherited systemic disease, a major manifestation of which is multiple neurofibromas (along with other tumour types).
Neurofibromatosis 1 (NF-2)	Bilateral acoustic neurofibromatosis NF-2	An inherited systemic disease characterised principally by bilateral schwannomas of the VIIIth cranial nerve.
Neurofibrosarcoma	See malignant peripheral nerve sheath tumour	
Neuromuscular hamartoma	Benign Triton tumour	Very rare benign tumour (probably malformation) of nerve.
Neurothekeoma	See dermal nerve sheath myxoma	
Neurothekeoma	See cellular neurothekeoma	
NF-1	See neurofibromatosis 1	
NF-2	See neurofibromatosis 2	
Nodular fasciitis		Reactive fibroblastic/myofibroblastic lesion, very rarely recurs.
Nodular subepidermal fibrosis	See fibrous histiocytoma	
Nodular tenosynovitis	See giant cell tumour of tendon sheath	
Non-chromaffin paraganglioma	See alveolar soft part sarcoma	Obsolete term.
Non-neural granular cell tumour		Heterogeneous group of rare granular cell tumours not of nerve sheath origin.

Tumour terminology Recommended terms are in **bold**	Synonyms	Comments
Nuchal fibroma		Benign fibrolipomatous lesion on the back of the neck.
Omental-mesenteric myxoid hamartoma	See inflammatory myofibroblastic tumour	
Ossifying fibromyxoid tumour		Usually benign, bone-forming tumour of uncertain histogenesis.
Osteolipoma		Benign lipoma with metaplastic bone.
Osteosarcoma	See soft tissue osteosarcoma	Malignant bone-forming neoplasm without other differentiation.
Pacinian neurofibroma	See Pacinian schwannoma	
Pacinian neuroma		Benign hyperplasia of Pacinian corpuscles.
Pacinian schwannoma	Pacinian neurofibroma	Benign nerve sheath tumour with focal Pacinian differentiation.
Palisaded encapsulated neuroma	See solitary circumscribed neuroma	
Palisaded myofibroblastoma	See intranodal myofibroblastoma	
Palmar fibromatosis	Dupuytren's contracture Dupuytren's disease	Locally aggressive fibroblastic lesion in the hand.
Papillary endothelial hyperplasia	Intravascular papillary endothelial hyperplasia Masson's tumour	Distinctive form of organising blood clot in a vessel or haemangioma.
Parachordoma		Very rare tumour, probably closely related to mixed tumour.
Paradoxical fibrosarcoma	See atypical fibroxanthoma	
Parosteal fasciitis		Variant of nodular fasciitis developing on the surface of a bone.
Pelvic lipomatosis	See lipomatosis	
Penile fibromatosis	See Peyronie's disease	
Pericytoma	See haemangiopericytoma	
Perineurial fibroma	See perineurioma	

Tumour terminology Recommended terms are in **bold**	Synonyms	Comments
Perineurioma	Extraneural perineurioma Intraneural perineurioma Storiform perineurial fibroma	Benign nerve sheath tumour showing perineurial cell differentiation.
Peripheral neuroepithelioma	See malignant peripheral primitive neuroectodermal tumour	
Peyronie's disease	Penile fibromatosis Plastic induration of penis	Benign but disfiguring fibroinflammatory condition of the penis.
Pigmented dermatofibrosarcoma protuberans	Bednár tumour Pigmented storiform neurofibroma	Variant of DFSP containing dendritic melanocytes.
Pigmented neuroectodermal tumour of infancy	See melanotic neuroectodermal tumour of infancy	
Pigmented storiform neurofibroma	See pigmented dermatofibrosarcoma protuberans	
Pigmented villonodular tenosynovitis	See diffuse-type giant cell tumour	
Pilar leiomyoma	Cutaneous leiomyoma Leiomyoma of arrector pili	Commonly painful skin tumour derived from arrector pili muscle. Frequently multiple.
Plane xanthoma	See xanthoma	
Plantar fibromatosis	Ledderhose's disease	Locally aggressive fibroblastic lesion in the sole of the foot.
Plastic induration of penis	See Peyronie's disease	
Pleomorphic adenoma	See mixed tumour	
Pleomorphic hyalinising angiectatic tumour		Uncommon low grade tumour with degenerative features.
Pleomorphic lipoma		Benign lipoma variant with bizarre giant cells; closely related to spindle cell lipoma.
Pleomorphic liposarcoma		High grade aggressive variant of liposarcoma.

Tumour terminology Recommended terms are in **bold**	Synonyms	Comments
Pleomorphic malignant fibrous histiocytoma	Fibroxanthosarcoma	Heterogeneous group of high grade sarcomas occurring mainly in adults. Commonly referred to as MFH.
Pleomorphic rhabdomyosarcoma		Rare histological variant of rhabdomyosarcoma occurring in adults. Associated with aggressive behaviour.
Plexiform fibrohistiocytic tumour		Uncommon fibrous histiocytoma variant, prone to recur, rarely metastasises.
Plexiform neurofibroma		Variant of neurofibroma pathognomonic of NF-1.
Plexiform schwannoma		Multinodular variant of benign schwannoma.
Polyvinylpyrrolidone granuloma	PVP granuloma	Reactive pseudoneoplastic process due to former use of plasma expander.
Port-wine stain		Birthmark composed of dilated blood vessels; usually does not regress.
Primitive neuroectodermal tumour	See malignant peripheral primitive neuroectodermal tumour	
Proliferative fasciitis		Variant of nodular fasciitis with plump ganglion-like cells.
Proliferative funiculitis		Variant of fasciitis occurring in spermatic cord.
Proliferative myositis		Variant of proliferative fasciitis occurring within skeletal muscle.
Psammomatous melanotic schwannoma		Variant of melanotic schwannoma especially associated with Carney's syndrome/complex.
Pseudosarcoma of skin	See atypical fibroxanthoma	
Pseudosarcomatous fibrous histiocytoma	See atypical benign fibrous histiocytoma	
PVP granuloma	See polyvinylpyrrolidone granuloma	
Pyogenic granuloma	See lobular capillary haemangioma	
Racemose haemangioma	See arteriovenous haemangioma	

Tumour terminology Recommended terms are in **bold**	Synonyms	Comments
Recklinghausen's disease (von)	See neurofibromatosis type 1	
Reticulohistiocytic granuloma	See reticulohistiocytoma	
Reticulohistiocytoma	Reticulohistiocytic granuloma	Usually solitary benign skin lesion composed of histiocytes.
Retiform haemangioendothelioma		Rare, recurring low grade vascular tumour with infrequent metastasis.
Retinal anlage tumour	See melanotic neuroectodermal tumour of infancy	
Rhabdoid tumour	See extrarenal rhabdoid tumour	
Rhabdomyofibrosarcoma		Very rare sarcoma with combined skeletal muscle and myofibroblastic differentiation.
Rhabdomyoma		Rare benign tumour showing skeletal muscle differentiation.
Rhabdomyomatous mesenchymal hamartoma		Exceedingly rare cutaneous malformation in infancy.
Rhabdomyosarcoma		Malignant tumour showing skeletal muscle differentiation, most common in first two decades of life.
Round cell liposarcoma		High grade, poorly differentiated histological variant of myxoid liposarcoma.
Salmon patch	See naevus flammeus	
Sarcoma		Malignant neoplasm showing connective tissue (mesenchymal) differentiation.
Sarcoma botryoides	See embryonal rhabdomyosarcoma	
Schwannoma	Neurilemmoma Neurinoma	Benign nerve sheath tumour, usually solitary, and only rarely associated with neurofibromatosis. Includes acoustic, ancient, cellular, and plexiform variants.
Sclerosing epithelioid fibrosarcoma		Rare histological variant of fibrosarcoma.

Tumour terminology Recommended terms are in **bold**	Synonyms	Comments
Sclerosing haemangioma		See Tumours of Skin (Non-Melanocytic) (Section 41).
Sclerosing liposarcoma		Histological variant of well differentiated liposarcoma.
Sclerotic fibroma	See storiform collagenoma	
Sequestrated meningocoele	See ectopic meningothelial hamartoma	
Sinusoidal haemangioma		Thin-walled histological variant of cavernous haemangioma.
Small cell tumour		Generic term for the small round cell tumours (e.g., rhabdomyosarcoma, MPNET, desmoplastic small round cell tumour) occurring in young patients.
Smooth muscle hamartoma	See congenital smooth muscle hamartoma	
Soft tissue chondroma	Chondroma Chondroma of soft parts Extraskeletal chondroma	Benign cartilaginous tumour, usually on a digit.
Soft tissue osteosarcoma	Extraosseous osteosarcoma Extraskeletal osteosarcoma Osteosarcoma	Osteosarcoma arising primarily in soft tissue; usually aggressive.
Solitary circumscribed neuroma	Palisaded encapsulated neuroma	Benign nerve sheath tumour, most common in "muzzle" area of face.
Solitary fibrous tumour	Localised fibrous tumour (Pleural fibroma)	Usually benign fibrous tissue tumour. Also found in the pleura. Approximately 10% are malignant.
Solitary myofibroma	Adult-type myofibroma Localised myofibromatosis	Usually cutaneous benign myoid nodule.
Spider naevus	Naevus araneus	Dilated blood vessel(s) in skin, usually acquired in adulthood.
Spindle cell haemangioendothelioma	Spindle cell haemangioma	Benign, often multifocal vascular tumour most common in skin of distal extremities.

Tumour terminology Recommended terms are in **bold**	Synonyms	Comments
Spindle cell haemangioma	See spindle cell haemangioendothelioma	
Spindle cell lipoma		Histological variant of lipoma showing distinctive spindle cell areas.
Spindle cell liposarcoma		Histological variant of well differentiated liposarcoma showing spindle cell morphology.
Spindle cell rhabdomyosarcoma		Histological variant of rhabdomyosarcoma. Associated with a good prognosis in children.
Sternomastoid tumour	See fibromatosis colli	
Stewart-Treves syndrome	See angiosarcoma	Angiosarcoma arising in chronic lymph oedema, classically post-surgical.
Storiform collagenoma	Circumscribed storiform collagenoma Sclerotic fibroma	See Tumours of Skin (Non-Melanocytic) (Section 41).
Storiform perineurial fibroma	See perineurioma	
Strawberry naevus	See capillary haemangioma	
Superficial angiomyxoma		Benign myxomatous skin lesion; prone to recur.
Symmetrical lipomatosis	See lipomatosis	
Synovial chondromatosis		Multinodular benign proliferation of cartilage occurring in tenosynovial tissue.
Synovial haemangioma		Haemangioma (usually cavernous) arising in synovium/joint.
Synovial lipoma	See lipoma arborescens	
Synovial sarcoma	Malignant synovioma (obsolete)	Soft tissue sarcoma with epithelial features, not truly related to synovium.
Synovioma, benign	See giant cell tumour of tendon sheath	Obsolete term.
Targetoid haemosiderotic haemangioma	See hobnail haemangioma	
Telangiectatic granuloma	See lobular capillary haemangioma	
Tendinous xanthoma		Clinical variant of xanthoma.

Tumour terminology Recommended terms are in **bold**	Synonyms	Comments
Tenosynovial fibroma	See fibroma of tendon sheath	
Tenosynovial giant cell tumour	See giant cell tumour of tendon sheath	
Thoracopulmonary small cell tumour	See malignant peripheral primitive neuroectodermal tumour	
Torticollis	See fibromatosis colli	
Traumatic neuroma	Amputation neuroma	Reactive proliferation at site of transected nerve.
Tuberous xanthoma		Clinical variant of xanthoma.
Tufted angioma	Angioblastoma of Nakagawa	Non-regressing variant of lobular capillary haemangioma.
Tumoural calcinosis	Calcifying bursitis Kikuyu bursa	Non-neoplastic deposition of calcific material. May be inherited or follow chronic trauma.
Vascular leiomyoma	See angioleiomyoma	
Vascular malformation		Benign vascular proliferation, which is probably developmental in origin; includes haemangioma and arteriovenous haemangioma.
Vegetant intravascular haemangioendothelioma	See intravascular papillary endothelial hyperplasia	
Venous haemangioma		Histological variant of haemangioma composed mainly of veins.
Verrucous haemangioma		Histological variant of haemangioma with overlying hyperkeratosis.
Villonodular tenosynovitis	See diffuse-type giant cell tumour	
von Recklinghausen's disease	See neurofibromatosis type I	
Well differentiated (WD) liposarcoma		Low grade variant of liposarcoma, recurs frequently but incapable of metastasis unless dedifferentiates; includes adipocytic, lipoma-like, sclerosing, and inflammatory variants. Atypical lipoma also belongs to the same category.

Tumour terminology Recommended terms are in **bold**	Synonyms	Comments
Xanthogranuloma	See juvenile xanthogranuloma	So-called juvenile xanthogranuloma also occurs in young adults.
Xanthoma	Eruptive xanthoma Tendinous xanthoma Tuberous xanthoma Plane xanthoma	Non-neoplastic deposition of lipid in soft tissue, often associated with hyperlipidaemia; includes eruptive, tendinous, and tuberous variants.

Section 43

Tumours of the Bone

J.R. Salisbury

Tumour terminology Recommended terms are in **bold**	Synonyms	Comments
Adamantinoma		Low grade malignant tumour predominantly affecting long bones, particularly the tibia.
Aggressive chondroblastoma		Rare variant of chondroblastoma characterised by a locally aggressive growth pattern and occasionally associated with pulmonary metastases.
Aggressive fibromatosis	See desmoplastic fibroma	
Aggressive osteoblastoma	Malignant osteoblastoma Osteosarcoma in situ	Controversial histological variant of osteoblastoma characterised by the presence of epithelioid osteoblasts. Recurrences are common but the tumour does not metastasise.
Aneurysmal bone cyst		Locally aggressive tumour-like lesion, which predominantly affects the long bones and arises most often in the first two decades.
Angiosarcoma	Haemangioendothelial sarcoma Haemangiosarcoma Malignant haemangioendothelioma	Rare, high grade tumour. Metastases to lung are common.
Askin's tumour	See Ewing's tumour/ PNET	A clinical variant of Ewing's tumour/ PNET presenting on the chest wall.
Benign chondroblastoma	See chondroblastoma	
Benign fibrous histiocytoma		Rare spindle cell tumour occurring in adults. Overlaps with metaphyseal fibrous defect.

Tumour terminology Recommended terms are in **bold**	Synonyms	Comments
Benign osteoblastoma	See osteoblastoma	
Bizarre parosteal osteochondromatous proliferation	BPOP Nora's lesion	Rare tumour-like lesion composed of ossifying cartilage. The hands and feet are most often affected. Recurrences are common.
Bone island	See osteoma	
BPOP	See bizarre parosteal osteochondromatous proliferation	
Brown tumour of hyperparathyroidism		Tumour-like lesion composed of spindle and giant cells with abundant haemosiderin pigment. It may be confused with giant cell tumour of bone.
Cartilage-capped exostosis	See osteochondroma	
Cartilaginous and vascular hamartoma (mesenchymoma)		Benign tumour-like lesion presenting on the chest wall of infants.
Cartilaginous exostosis	See osteochondroma	
Central low grade osteosarcoma		Histological variant of osteosarcoma. Fibrosarcoma-like tissue with coarse trabeculae of immature bone remiscent of fibrous dysplasia.
Chloroma	See granulocytic sarcoma	
Chondroblastic osteosarcoma		Histological variant of osteosarcoma. A dominant proportion of the tumour must be chondroblastic.
Chondroblastoma	Benign chondroblastoma Codman's tumour Epiphyseal chondroblastoma Epiphyseal chondromatous giant cell tumour (obsolete)	Benign tumour of primitive cartilage, which most often arises in the epiphysis of long bones. Patients in the second decade are typically affected. Variants include aggressive chondroblastoma and cystic chondroblastoma.
Chondroid chordoma		Histological variant of chordoma showing cartilaginous differentiation and typically presenting in the spheno-occipital region.

Tumour terminology Recommended terms are in **bold**	Synonyms	Comments
Chondroma		Benign tumour of cartilage. Clinical variants include enchondroma, periosteal/juxtacortical chondroma, and soft tissue chondroma.
Chondrometaplasia	See synovial chondromatosis	
Chondromyxoid fibroma		Rare, benign, cartilaginous tumour, which most often presents in the metaphysis of long bones or the small bones of the feet. Local recurrence is common.
Chondrosarcoma		Malignant tumour of hyaline cartilage, which may arise in a central (pelvis, ribs, and shoulder girdle) or peripheral (often developing in a pre-existent osteochondroma) location. Prognosis is particularly related to the cytological grade. Variants include clear cell, dedifferentiated, mesenchymal, myxoid, and periosteal chondrosarcoma.
Chondrosarcoma with additional mesenchymal component	See dedifferentiated chondrosarcoma	
Chordoma		Rare, low grade malignant tumour derived from remnants of the notochord and presenting most often in the sacrococcygeal and spheno-occipital regions. Recurrences are common. Chondroid chordoma is a histological variant.
Chordoma periphericum	See parachordoma	
Circumscribed osteoblastoma	See osteoid osteoma	
Clear cell chondrosarcoma		Low grade, histological variant of chondrosarcoma, usually affecting the ends of long bones. Sometimes associated with contiguous aneurysmal bone cyst.
Codman's tumour	See chondroblastoma	
Congenital fibromatosis	See infantile myofibromatosis	
Congenital melanocarcinoma	See melanotic neuroectodermal tumour of infancy	

Tumour terminology Recommended terms are in **bold**	Synonyms	Comments
Cortical fibrous dysplasia	See osteofibrous dysplasia	
Cortical osteoblastoma	See osteoid osteoma	
Cystic chondroblastoma		Variant of chondroblastoma characterised by the juxtaposition of an aneurysmal bone cyst.
Dedifferentiated chondrosarcoma	Chondrosarcoma with addition mesenchymal component.	Variant of chondrosarcoma combining a usually low grade lesion juxtaposed with a high grade poorly differentiated sarcoma. The prognosis is poor.
Desmoid tumour of bone	See desmoplastic fibroma	
Desmoplastic fibroma	Aggressive fibromatosis Desmoid tumour of bone	This is the osseous equivalent of fibromatosis. Recurrences are common.
Diaphyseal aclasia	See osteochondromatosis	
Dyschondroplasia	See multiple enchondromatosis	
Ehrenfried's hereditary deforming chondrodysplasia	See osteochondromatosis	
Enchondroma		Clinical variant of chondroma, which most often presents in the small bones of the hands and feet.
Endothelial myeloma	See Ewing's tumour/ PNET	Obsolete term.
Enostoma	See osteoma	
Enostosis	See osteoma	
Eosinophilic granuloma	See Langerhans cell histiocytosis	
Epiphyseal chondroblastoma	See chondroblastoma	
Epiphyseal chondromatous giant cell tumour	See chondroblastoma	Obsolete term.
Epithelioid angiosarcoma	See haemangioendothelioma	
Epithelioid haemangioendothelioma	See haemangioendothelioma	

Tumour terminology Recommended terms are in **bold**	Synonyms	Comments
Epithelioid haemangioma	See haemangioendothelioma	
Epithelioid osteosarcoma		Histological variant of osteosarcoma. Epithelioid cells arranged in compact groups and sheets within, which are found delicate trabeculae of osteoid.
Ewing's sarcoma	See Ewing's tumour/ PNET	
Ewing's tumour/PNET	Askin's tumour Endothelial myeloma (obsolete) Ewing's sarcoma Malignant neuroectodermal tumour Malignant neuroepithelioma of bone	Rare primitive neuroectodermal tumour (PNET) arising predominantly in long bones and affecting people in the second decade. Most tumours are associated with a reciprocal translocation 11:22 (q24; q12) and respond dramatically to high-dose irradiation and multi-drug chemotherapy.
Exostosis	See osteochondroma	
Fibroblastic osteosarcoma		Histological variant of osteosarcoma. A dominant proportion of the tumour must be fibroblastic.
Fibrocartilaginous dysplasia		Histological variant of fibrous dysplasia characterised by the presence of cartilage.
Fibrocartilaginous mesenchymoma of infancy		Rare hamartoma affecting the metaphysis of long bones.
Fibrohistiocytic/ malignant fibrous histiocytoma-like osteosarcoma		Histological variant of osteosarcoma. Cellular fibroblastic tissue with an admixture of mononuclear cells results in an appearance similar to pleomorphic malignant fibrous histiocytoma.
Fibroma	See metaphyseal fibrous defect	
Fibromatosis hyalinica multiplex	See juvenile hyaline fibromatosis	
Fibro-osseous dysplasia	See osteofibrous dysplasia	
Fibrosarcoma		Rare malignant fibroblastic tumour usually presenting in the metaphysis of long bones.

Tumour terminology Recommended terms are in **bold**	Synonyms	Comments
Fibrous cortical defect	See metaphyseal fibrous defect	
Fibrous dysplasia		Tumour-like lesion affecting children or young adults. Multiple lesions may be associated with lentigines and precocious puberty (Albright's syndrome).
Fibrous xanthoma	See metaphyseal fibrous defect	
Fibroxanthoma	See metaphyseal fibrous defect	
Ganglion cyst	See juxta-articular bone cyst	
Genuine osteoblastoma	See osteoblastoma	
Giant cell (reparative) granuloma		Tumour-like reactive lesion, which presents in the jaw and may be confused with giant cell tumour of bone and brown tumour of hyperparathyroidism.
Giant cell tumour of bone	Osteoclastoma	Usually benign tumour rich in osteoclast-like giant cells. Recurrences are common; 5–10% undergo sarcomatous transformation, sometimes following radiotherapy.
Giant osteoid osteoma	See osteoblastoma	Obsolete term.
Glomangioma		See Tumours of Soft Tissue (Section 42).
Glomus tumour		See Tumours of Soft Tissue (Section 42).
Granulocytic sarcoma		See Tumours of the Bone Marrow and Leukaemia (Section 23).
Haemangioendothelial sarcoma	See angiosarcoma	
Haemangioendothelioma		A vascular tumour of variable biological potential characterised by the presence of epithelioid endothelial cells. The most benign end of the spectrum is sometimes classified as epithelioid haemangioma. Intermediate tumours are known as epithelioid haemangioendothelioma and the most malignant as epithelioid angiosarcoma. Most bone tumours are multifocal and characterised by an aggressive growth pattern. Metastases are rare.

Tumour terminology Recommended terms are in **bold**	Synonyms	Comments
Haemangioma		Rare benign vascular lesion. Many are hamartomatous rather than tumours.
Haemangiopericytoma		Extremely rare malignant tumour. Cell of origin is uncertain. It probably represents a heterogeneous condition.
Haemangiosarcoma	See angiosarcoma	
Hand-Schuller-Christian disease	See Langerhans cell histiocytosis	
High grade surface osteosarcoma		Very rare, highly malignant osteoblastic lesion arising on the bone surface.
Histiocytic xanthogranuloma	See metaphyseal fibrous defect	
Histiocytosis X	See Langerhans cell histiocytosis	Obsolete term.
In situ osteosarcoma	See aggressive osteoblastoma	
Infantile fibrosarcoma of bone		Exceptionally rare bone tumour. Most examples of this tumour arise in the soft tissues.
Infantile myofibromatosis	Congenital fibromatosis	Primary solitary bone lesions are very rare. Multifocal disease quite often involves the skeleton. See Tumours of Soft Tissue (Section 42).
Intracortical osteosarcoma		The rarest variant of osteosarcoma. Most are sclerotic.
Intraosseous ganglion	See juxta-articular bone cyst	
Ivory osteoma	See osteoma	
Juvenile bone cyst	See solitary bone cyst	
Juvenile hyaline fibromatosis	Fibromatosis hyalinica multiplex	See Tumours of Soft Tissue (Section 42).
Juxta-articular bone cyst	Ganglion cyst Intraosseous ganglion Synovial cyst	Intraosseous equivalent of ganglion cyst.
Juxtacortical chondroma	See chondroma	
Juxtacortical chondrosarcoma	See parosteal chondrosarcoma	

Tumour terminology Recommended terms are in **bold**	Synonyms	Comments
Juxtacortical osteosarcoma	See parosteal osteosarcoma	
Langerhans cell granulomatosis	See Langerhans cell histiocytosis	
Langerhans cell histiocytosis	Histiocytosis X (obsolete) Langerhans cell granulomatosis Reticuloendotheliosis (obsolete)	Proliferative lesion of Langerhans cells of variable biological potential ranging from completely benign (eosinophilic granuloma) or multifocal (Hand-Schuller-Christian disease) to a potentially lethal multisystem variant (Letterer-Siwe disease).
Leiomyoma		Extremely rare. See Tumours of Soft Tissue (Section 42).
Leiomyosarcoma		Extremely rare. See Tumours of Soft Tissue (Section 42).
Letterer-Siwe disease	See Langerhans cell histiocytosis	
Lipoma		Extremely rare in bone. See Tumours of Soft Tissue (Section 42).
Liposarcoma		Extremely rare in bone. See Tumours of Soft Tissue (Section 42).
Lymphangioma		Bone lesions are extremely rare and are often multiple. See Tumours of Soft Tissue (Section 42).
Lymphosarcoma of bone	See malignant lymphoma of bone.	Obsolete term.
Maffucci's syndrome		Skeletal osteochondromatosis (multiple osteochondromas) associated with soft tissue angiomas. The incidence of malignancy in Maffucci's syndrome is estimated to be 23%.
Malignant fibrous histiocytoma		High grade pleomorphic sarcoma showing no evidence of osteoid or chondroid formation. Probably represents the endpoint for multiple anaplastic tumours of variable histogenesis and, as such, denotes a heterogeneous entity.
Malignant haemangioendothelioma	See angiosarcoma	

Tumour terminology Recommended terms are in **bold**	Synonyms	Comments
Malignant lymphoma of bone	Lymphosarcoma of bone (obsolete) Parker-Jackson reticulosarcoma (obsolete) Reticulosarcoma of bone (obsolete)	See Tumours of the Lymph Nodes and Spleen (Section 24).
Malignant mesenchymoma	Osteoliposarcoma	Extremely rare high grade sarcoma showing divergent differentiation.
Malignant neuroectodermal tumour	See Ewing's tumour/ PNET	
Malignant neuroepithelioma of bone	See Ewing's tumour/ PNET	
Malignant osteoblastoma	See aggressive osteoblastoma	
Malignant small cell tumour of bone	See Ewing's tumour/ PNET	
Mastocytosis		Involvement of bone is common in systemic mastocytosis. It has no prognostic significance.
Medullary osteoma	See osteoma	
Melanotic adamantinoma	See melanotic neuroectodermal tumour of infancy	
Melanotic anlage tumour	See melanotic neuroectodermal tumour of infancy	
Melanotic hamartoma	See melanotic neuroectodermal tumour of infancy	
Melanotic neuroectodermal tumour of infancy	Congenital melanocarcinoma Melanotic adamantinoma Melanotic anlage tumour Melanotic hamartoma Melanotic progonoma Pigmented epulis (of infancy) Pigmented neuroectodermal tumour of infancy Retinal anlage tumour Retinal choristoma	The maxilla is the most common site of origin of this rare tumour. See Tumours of Soft Tissue (Section 42).

Tumour terminology Recommended terms are in **bold**	Synonyms	Comments
Melanotic progonoma	See melanotic neuroectodermal tumour of infancy	
Mesenchymal chondrosarcoma		Histological variant of chondrosarcoma, which may arise in the soft tissues and other sites in addition to bone. It is usually associated with a poor prognosis.
Metaphyseal fibrous defect	Fibroma Fibrous cortical defect Fibrous xanthoma Fibroxanthoma Histiocytic xanthogranuloma Non-ossifying fibroma Non-osteogenic fibroma	Tumour-like lesion presenting in the metaphysis of long bones. Usually affects patients in the first two decades and often represents an incidental finding on X-ray examination.
Multiple cartilaginous exostosis	See osteochondromatosis	
Multiple enchondromatosis	Dyschondroplasia Ollier's disease	Multiple benign enchondromas often in a unilateral distribution and associated with a significant risk of developing chondrosarcoma.
Myeloma		A malignant tumour of plasma cells. See lymphoproliferative and haemopoietic tumours See Tumours of the Bone Marrow and Leukaemia (Section 23).
Myositis ossificans		A tumour-like lesion, which arises in skeletal muscle usually following trauma. It is characteristically zoned, being composed of spindle cells in the middle and trabecular bone at the periphery.
Myxoid chondrosarcoma		Histological variant of chondrosarcoma, which arises most often in the soft tissues. See Tumours of Soft Tissue (Section 42).
Neurilemmoma	Neurinoma Schwannoma	Primary lesions in bone are exceedingly rare. See Tumours of Soft Tissue (Section 42).
Neurinoma	See neurilemmoma	
Neurofibroma		Primary lesions in bone are exceedingly rare. See Tumours of Soft Tissue (Section 42).

Tumour terminology Recommended terms are in **bold**	Synonyms	Comments
Non-ossifying fibroma	See metaphyseal fibrous defect	
Non-osteogenic fibroma	See metaphyseal fibrous defect	
Nora's lesion	See bizarre parosteal osteochondromatous proliferation	
Ollier's disease	See multiple enchondromatosis	
Ossifying fibroma	See osteofibrous dysplasia	
Osteoblastic osteosarcoma		Histological variant of osteosarcoma.
Osteoblastoma	Benign osteoblastoma Genuine osteoblastoma Giant osteoid osteoma (obsolete) Spongious osteoblastoma	Benign or locally aggressive tumour showing considerable overlap with osteoid osteoma. Recurrences are seen in up to 15% of cases.
Osteocartilaginous exostosis	See osteochondroma	
Osteochondroma	Cartilage-capped exostosis Cartilaginous exostosis Osteocartilaginous exostosis	Common tumour-like lesion most often presenting in the metaphysis of the long bones and representing a misplaced epiphyseal plate. Usually affects adolescents and young adults. Chondrosarcoma is a rare complication. Osteochondromatosis is a clinical variant.
Osteochondromatosis	Multiple cartilaginous exostosis Ehrenfried's hereditary deforming chondrodysplasia Diaphyseal aclasia	A rare syndrome of multiple osteochondromas. Malignant change may affect up to 10% of patients.
Osteoclastoma	See giant cell tumour of bone	
Osteoclast-rich osteosarcoma		Histological variant of osteosarcoma.

Tumour terminology Recommended terms are in **bold**	Synonyms	Comments
Osteofibrous dysplasia	Cortical fibrous dysplasia Fibro-osseous dysplasia Ossifying fibroma	Variant of fibrous dysplasia, predominantly involving the cortex of the tibia and fibula.
Osteogenic sarcoma	See osteosarcoma	Histological variant of osteosarcoma.
Osteoid osteoma	Circumscribed osteoblastoma Cortical osteoblastoma	Rare benign tumour most often affecting the metaphysis of long bones. Severe pain, relieved by aspirin, is characteristic feature.
Osteoliposarcoma	See malignant mesenchymoma	
Osteoma	Bone island Enostoma Enostosis	Localized overgrowth of mature bone. The facial bones and sinuses are most often affected. Variants include ivory osteoma and medullary osteoma.
Osteosarcoma	Osteogenic sarcoma	Most common primary malignant bone tumour. The lower end of the femur, the upper end of the tibia, and fibula are most often affected. Patients are most often children or adolescents. A second peak occurs in the elderly in association with Paget's disease. Variants include central low grade osteosarcoma, chondroblastic, epithelioid, fibroblastic, fibrohistiocytic/malignant fibrous histiocytoma-like, high grade surface osteosarcoma, intracortical, osteoblastic, osteoclast-rich, Paget's disease, parosteal osteosarcoma, post-irradiation, small cell, and Telangiectatic osteosarcoma.
Osteosarcoma in situ	See aggressive osteoblastoma	
Paget's disease-associated osteosarcoma		There must be evidence of Paget's disease of bone must (this may be radiological).
Parachordoma		Extremely rare chordoma-like tumour, not in the midline.
Parker-Jackson reticulosarcoma	See malignant lymphoma of bone	Obsolete term.
Parosteal desmoid	See periosteal desmoid	

Tumour terminology Recommended terms are in **bold**	Synonyms	Comments
Parosteal osteosarcoma	Juxtacortical osteosarcoma	Variant of osteosarcoma, closely applied to outer surface of the cortex. The tumour is characterised by a protracted natural history. It is associated with a considerable risk of recurrence and progression if primary surgery is inadequate.
Periosteal chondroma		Histological variant of chondroma occurring on the surface of a long bone.
Periosteal chondrosarcoma	Juxtacortical chondrosarcoma	Rare variant of chondrosarcoma arising on the surface of the bone, particularly the femur.
Periosteal desmoid	Parosteal desmoid	A non-neoplastic proliferation of fibrous tissue affecting the distal femur of young children.
Periosteal osteosarcoma		Variant of osteosarcoma resting on the outer surface of the cortex. There is a large cartilage component. Prognosis is fair.
Peripheral neuroblastoma of bone	See Ewing's tumour/PNET	
Pigmented epulis (of infancy)	See melanotic neuroectodermal tumour of infancy	
Pigmented neuroectodermal tumour of infancy	See melanotic neuroectodermal tumour of infancy	
Pigmented villonodular synovitis		Synovial equivalent of giant cell tumour of tendon sheath. Most often affects the knees, followed by the hips. Recurrences are common. Malignant transformation is exceptional.
Plasmacytoma	Solitary myeloma	See Tumours of the Lymph Nodes and Spleen (Section 24).
Post-irradiation osteosarcoma		Variant of osteosarcoma. Sufficient radiation to site (<60 Gy). Latent period of 5–30 years.
Primitive malignant neuroectodermal tumour of bone	See Ewing's tumour/PNET	

Tumour terminology Recommended terms are in **bold**	Synonyms	Comments
Pseudomalignant osteoblastoma		Controversial histological variant of osteoblastoma characterised by nuclear pleomorphism. A term to be avoided.
Reticuloendotheliosis	See Langerhans cell histiocytosis	Obsolete term.
Reticulosarcoma of bone	See malignant lymphoma of bone	Obsolete term.
Retinal anlage tumour	See melanotic neuroectodermal tumour of infancy	
Retinal choristoma	See melanotic neuroectodermal tumour of infancy	
Rosai-Dorman disease	See sinus histiocytosis with massive lymphadenopathy	
Schwannoma	See neurilemmoma	
Simple bone cyst	See solitary bone cyst	
Sinus histiocytosis with massive lymphadenopathy	Rosai-Dorfman disease	Bone involvement is uncommon. See lymphoproliferative and haemopoietic tumours. See Tumours of the Lymph Nodes and Spleen (Section 24).
Small cell osteosarcoma		Histological variant of osteosarcoma with small uniform cells. Same sites and prognosis as conventional osteosarcoma.
Soft tissue chondroma		See Tumours of Soft Tissue (Section 42).
Solitary bone cyst	Juvenile bone cyst Simple bone cyst Unicameral bone cyst	Tumour-like lesion, which usually presents in the proximal femur and proximal humerus. Young boys are most often affected.
Solitary myeloma	See plasmacytoma	
Spongious osteoblastoma	See osteoblastoma	
Synovial chondromatosis	Chondrometaplasia	Rare tumour-like condition consisting of multiple foci of chondroid metaplasia. The synovium of the knee joint is most commonly involved. There is a predilection for young males. It does not recur following synovectomy.

Tumour terminology Recommended terms are in **bold**	Synonyms	Comments
Synovial cyst	See juxta-articular bone cyst	
Telangiectatic osteosarcoma		Histological variant of osteosarcoma. Large, thin-walled vascular spaces dominate the tissue. At the extreme, it can be difficult to identify the osteoblastic component. This represents an aggressive lethal variant that is controlled by chemotherapy.
Unicameral bone cyst	See solitary bone cyst	

Section 44

Tumours of the Jaws and Teeth

F. Bonetti
W.M. Tilakaratne
P.R. Morgan
G.M. Mariuzzi

Tumour terminology Recommended terms are in **bold**	Synonyms	Comments
Adamantinoma	See ameloblastoma	Obsolete term.
Adenoameloblastoma	See adenomatoid odontogenic tumour	Obsolete term.
Adenomatoid odontogenic tumour	Adenoameloblastoma (obsolete) Ameloblastic adenomatoid tumour (obsolete) Glandular adamantinoma Pseudoadenoma adamantium (obsolete)	Benign tumour, which commonly presents as a dentigerous cyst.
Ameloblastic adenomatoid tumour	See adenomatoid odontogenic tumour	Obsolete term.
Ameloblastic carcinoma		This is a very rare tumour showing an ameloblastoma-like histological pattern but with cytological and behavioural features of malignancy.
Ameloblastic fibrodentinoma	Dentinoma (obsolete)	This is a very rare benign tumour similar to ameloblastic fibro-odontoma showing dentine but not enamel formation.
Ameloblastic fibrodentinosarcoma		This is an extremely rare malignant tumour resembling ameloblastic fibrosarcoma but also containing dentine-like tissue.

Tumour terminology Recommended terms are in **bold**	Synonyms	Comments
Ameloblastic fibroma	Soft mixed odontogenic tumour Soft mixed odontoma	This is a rare usually benign tumour, which occurs most often in children. It is composed of a mixture of ameloblastoma-like epithelium and odontogenic ectomesenchymal stroma. On occasion it may show locally aggressive behaviour or even malignant transformation.
Ameloblastic fibro-odontoma	Ameloblastic odontoma (obsolete)	This rare tumour is similar to ameloblastic fibroma but also shows dentine and enamel formation.
Ameloblastic fibro-odontosarcoma		This is an extremely rare malignant tumour resembling ameloblastic fibrosarcoma but also containing dentine and enamel.
Ameloblastic fibrosarcoma	Ameloblastic sarcoma	This is a very rare tumour, which sometimes arises as a consequence of malignant change in ameloblastic fibroma.
Ameloblastic odontoma	See ameloblastic fibro-odontoma	Obsolete term, which in the past was also used as a synonym for odontoameloblastoma.
Ameloblastic sarcoma	See ameloblastic fibrosarcoma	
Ameloblastoma	Adamantinoma (obsolete)	This is the most common odontogenic tumour. It is usually slowly growing and associated with a locally infiltrative growth pattern. A number of histological variants are recognised, including plexiform, follicular, acanthomatous, granular cell, basaloid, desmoplastic, and papillary keratoameloblastoma.
Aneurysmal bone cyst		See Tumours of the Bone (Section 43).
Benign cementoblastoma	True cementoma	This benign tumour histologically resembles osteoblastoma. It is usually found attached to the apex of a premolar or molar tooth.
Calcifying epithelial odontogenic tumour	Pindborg tumour	This rare tumour is benign but sometimes shows an infiltrative growth pattern. Although there is epithelial cell atypia, mitoses are not usually present. Despite its name, calcification is not invariable.

Tumour terminology Recommended terms are in **bold**	Synonyms	Comments
Calcifying odontogenic cyst	Cystic keratinising tumour (obsolete) Gorlin's cyst	This is a benign tumour, which sometimes has an infiltrative growth pattern. It shows some of the features of ameloblastoma but there are also keratinising "ghost cells" present.
Cementifying fibroma	See cemento-ossifying fibroma	
Cementoma		Collective term for tumour or tumour-like cementum-forming lesions.
Cemento-ossifying fibroma	Cementifying fibroma Ossifying fibroma	Encapsulated benign fibro-osseous neoplasm.
Central giant cell granuloma	Giant cell granuloma Giant cell reparative granuloma (obsolete)	This benign tumour is richly vascular and contains numerous giant cells. It is histologically indistinguishable from "brown tumour" of hyperparathyroidism. Recurrences may sometimes develop.
Central granular cell tumour of the jaws	See granular cell odontogenic tumour	
Cherubism	Familial fibrous dysplasia (obsolete) Familial multilocular cystic disease of the jaws (obsolete)	Genetic condition with gross but self-limiting symmetrical, jaw swellings.
Clear cell odontogenic carcinoma	Clear cell odontogenic tumour	This is a very rare tumour. The clear cells disguise the odontogenic origin. It is associated with an infiltrative growth pattern and commonly metastasises.
Clear cell odontogenic tumour	See clear cell odontogenic carcinoma	
Complex composite odontoma	See complex odontoma	Obsolete term.
Complex odontoma	Complex composite odontoma (obsolete)	Developmental malformation showing haphazard formation of dental hard tissues.
Composite odontoma		Collective term for complex and compound odontomas, rarely used nowadays.
Compound composite odontoma	See compound odontoma	

Tumour terminology Recommended terms are in **bold**	Synonyms	Comments
Compound odontoma	Compound composite odontoma	Tumour-like developmental malformation characterised by the formation of multiple tooth-like structures.
Cystic keratinising tumour	See calcifying odontogenic cyst	Obsolete term.
Dens in dente	See dens invaginatus	
Dens invaginatus	Dens in dente Gestant odontoma (obsolete) Invaginated odontome	Tumour-like developmental abnormality.
Dentinogenic ghost cell tumour	See odontogenic ghost cell tumour	
Dentinoma	See ameloblastic fibrodentinoma	Obsolete term.
Dilated odontoma		Far end of spectrum of dens invaginatus.
Enamel drop	See enamel pearl	Obsolete term.
Enamel pearl	Enamel drop (obsolete) Enameloma (obsolete)	Rare tumour-like nodule composed of enamel and dentine.
Enameloma	See enamel pearl	Obsolete term.
Eosinophilic granuloma		See Tumours of the Bone (Section 43).
Familial fibrous dysplasia	See cherubism	Obsolete term.
Familial multilocular cystic disease of the jaws	See cherubism	Obsolete term.
Fibrous dysplasia		A developmental, sometimes multiple, tumour-like fibro-osseous lesion. Very rarely may undergo malignant transformation.
Florid cemento-osseous dysplasia		Tumour-like multiple, periapical cementum-forming lesions.
Focal cemento-osseous dysplasia		Common tumour-like fibro-osseous lesion.
Gestant odontoma	See dens invaginatus	Obsolete term.
Giant cell granuloma	See central giant cell granuloma	

Tumour terminology Recommended terms are in **bold**	Synonyms	Comments
Giant cell reparative granuloma	See central giant cell granuloma	Obsolete term.
Giant cell tumour of bone		Debatable entity in the jaws. More aggressive than central giant cell granuloma but rarely malignant.
Gigantiform cementoma		Familial variant of florid cemento-osseous dysplasia. Commonly affects all quadrants.
Glandular adamantinoma	See adenomatoid odontogenic tumour	
Gorlin's cyst	See calcifying odontogenic cyst	
Granular cell ameloblastic fibroma	See granular cell odontogenic tumour	
Granular cell odontogenic fibroma	See granular cell odontogenic tumour	
Granular cell odontogenic tumour	Central granular cell tumour of the jaws

Granular cell odontogenic fibroma | Very rare, benign odontogenic tumour with low recurrence rate. |
Histiocytosis X		See Tumours of the Bone (Section 43).
Invaginated odontome	See dens invaginatus	
Langerhans cell histiocytosis		See Tumours of the Bone (Section 43).
Malignant ameloblastoma		Malignant odontogenic neoplasm with some features of ameloblastoma.
Melanoameloblastoma	See pigmented neuroectodermal tumour of infancy	Obsolete term.
Melanotic progonoma	See pigmented neuroectodermal tumour of infancy	Obsolete term.
Myxoma	See odontogenic myxoma	
Odontoameloblastoma		Very rare tumour similar to ameloblastoma but with the formation of dentine and enamel.

Tumour terminology Recommended terms are in **bold**	Synonyms	Comments
Odontogenic carcinoma		Generic term for any carcinoma arising from odontogenic epithelium, pre-existing cyst, or tumour.
Odontogenic carcinosarcoma		Extremely rare malignant tumour resembling ameloblastic fibrosarcoma in which the epithelial component is also cytologically malignant.
Odontogenic cyst		A heterogeneous group of cystic lesions sharing a common feature of an odontogenous epithelial lining.
Odontogenic fibroma		Rare benign odontogenic tumour with good prognosis and low recurrence rate.
Odontogenic ghost cell tumour	Dentinogenic ghost cell tumour	A rare tumour with variable behaviour.
Odontogenic keratocyst	Primordial cyst (obsolete)	A common jaw cyst with a high recurrence rate.
Odontogenic myxoma		A rare multiloculated benign tumour.
Odontoma	See complex odontomas See compound odontomas	
Ossifying fibroma	See cemento-ossifying fibroma	
Osteogenic sarcoma		See Tumours of the Bone (Section 43).
Periapical cemental dysplasia	Periapical fibrous dysplasia	Symptomless multiple tumour-like cemento-osseous lesions found most commonly around the roots of lower incisor teeth.
Periapical fibrous dysplasia	See periapical cemental dysplasia	
Pigmented neuroectodermal tumour of infancy	Melanoameloblastoma (obsolete) Melanotic progonoma (obsolete) Retinal anlage tumour (obsolete)	A rare benign but occasionally aggressive neoplasm of neural crest origin with a significant recurrence rate.
Pindborg tumour	See calcifying epithelial odontogenic tumour	

Tumour terminology Recommended terms are in **bold**	Synonyms	Comments
Primary intraosseous carcinoma		A squamous cell carcinoma of jaws of presumed odontogenic rather than mucosal origin.
Primordial cyst	See odontogenic keratocyst	Obsolete term.
Pseudoadenoma adamantium	See adenomatoid odontogenic tumour	Obsolete term.
Retinal anlage tumour	See pigmented neuroectodermal tumour of infancy	Obsolete term.
Soft mixed odontogenic tumour	See ameloblastic fibroma	
Soft mixed odontome	See ameloblastic fibroma	
Squamous odontogenic tumour		A rare benign but sometimes locally infiltrative odontogenic tumour with a low recurrence rate.
True cementoma	See benign cementoblastoma